Aging *and* Communication

SECOND EDITION

Edited by
Mary Ann Toner
Barbara B. Shadden
Michael B. Gluth

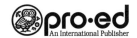

pro·ed
An International Publisher

8700 Shoal Creek Boulevard
Austin, Texas 78757
800/897-3202   Fax: 800/397-7633
www.proedinc.com

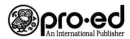

© 2011, 1997 by PRO-ED, Inc.
8700 Shoal Creek Boulevard
Austin, Texas 78757-6897
800/897-3202   Fax 800/397-7633
www.proedinc.com

Library of Congress Cataloging-in-Publication Data

Aging and communication / edited by Mary Ann Toner, Barbara B. Shadden,
Michael B. Gluth.—2nd ed.
      p. cm.
   ISBN 978-1-4164-0494-1
   1. Communicative disorders in old age—Treatment. 2. Older
people—Communication. I. Toner, Mary Ann, 1954– II. Shadden, Barbara B.
(Barbara Bennett) III. Gluth, Michael B. IV. Title.

   RC429.A35 2011
   618.97'6855—dc22

                                                    2011000452

Art director: Jason Crosier
Designer: Lissa Hattersley
This book was designed in Myriad Pro and Fairfield LH

Printed in the United States of America
1   2   3   4   5   6   7   8   9   10   20   19   18   17   16   15   14   13   12   11

Aging and Communication

Contents

For Clinicians by Clinicians

This book, *Aging and Communication*, is the second edition of the ninth volume in the For Clinicians by Clinicians series of texts on the diagnosis and clinical management of speech, language, voice, and swallowing disorders. Each text provides a contemporary perspective on one major disorder or clinical area and is designed for use in clinical methodology courses, in continuing education programs, and as a clinical practice resource. Authors have been selected who represent a broad spectrum of clinical interests and theoretical positions and who hold the common belief that their viewpoints, experiences, and successes should be shared in order to provide a forum for clinicians by clinicians.

Michael P. Cannito, *Series Editor*

Contributors

William M. Buron, PhD, RNC, FNP-BC
Assistant Professor
Eleanor Mann School of Nursing
University of Arkansas
Fayetteville, AR

Colin L. W. Driscoll, MD
Consultant
Department of Otorhinolaryngology, Mayo Clinic and Mayo
    Foundation
Associate Professor, Mayo Medical School
Rochester, MN

Karee E. Dunn, PhD
Clinical Assistant Professor
Educational Statistics and Research Methods
College of Education and Health Professions
University of Arkansas
Fayetteville, AR

Alan D. Gluth
Partner
Ryan Sanders and Gluth, LLP
Certified in Estate Planning and Probate Law, Texas Board of
    Legal Specialization
Certified in Estate Planning, Trusts, and Probate Law, New
    Mexico Board of Legal Specialization
El Paso, TX

Michael B. Gluth, MD
Assistant Professor
Division of Otology and Neurotology
Department of Otolaryngology–Head and Neck Surgery
University of Arkansas for Medical Sciences
Little Rock, AR

Amy Hunter, AuD, CCC-A
Audiologist
Ear, Nose, & Throat Center of the Ozarks
Springdale, AR

Lance A. Manning, MD
Otolaryngology–Head and Neck Surgery
Ear, Nose, & Throat Center of the Ozarks
Springdale, AR

Barbara B. Shadden, PhD, CCC-SLP
Professor
University of Arkansas
Department of Rehabilitation, Human Resources and
   Communication Disorders
Fayetteville, AR

C. Blake Simpson, MD
Professor
Director, University of Texas Voice Center
Department of Otolaryngology–Head and Neck Surgery
University of Texas Health Science Center
San Antonio, TX

Leah Skladany, PhD, CCC-SLP
Associate Professor
Department of Speech Pathology and Audiology
University of Nevada School of Medicine
Reno, NV

Mary Ann Toner, PhD, CCC-SLP
Associate Professor
Department of Rehabilitation, Human Resources and
   Communication Disorders
University of Arkansas
Fayetteville, AR

Mary Ann Westphal, MA, JD
Attorney
Fayetteville, AR

Gillian Woods, PhD
Licensed Psychological Examiner
Senior Health Education/Outreach Coordinator
Washington Regional Medical System
Pat Walker Center for Seniors
Fayetteville, AR

Gina L. Youmans, PhD, CCC-SLP
Assistant Professor
Communication Sciences and Disorders
Long Island University
Brooklyn, NY

Scott R. Youmans, PhD, CCC-SLP
Assistant Professor
Communication Sciences and Disorders
Long Island University
Brooklyn, NY

CHAPTER I

Communication and Aging

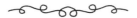

Mary Ann Toner, Barbara B. Shadden,
and Michael B. Gluth

TONER, SHADDEN, AND GLUTH begin by challenging clinicians to examine their own perceptions of and biases about aging and the elderly. After asking readers to examine their personal perspectives, the authors introduce basic text concepts and provide demographics in the form of questions about common aspects of aging and the elderly. Chapter 1 next highlights the diversity of research approaches used to study aging and the complexity of aging phenomena. The central text concepts of primary, secondary, and tertiary aging are defined. Professionals working with the elderly and in diverse healthcare settings are identified, and the potential impact of stereotypical ways of communication (e.g., elderspeak) is noted. Chapter 1 ends with an overview of the content of the book chapters.

Most people know that the elderly population is growing and the burden on the healthcare system is increasing. In the next 20 years, the older population will grow to become approximately 20% of the American population. Statistics describing the elderly population are available at www .agingstats.gov. Effective service delivery for this rapidly growing portion of our population will require a larger body of professionals who have a thorough understanding of the characteristics of aging and the healthcare issues involved. Quality care is not determined by the clinician's technical skills alone. The clinician's ability to interact and communicate appropriately with older clients is an essential factor for optimal care. In this first chapter, therefore, we attempt to personalize your reading experience by asking you to reflect on your own views of aging and the elderly.

What Is Your Perspective on Aging?

How do you really feel about aging and elderly people? What are the first words that come to your mind when you hear the words *old people*? Do the words tend to be negative: *sick, weak, death*, or *Alzheimer's*? Do you picture nursing homes and canes? Are you ever tempted to say things like "They're too old to care," "All old people do that," "That's wasted on somebody that old"? Alternatively, are you more prone to words like *stability, grandchildren, relaxation, vacationing*, and *wisdom*? Do you find yourself asking older people for advice and input, or do you become annoyed when they relate stories about things that happened to them? Do you discount the value of knowing anything that happened before you were born, or do you find it interesting to learn about past events and people? Your responses to these questions may tell you something about how you feel about aging and how you will approach elderly patients.

Recognizing your personal biases is particularly important in working with older adults. Many clinicians have biases about aging, age-related disorders, and what the elderly should or should not be doing. Some of these biases are negative, in terms of the diminished value attributed to the older adult or certain stereotypes of limited capacity that are associated with aging. Negative biases may influence decisions about the length or nature of intervention and determinations of prognosis. Positive biases also exist. The "Isn't she a sweet little old lady?" perspective does not further the therapeutic process, and denial of very real aspects of aging and decline may prevent development of a reasonable and practical treatment program. All biases affect the way clinicians talk and interact with older clients.

Some healthcare professionals may fear what is happening to the older person, perhaps due to personal experiences with older family members. Overpersonalizing can be positive ("You remind me of my grandmother") but still inappropriate. Professionals may feel that they need to control the client and caregiver, or they may have preconceived ideas about what the elderly client and caregiver should want, do, and feel. The clinician must be careful not to assume anything simply because a client or caregiver is old.

Stereotypes, biases, and fears are exacerbated when the practitioner has little or no understanding of normal aging and the complex variability associated with the aging process and with older adults. Healthcare professionals working with the elderly should acknowledge their biases and stereotypes, as well as their strengths and weaknesses concerning their knowledge of normal aging. They need to be aware of the factors in their personal background and training that may influence the way they treat their elderly clients.

The culture itself is biased. It isn't a good thing to be old, and aging certainly isn't easy. Numerous physical, emotional, and financial challenges confront the elderly person. The challenge of dealing with healthcare professionals who are governed by bias instead of knowledge should not be added to the elderly person's burden.

What Do You Know About Aging?

Even if you have a positive, realistic attitude toward aging, you may be biased by common myths. Answer the following questions to see if you know some of the basic "truths" about aging.

1. **Does cultural background affect aging and the response to it?** Cultural influences do affect attitudes about aging, but those effects interact with socioeconomic influences and life experiences. Expectations of old age are strongly influenced by life experiences, and life experiences are obviously influenced by both culture and socioeconomic status. One study reported that various cultural groups had similar concerns about their future but ranked them differently (Condon, 2003). White, Black, and Hispanic elderly people ranked "loss of independence due to physical deterioration" and "being a victim of crime other than fraud" as their number one and two concerns. The Black and Hispanic elderly respondents rated "becoming a financial burden" as their third concern, whereas White elderly people ranked it fifth. Black elderly respondents did not rank "going to a nursing home" in their top five concerns, but it was ranked fourth by Whites and fifth by Hispanics.

2. **Is becoming senile a natural part of aging?** The elderly do experience changes in cognitive functioning, but those changes are generally mild and do not interfere significantly with daily functioning. A significant cognitive problem is a sign of a disorder, but people should not assume that every change is a sign of Alzheimer's disease. Many factors are

associated with a decline in cognitive functioning, and often the declines are reversible with appropriate identification and intervention.

3. **Is it safe for older people to exercise?** The *Older Americans 2008: Key Indicators of Well-Being* report indicates that in the period from 2004 to 2006, 74% of people over the age of 65 rated their health as good or excellent, with the percentage being higher for Whites than Blacks or Hispanics (Federal Interagency Forum on Aging-Related Statistics, 2008). People who exercise as young and middle-age adults are likely to continue to exercise into their later years. Exercise in the elderly helps maintain both physical health and cognitive abilities. Motivation to exercise may actually increase in later years, when people have greater awareness of its benefits for bone health, cardiac functioning, and respiratory health. It is never too late to begin an appropriate exercise program to slow or reverse some effects of aging.

4. **Do people experience fewer negative emotions as they get older?** Personality does not change significantly, but there is evidence that negative emotions decline as one ages. The decline is strongest up to age 65, and then it decreases more slowly up to the age of 80 (Charles, Reynolds, & Gatz, 2001). It appears that older people develop coping skills that allow them to respond less emotionally to negative experiences.

5. **Does aging affect everyone in the same way?** The expression of aging in any individual reflects a combination of influences including genetic, health, and socioeconomic ones. Basic physiological changes are expected in all people as they become older, but the age at which those changes appear varies widely. People born into families with healthy, active elderly members are more likely to show effects of aging at later ages than are those born into families with members that became frail or died at relatively early ages. Activities and experiences in early life, however, can counteract some genetic influences. For example, people from a family filled with healthy elders are more likely to show early signs of aging if they smoked from an early age, never exercised, and had a poor diet.

6. **Are older people motivated to learn new things?** The older generation is more educated than ever and is capable

of learning new information and new skills. Awareness that active learning helps maintain cognitive ability adds to the motivation of many elderly people. Older individuals are more self-directed in their learning than are their younger counterparts. Although they are more likely to disregard information that does not appear relevant to them, they are skilled at acquiring information that answers questions of interest. Their experience also allows them to associate and apply information they learn.

7. **Are older people a financial burden on society?** The majority of people over age 65 do receive income from Social Security; however, it accounts for less than half of the income reported by over 60% of that group. Data reported in *Older Americans 2008: Key Indicators of Well-Being* (Federal Interagency Forum on Aging-Related Statistics, 2008) indicate that one third of the elderly receive income from continued employment. They also report income from pensions and assets. Less than 10% of the elderly live at or below the poverty level, with more than 78% reporting incomes at or above 150% of the poverty level. The nation's economy definitely affects income for the elderly, so times of economic hardship for the country are also times of increased hardship for the elderly. Income statistics vary significantly for different races and educational levels, but most elderly people "pay their own way."

8. **Do most elderly individuals end up in nursing homes or under the care of professional caregivers?** Most elderly people who require long-term care receive that care at home, not in an institutional setting. Spector, Fleishman, Pezzin, and Spillman (2000) reported that only 5% of the elderly live in nursing homes. Most individuals over 65 are able to care for themselves and live independently. The majority of elderly individuals live with a spouse, although elderly women are more likely to live alone than are elderly men. When care is needed, it is usually provided by a family member or friend. Often, the caregiver is an elderly spouse who also has health problems.

9. **Do older people have trouble understanding what you say and find it easier if you speak louder, exaggerate your speech, and use simple words?** The senses, including hearing, do decline somewhat, but a significant

impairment is not attributable to normal aging. Speaking loudly is not an appropriate communication strategy; it may actually decrease understanding. It is also not appropriate to make language oversimplistic. Healthy older people have no problem understanding language if they can hear the speaker. Oversimplification of language and use of an exaggerated speaking style may suggest more about the speaker than the listener.

10. **Do older people know what to expect as they age?** The elderly are as uninformed as the rest of the population about the actual effects of normal aging. When they do experience a problem, the elderly often attribute signs of disease to the unavoidable effects of aging. As a result, they may assume nothing can be done and choose not to seek medical help. It is also easier to recognize when others are "getting old" than to recognize the same signs in oneself. Although people are aware they are getting older, they may not feel they are "old" as long as they are relatively healthy and independent.

When Is Someone Old?

It is almost impossible to define what we mean when we talk about aging or the elderly. In a college class on communication and aging, students were asked how they would define getting old. There were almost as many answers as there were students. We often call someone old when they reach a certain age, but that age is a moving target. For example, the American Association of Retired Persons begins membership at age 50. Senior citizen discounts may not take effect until 55 or 60. One becomes eligible for Social Security at age 62, but full retirement age varies from 65 to 67 years of age, depending on the year of birth. The highest benefits are currently not paid until age 70. Even if we could agree on one chronological age as the starting point for becoming "old," people are living longer and there is more than one generation of elderly individuals. Although some references use descriptions such as *young-old, middle-old,* and *old-old,* there is no standard agreement on the chronological ages assigned to each category.

One's physical condition cannot be predicted based solely on chronological age; therefore, some people suggest that aging should be defined in terms of biological or health status. Some people show very few signs of aging into their 80s, while others the same age have multiple impairments.

Attempts have been made to quantify biological aging in terms of measures such as strength, respiratory capacity, cardiac function, or even cellular changes. Although all of these physical markers are useful, they fail to capture the full sense of aging.

Sometimes, being seen as old is a by-product of the roles played by each individual. For example, retirement means loss of the role of productive worker and can signal old age to some people. Not surprisingly, it may be difficult for some aging adults to adjust well to retirement. Becoming a grandparent may also be a marker of old age. How often do you hear someone say, "I can't believe you're a grandmother; you seem so young"? Some of these old-age roles are signs of moving forward through somewhat predictable life stages, which can become another sign of aging.

In recent years, aging has often been characterized in terms of daily functioning, independence, and well-being. Terms such as *aging well, aging productively*, and *successful aging* are used to indicate that an elderly person is making appropriate adaptations to remain healthy, active, and well-adjusted. Some individuals continue to show only minor effects of aging well into their eighth and ninth decades. These people are sometimes referred to as "geriatric supermen."

How Do We Learn About Aging and the Elderly?

Older adults and the aging process have been studied in a variety of ways. Some researchers compare groups of young and old people on a particular task in order to understand differences between age groups. These are called cross-sectional studies. Other researchers use longitudinal designs, which track a group of adults across the lifespan. These longitudinal studies provide important information about how a cohort of individuals from a specific generation develop and change over time. The term *cohort* is used to refer to a group of people who have lived through similar historical, social, and economic experiences because they were born around the same time.

One challenge in studying normal aging is the fact that the elderly are such a heterogeneous group, making it difficult to draw conclusions about what is "normal" aging. Another challenge stems from the fact that researchers like to control characteristics of the subjects in their studies. If people who have health problems, demonstrate a sensory impairment, or take prescription medications are excluded from participation as subjects, it is difficult to feel comfortable calling the remaining subjects typical of the elderly population. Sometimes, researchers end up using subjects who resemble geriatric supermen more closely than the majority of older persons.

Research tools continue to evolve over time. One exciting development in our efforts to understand aging involves the use of sophisticated research tools such as functional magnetic imaging and evoked cortical potentials. Functional magnetic resonance imaging (fMRI) is a minimally invasive imaging technique that allows measurement of changes in blood flow in the brain during brain activation. It allows investigators to determine which cortical regions are engaged during specific cognitive activities. Evoked cortical potential measures how the nervous system responds to an incoming stimulus. It provides information about where and when responses occur and the amplitude of the responses. These tools allow us to combine measures of behavior with analyses of underlying brain activity. The resulting data help us understand what is and is not normal in the aging brain, as well as how the brain compensates for age-related changes.

What Makes Aging So Complex?

It should already be clear that defining aging and understanding the elderly is not a simple task. One part of the challenge for professionals is to understand the difference between normal aging and disordered processes. If we expect the elderly to have difficulty in speaking, understanding, thinking, and swallowing, we are likely to overlook the early signs of disorders that should be identified and treated. On the other hand, if we assume that all signs of aging indicate disorder, we may inappropriately recommend intervention for a "normal" person.

Various models or theories describe the aging process and the variables that influence that process. Some of these models are discussed in Chapters 7 and 9. To facilitate understanding of the important distinctions between normal and abnormal aging, the chapters of this book use a model that describes primary, secondary, and tertiary aging factors (Granieri, 1990).

Primary aging factors are the result of the normal aging process and are expected to appear in many older adults. Primary changes may be relatively neutral (e.g., gray hair), or they may alter functions. However, they do not pose a significant threat or interfere in any major way with daily activities. As we age, we draw upon our "reserve capacity" to allow us to adapt to the effects of aging. As the degree of primary aging increases, reserve capacity is reduced and the risk of disease, injury, or disorder is increased.

The prefix *presby-* denotes old age. It should not be confused with the prefixes that suggest abnormality or illness (e.g., *dys-*, *dis-*). Technically, *presby-* does not indicate a disorder but instead the natural changes that take place. There is no general agreement on the use of this prefix in areas affecting communication disorders. Some sources use the prefix to denote changes related to the normal aging process that are not clinically significant. Others use the prefix to describe a clinically significant problem that is related to the aging process. For example, in the current text, *presbycusis* (hearing) is described as an age-related decline that may benefit from some clinical intervention, whereas *presbyphagia* (swallowing) is used to describe changes that the elderly adapt to without significant impairment of daily functioning.

study of disease

Secondary aging factors represent pathologies. Elderly people are more prone to diseases and disorders such as stroke, heart disease, arthritis, and sensory impairments; they are also likely to suffer from more than one condition. Additionally, medications, surgeries, and treatments that address the elderly person's medical problems may add to the impairments experienced.

loss of mobility

Tertiary aging factors are those that result from social, psychological, and environmental changes. The social and support network of the elderly client is often reduced due to retirement, death of peers, children moving away, and loss of mobility. Elderly couples may be on a fixed income, with illness further reducing their financial resources. When these factors combine, it is not unusual for the older person to experience depression. If both the client and the spouse are elderly, the aging factors affecting each can contribute to further declines.

can ct ut

C

Who Cares for the Elderly?

When an elderly person's health declines, someone must provide assistance to meet his or her daily needs. Most elderly persons are cared for in the home, with spouses or adult children providing much of the necessary assistance. Some of these children are themselves senior citizens. The care provided by family members is often called "informal caregiving" because caregivers are not trained for this role and do not receive reimbursement. Most of the caregiving in the United States is informal. It is not unusual for these older caregivers to assume responsibility for more than one aging family member (e.g., a parent and a spouse). The impact of caregiving on the physical and emotional health of any family member should not be underestimated, but serving as a caregiver is especially risky for the elderly, who are likely to suffer from chronic health problems themselves.

It is essential that healthcare professionals understand the needs of primary caregivers, the burdens placed on them by the older care recipient, and their response to the stress of changes in roles and added responsibilities. Caregiver stress is influenced by many variables; stress is particularly increased by change in the caregiver's life. Areas of change are multiple: role reversal, social network reduction, altered living environment, and strained financial status. Financial strains can be particularly difficult to manage when a caregiver must leave a job because of caregiving responsibilities or when a caregiver tries to juggle work and caregiving simultaneously.

Relationship to the client can also be a factor in stress. Spouses suffer the most stress, and "favored" children report more stress but less burden than do "problem" children (Cantor, 1983; Henderson, 1994). Caregivers with limited family ties and those who are not "raised" to be caregivers experience higher stress levels. Female caregivers feel more emotional stress than do male caregivers, which may be due in part to females being less likely to seek help from other family members and more likely to quit their jobs instead of hiring outside help.

Degree of caregiver stress has also been found to vary with the type of disorder demonstrated by the client. Although we often think of the greatest burden being experienced by those who provide physical care, the level of caregiver stress is actually greater when the disorder is characterized by cognitive changes and declines in communication ability. Caregivers of clients with dementia often feel that their social network is reduced and experience feelings of isolation.

The issues confronting the caregiver are obviously multiple and complex. Consequences of resulting stress can be devastating, with numerous possible physical effects (Pruchno & Resch, 1989). The autoimmune system of the caregiver is often affected, making him or her more vulnerable to disease. If stress is ongoing, the body will always be mobilized for crisis responses. As a result, stress may contribute to chronic fatigue, heart attacks, headaches, ulcers, obesity, and high blood pressure.

Psychologically, spouses are often plagued by concerns about their future financial condition and their ability to continue to care for the client. Cost of institutional placement is often prohibitive and may exhaust a couple's savings in only a few months. If placement in a nursing home is required, spouses may be required to divest themselves of most of their assets to qualify for Medicaid funding. Elderly caregivers may not be receiving available financial help because they do not know it is available, do not know how to apply for it, or feel that it carries a social stigma.

Who Works with Older Adults?

The complexity of aging requires the involvement of a number of health-care professionals to help maintain optimal functioning of the elderly person. Because the elderly are more likely to experience multiple health problems, they are also more likely to be under the care of more than one medical specialist.

Most elderly patients have a primary healthcare provider. Primary care providers serve elderly clients with a wide range of needs. Their clients include the geriatric supermen as well as those in the poorest heath. In addition to the primary healthcare provider, older adults and their families may see social workers, counseling and psychiatric professionals, physical therapists or occupational therapists, and other care providers. Most healthcare professions have developed specialized fields of study in geriatrics or gerontology, but much more training is needed to ensure a workforce knowledgeable enough to work with the elderly.

When an elderly person experiences a communication or swallowing problem, it is likely that his or her first contact in the healthcare system will be with a primary care provider. It is the responsibility of the primary care provider to refer elderly patients to appropriate medical specialists or rehabilitation professionals. It is not uncommon, however, for a speech–language pathologist or audiologist to be the first contact an elderly client makes for a potentially serious health problem. For that reason, communication disorders professionals must have a clear understanding of both normal and pathological aging factors and be prepared to provide information regarding previously unidentified medical issues.

The elderly are seen in a variety of healthcare settings. The characteristics of each setting and the needs of individual clients influence which healthcare professionals are available and the types of services that can be provided. In some settings, healthy elderly people may be seen only for services that maintain their health, such as hearing screenings at health fairs. In contrast, those individuals whose health is compromised may be served in settings such as acute care, outpatient clinics, short- and long-term rehabilitation settings, or home healthcare. In recent years, more facilities have been providing healthcare specifically targeting the unique needs and characteristics of the elderly.

Regardless of setting or profession, healthcare providers need to communicate effectively and appropriately with aging clients. Unfortunately, given common biases about aging and the elderly, professionals often fall into a pattern of communication called *elderspeak*. Elderspeak essentially involves talking down to an older person just because he or she appears to be old. This behavior will be discussed further in the final chapter of this text, but it is important to note here that use of elderspeak can interfere with effective clinical interaction and service delivery.

What Is This Book About?

The expanding elderly population is expected to require the services of an increasing number of healthcare professionals with more specialized knowledge. Communication is critical to quality of life and to accessing services; therefore, speech–language pathologists and audiologists are among the professionals who will be serving more elderly clients. The intent of this book is to provide clinicians and students in communication disorders with an overview of normal and pathological aging and the services commonly provided to the elderly. This text is not designed to be a comprehensive discussion of the assessment and treatment of disorders, nor does it provide an exhaustive review of the research literature. It highlights those factors that are most pertinent to the care of the elderly population.

Professions vary in their approach to aging issues and use language that is distinctive when discussing those issues. Differences in perspective also exist between the various specialties within the field of communication disorders. Additionally, emphasis may differ based on work setting. For example, academically oriented and clinically based professionals are likely to relate differently to the details of reimbursement. To facilitate multidisciplinary interactions, it is helpful for healthcare professionals to become familiar with these differing viewpoints. In this text, contributions from authors representing a variety of professions, specialties, and work settings make these differences clear.

How Is the Book Organized?

This is the second edition of *Aging and Communication: For Clinicians by Clinicians*. A number of changes have been made to make the book more clinician-friendly and inclusive of other disciplines. To begin, a nurse practitioner provides an overview of physical aging in Chapter 2. It is sometimes difficult for professionals to understand where normal aging ends and pathological aging begins. For that reason, aspects of communication and swallowing are approached from the perspective of primary, secondary, and tertiary aging, as defined earlier in this chapter. Chapter 3 combines otolaryngology and audiology viewpoints on aging of the hearing mechanism. Speech and voice are presented from a medical perspective in Chapter 4 and from a speech–language pathology perspective in Chapter 5. The differing approaches to diagnosis and treatment of speech disorders in the elderly are provided, with the physicians emphasizing diagnosis of organic pathologies that determine medical and surgical interventions and the speech–language pathologists emphasizing functional, perceptual, and acoustic characteristics that influence speech interventions. Chapter 6 provides a comprehensive view of aging and swallowing, with an emphasis on the role of the speech–language pathologist.

In considering aging of the cognitive and linguistic systems, primary and tertiary aspects are addressed separately from secondary aspects. Chapter 7 discusses primary and tertiary aspects of cognitive aging. Chapter 8 discusses secondary aspects of cognitive aging, including Alzheimer's disease. Chapter 9 describes aging of the linguistic system. Chapter 10 describes language assessment and intervention. This organization facilitates discussion of primary and tertiary aging issues of interest to practitioners from many fields separately from the detailed discussion of assessment and intervention strategies relevant to the practice of speech–language pathology.

The text concludes with chapters that introduce broader considerations in working with older adults. Chapter 11 takes on the challenge of end-of-life decision making and care. Chapter 12 examines clinical interactions with aging adults and makes recommendations for more effective counseling and communication.

At the end of each relevant chapter, information regarding reimbursement for speech–language pathology and audiology services is provided. The coding systems used to obtain reimbursement are discussed. These systems include the following:

- Current Procedural Terminology (CPT; American Medical Association [AMA], 2009a): These codes indicate procedures conducted during a contact with a client.
- Healthcare Common Procedure Coding System (HCPCS; AMA, 2009b): Services not included in the CPT system are specified by the HCPCS codes. These codes may be used when devices or equipment are required.

- International Classification of Diseases–Clinical Modification, 9th Revision (ICD-9-CM; National Center for Health Statistics [NCHS], 2009): The disorder or diagnosis is identified using ICD-9-CM codes. The 10th revision of the codes (ICD-10-CM) is scheduled to go into effect in 2013 (NCHS, 2010).

These are not static coding systems. They are updated to reflect advances in diagnostic and treatment procedures. Professionals should not assume that all of their services will be covered by Medicare or by many private insurance policies. Reimbursement issues may dictate which services are provided; therefore, it is essential for speech–language pathologists and audiologists to understand how to obtain funding for needed services and be able to provide that information to their elderly clients. The American Speech-Language-Hearing Association provides extensive reimbursement information for speech–language pathologists and audiologists, including current diagnostic and procedural codes.

Finally, each chapter concludes with Key Points that capture the most important "take-home" messages. Collectively, these chapters provide students and clinicians with an overview of aspects of aging, common communication and swallowing problems, and clinical management approaches.

Key Points

This chapter addressed common questions, myths, and biases about aging. Several factors that contribute to the heterogeneity of the aging population were discussed. An overview of the topics and organization of the book was provided. Key points in this chapter included the following:

- Personal perspectives on aging may affect interactions with the elderly.
- Culture and personal experiences influence perceptions of older people.
- Cognitive abilities change, but older people are motivated to learn new information and skills. Dementia is not part of normal aging.
- Most older people report that they are in good health. They also experience fewer negative emotions.
- The majority of older people live at home and above the poverty level.

- Effective communication with older people does not require loud, slow, simple speech.
- There is no simple or agreed-upon definition of *old*.

References

American Medical Association. (2009a). *Current procedural terminology (CPT) 2010*. Chicago: American Medical Association.

American Medical Association. (2009b). *Healthcare common procedure coding system 2010: Level II*. Chicago: American Medical Association.

Cantor, M. H. (1983). Strain among caregivers: A study of experience in the United States. *The Gerontologist, 23*, 597–604.

Charles, S. T., Reynolds, C. A., & Gatz, M. (2001). Age-related differences and change in positive and negative affect over 23 years. *Journal of Personality and Social Psychology, 80*, 136–151.

Condon, K. M. (2003). *Culture and aging: Cultural differences in expression of need by elders*. Paper presented at the annual meeting of the American Sociological Association, Atlanta, GA. Retrieved May 26, 2009, from http://www.allacademic.com/meta/p107844_index.html

Federal Interagency Forum on Aging-Related Statistics. (March, 2008). *Older Americans 2008: Key indicators of well-being*. Washington, DC: U.S. Government Printing Office.

Granieri, E. (1990). Nutrition and the older adult. *Dysphagia, 4*, 196–201.

Henderson, J. N. (1994). Caregiving issues in culturally diverse populations. *Seminars in Speech and Language, 15*, 216–224.

National Center for Health Statistics. (2009). *International classification of diseases, 9th revision, clinical modification*. Retrieved March 3, 2009, from http://www.cdc.gov/nchs/icd/icd9cm.htm

National Center for Health Statistics. (2010), *International classification of diseases, 10th revision, clinical modification*. Retrieved March 3, 2009, from http://www.cdc.gov/nchs/icd/icd10cm.htm

Pruchno, R. A., & Resch, N. L. (1989). Caregiving spouses: Physical and mental health perspective. *Journal of American Geriatrics Society, 37*, 697–705.

Spector, W. D., Fleishman, J. A., Pezzin, L. E., & Spillman, B. C. (2001). *The characteristics of long-term care users* (AHRQ Research Report No. 00-0049). Rockville, MD: Agency for Healthcare Research and Quality.

I know vocab

Getting Old: Physical Aging

William M. Buron

BURON BEGINS HIS DISCUSSION by placing physical aging on a continuum from poor to excellent health and acknowledges the many factors that affect each individual's physical aging. Primary and secondary aging effects on physical systems are explored. Emphasis is placed on the impact of aging on daily functioning. Buron then outlines assessment needs and challenges, describing the components of a comprehensive geriatric assessment, common laboratory tests, and issues related to medications. Buron also introduces the reader to common risks confronted by the elderly, including risk of falls, failure to thrive, and elder abuse or neglect. The chapter closes with a discussion of key elements in aging well physically, along with obstacles to doing so.

Physical decline, poor health, and increasing physical dependence are some of the most common negative stereotypes about growing old. Although it is true that some older adults experience these characteristics, severe acquired chronic illness and associated disability are not inevitable. The process of aging actually begins at an early age, and many body systems begin to decline after early adulthood. Further, the rate of physical aging and the particular systems affected vary widely among individuals based on a number of positive and negative genetic, lifestyle, and environmental factors.

A broad perspective on physical aging places it on a continuum from normal healthy aging to poor health, with many factors influencing health status, as shown in Figure 2.1. For example, poor health can be the product of a specific illness, such as diabetes. In the presence of negative factors such as poor diet, limited activity, or lack of support from others, this specific

if you do good things for your body, you will have less problems

illness can lead to severe physical challenges, increasing dependence, and ultimately morbidity or mortality. In contrast, with good social supports, modified diet, exercise, and appropriate medications, individuals can limit the negative health effects of diabetes. While it is not possible to eliminate the reality of primary and secondary physical aging, it should be the goal of each healthcare provider to proactively assist in the promotion of aging well, starting at a relatively early stage of adulthood.

primary

As we age, most of us would like to remain healthy as long as possible. To do so, we have to deal with both primary and secondary physical changes that accompany aging. As stated in Chapter 1, primary aging changes are those that occur as a normal consequence of physical aging. For example, hair becomes gray, eyes lose near vision, the heart loses efficiency, and muscle mass decreases. *Secondary aging* refers to common disease conditions that occur with increased frequency as we grow older. These diseases include atherosclerosis, arthritis, stroke, and dementia.

This chapter provides an overview of physical changes that accompany aging, basic considerations in assessing the health of older adults, and approaches to promoting healthy aging. Emphasis is placed on evaluating physical systems and on ways to reduce the negative effects of physical aging on quality of life.

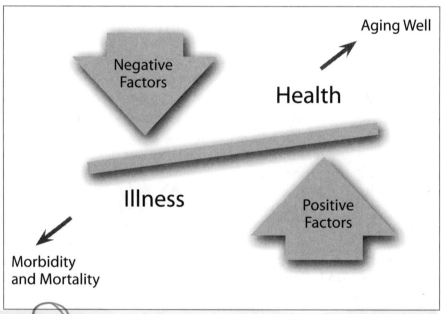

Figure 2.1. The delicate balance between aging well and morbidity and mortality.

Why Communication Disorders Professionals Need to Understand Physical Aging

Aspects of physical aging can directly or indirectly affect one's ability to communicate. Some of these effects are relatively obvious. For example, vision affects reading, which is an important source of information, a means of maintaining contact with others, and a potential source of pleasure. Other effects of physical aging on communication are less obvious. If older adults must deal with chronic pain on a daily basis, they may have less energy for interpersonal interactions or may be less likely to engage in social activities in the community. Because communication is a critical tool in accessing healthcare, obtaining appropriate services, and informing caregivers, any limitations of it can have a significant impact on patient care outcomes and quality of life. Without a clear understanding of the nature of physical changes, professionals might misinterpret assessment findings as pathological (secondary) instead of normal consequences of primary physical aging.

Impact of Primary and Secondary Physical Aging

Satisfaction with health is linked to physical changes that accompany aging. Specifically, primary aging affects physical systems in ways that may place older adults at risk for loss of independence in daily activities and reduced quality of life. For example, considering primary aging, older adults typically experience a loss of organ reserve capacity. This loss is especially apparent in the functioning of the heart and lungs. The heart tends to lose efficiency due to a reduction in contractile strength, and blood pressure may increase due to diminished elasticity of the arteries. Additionally, progressive muscular rigidity in the respiratory system can lead to ineffective breathing and diminished vital capacity. As a result, older adults may react to these changes by avoiding participation in strenuous activities that tend to stress the heart and lungs. Conversely, a trend to limit vigorous physical activity can then lead to deconditioning and additional declines in reserve capacity. Eventually this chronic cycle can lead to dyspnea, angina, and fatigue with little activity, thereby negatively affecting quality of life.

Primary aging changes in the gastrointestinal and urinary systems also can contribute to a loss of independence and reduced quality of life. A normal reduction in gastrointestinal motility with age can lead to constipation.

independence : Bowel problem

A reduction in bladder capacity, combined with weakened bladder and perineal muscles, may result in incontinence in women. Men often experience prostate enlargement, which can lead to urinary frequency and dribbling.

Secondary aging further increases these risks for lost independence and reduced quality of life. *Secondary physical aging* refers to labeled healthcare diagnoses that indicate health problems (i.e., chronic physical conditions and diseases). Older adults differ from younger adults in terms of the specific health problems they typically experience as well as the chronicity of the problems and their impact on daily functioning.

Some of the more common and most costly chronic health problems that affect the elderly include heart disease, stroke, cancer, diabetes, hearing loss, arthritis, osteoporosis, and hypertension. According to the Centers for Disease Control and Prevention (CDC), almost half of all Americans are living with at least one chronic condition, and this figure rises to 80% in the population over age 65 (CDC, 2008a; CDC and The Merck Company Foundation, 2007). The most common causes of death (from higher to lower rate of occurrence) are heart disease, malignant neoplasm, cerebrovascular disease, and chronic respiratory conditions (CDC, 2008a). The prevalence of common chronic health conditions differs by gender, race, and ethnicity. Seventy-five percent of the nation's $2 trillion healthcare costs can be attributed to chronic disease (CDC, 2008a).

Table 2.1 provides an overview of the common changes and diseases associated with primary and secondary aging, organized by system.

What is perhaps most important about physical aging is that primary and secondary changes may limit an individual's ability to function independently. Usually, physical functioning is described in terms of ADLs (activities of daily living) or IADLs (instrumental activities of daily living). ADLs include activities such as sitting, standing, and using the toilet. IADLs describe functional activities that are a bit more skilled, such as driving and cooking a meal. More than 40% of people over the age of 65 report at least one limitation in ADLs or IADLs, and women experience more functional challenges than men do. For example, 19% of men and 32% of women in this age group could not perform any key physical indicators (e.g., reaching over one's head or walking two blocks). By age 85, more than half of women cannot perform these activities (Federal Interagency Forum on Aging-Related Statistics, 2008).

Restrictions in independent functioning increase the need for potentially costly caregiving. As noted in Chapter 1, much of the burden of care falls on informal caregivers, defined as family or friends who take on the responsibility of meeting the needs of aging individuals without any

Memorize

TABLE 2.1
Changes and Diseases Associated with
Primary and Secondary Aging

System	Primary aging changes	Secondary aging changes
Eyes/vision	• Presbyopia (loss of near vision) • Reduced tearing • Reduced pupil size • Poorer night vision • More "floaters" • Lens enlargement, less transparency • Decrease in color vision	• Cataracts • Glaucoma • Macular degeneration
Somesthetic	Increase in pain/temperature/touch thresholds	
Hearing	See Chapter 3	See Chapter 3
Taste/smell	See Chapter 6	See Chapter 6
Skin	• Loss of elasticity • Wrinkling • Reduced moisture • Hair thinning • Facial hair in females • Reduction of subcutaneous fat • Reduction in sweat glands	• Bedsores • Skin shearing • Bruising • Shingles
Respiratory	• Reduced vital capacity • Increased residual volume • Loss of elasticity of lung tissue • Reduction in cilia • Reduction in alveoli (oxygen uptake)	• Chronic obstructive pulmonary disease (COPD) • Pneumonia
Cardiovascular	• Loss of cardiac muscle bulk and elasticity • Decreased heart rate • Increased stroke volume • Increased systolic pressure • Heart valves more sclerotic • Stiffening and narrowing of arteries • Decline in barorecepter reflex	• Congestive heart failure • Coronary artery disease • Stroke • Heart attack • Hypertension
Gastro-intestinal	• Reduced motility • Reduction of secretions • Reduction of metabolism in liver	• Cancer, especially colon • Diverticula • Fecal impaction

(continues)

TABLE 2.1 *(continued)*

System	Primary aging changes	Secondary aging changes
Urinary/renal	• Decrease in kidney size and function • Weakening of bladder muscles • Slower drug clearance	• Incontinence • Urinary tract infection • Renal failure • Benign prostate hypertrophy
Neurological	• Loss of neurons • Slower transmission • Poorer regulation of temperature due to hypothalamic changes • Reduction in REM sleep • Decline in balance	• Alzheimer's disease • Dementia • Balance disorders • Parkinson's disease
Muscular/ skeletal	• Loss of muscle • Increase of adipose tissue • Loss of bone minerals • Decrease in height due to compression of vertebral column • Decreased weight due to loss of muscle mass • Loss of elasticity of muscles, ligaments, etc. • Loss of joint flexibility	• Arthritis • Bursitis • Fractures, dislocations • Osteoporosis • Rheumatism • Spinal stenosis • Tendonitis

compensation. Often, caregivers themselves are also aging and may be experiencing their own health challenges.

Clearly, disorders affecting physical systems require medical evaluation and treatment. What may be less obvious is the increased need for monitoring primary aging changes and for developing programs of disease prevention or health promotion for the elderly to maximize daily functioning and quality of life.

Assessment for Prevention and Treatment of Secondary Aging

Prior to determining the healthcare needs of older adults as a result of primary and secondary aging, healthcare providers should recognize the importance of a thorough geriatric assessment. Only then will healthcare be comprehensive enough to meet the complex needs of the whole aging person.

Comprehensive Geriatric Assessment and Routine Annual Examinations

All adults over the age of 65 should have an assessment to identify the presence of characteristics associated with secondary aging. This in-depth assessment of older adults is often referred to as a comprehensive geriatric assessment (CGA). This assessment has its own Healthcare Common Procedure Coding System (HCPCS) Code, defined as a "comprehensive geriatric assessment and treatment planning performed by assessment team" (HCPCS, n.d.).

The CGA differs from a routine annual adult exam in many ways. First, the assessment is interdisciplinary and multidimensional. In addition to physical health, it includes an evaluation of mental health, cognitive health, and socioenvironmental factors. There is a strong emphasis on function and quality of life.

The goal of the CGA is to provide not only a broader understanding of daily functioning and quality of life but also opportunities to develop better plans for treatment and follow-up, improved access to coordinated care, long-term-care needs (if any), and best use of resources. Considering the complex nature of the exam, the evaluation must include more than standard physical examinations of all bodily systems, a review of current medications, and an extended history. According to *The Merck Manual of Geriatrics* (Beers & Berkow, 2000), the CGA should also include consideration of the following domains:

- *Functional ability.* This domain includes a comprehensive assessment of ADLs and IADLs. The Activities of Daily Living Scale (Katz, Ford, Moskowitz, Jackson, & Jaffe, 1963) and the Instrumental Activities of Daily Living Scale (Lawton & Brody, 1969) are considered appropriate tools for this assessment. If deficits are discovered, additional information about the patient's socioenvironmental living conditions should be assessed. The interdisciplinary team must recognize that a need for help with ADLs and IADLs increases dependency on others, which may lead to caregiver stress, abuse, and neglect.
- *Physical health.* An examination of physical health must be geriatric-focused. For example, an emphasis should be placed on vision, hearing, continence, gait, and balance. The Tinetti Balance and Gait Evaluation (Tinetti, 1986) is a common tool for assessing physical health.

- *Cognitive and mental health*. A variety of tools may be used for cognitive and mental health assessment. The Mini-Mental State Examination (MMSE; Folstein, Folstein, & McHugh, 1975) is one tool used to screen major aspects of cognitive function. Depression is often assessed with the Geriatric Depression Scale (GDS; Yesavage et al., 1982–1983) or the Center for Epidemiological Studies Depression Scale (CES-D; Radloff, 1977). Specific psychiatric symptoms (e.g., paranoia, delusions, and behavior abnormalities) are rarely included in the rating scales and are best evaluated by a psychiatrist in this comprehensive, interdisciplinary assessment model.
- *Socioenvironmental situation*. The socioenvironmental assessment should include a focus on the social network, resources for support, and environmental safety. This assessment helps guide the best treatment approach.

Best-practice models for the CGA assessment may include a variety of approaches, and they continue to evolve with time. Potential benefits of the CGA include more precise diagnosis, treatment, counseling, education, and various aspects of support (Aminzadeh et al., 2005).

In addition to the need for a comprehensive geriatric assessment and annual follow-up examinations, older adults should be routinely screened for a variety of physical conditions often associated with secondary aging (Spalding & Sebesta, 2008). Screening tests are usually included as part of the CGA or annual follow-up. They may be completed at the time of the exam or ordered later on an outpatient basis. A list of standard, routine screening recommendations is included in Table 2.2. Senior health fairs provide opportunities for similar screenings. Unfortunately, these screenings are often limited in scope and should not replace the CGA and annual physical exams. Lab exams may be ordered for a routine screening or to rule out a condition or disease process in response to actual symptoms. Health professionals should screen as needed for conditions or diseases that may manifest in physical changes, loss of functional abilities, or psychosocial changes (e.g., depression).

Laboratory Assessment

Some of the conditions frequently experienced by the elderly may be indicated by common blood and urine tests performed during the CGA or the routine annual examination. These conditions include cardiovascular

TABLE 2.2

Routine Screening Recommendations for Older Adults

Disease	Screening or intervention	Target group
Abdominal aortic aneurysm	• Ultrasound	• One time for men ages 65–75
Breast cancer	• Screening mammography	• Women, every 1–2 years beginning at 40 years of age; when life expectancy is 5 years or more
Colorectal cancer	• Fecal occult blood • Colonoscopy • Flexible sigmoidoscopy	• Annual, beginning at age 50 • Every 10 years • Every 5 years
Coronary heart disease (CHD)	• Tobacco use • Annual cholesterol screening • Discuss aspirin prophylaxis therapy for those at risk for CHD	• All • Men age 35 and older, women 45 and older, and anyone at risk for CHD
Diabetes mellitus	• Routine screening	• Every 3 years in asymptomatic persons starting at age 45; earlier than age 45 in overweight persons with at least one risk factor (cardiovascular disease, African American or Hispanic, sedentary lifestyle)
Hearing impairment	• Routine screening	• All, by questioning about patient's hearing
Hypertension	• Routine screening	• All
Obesity	• Routine screening	• All
Osteoporosis	• Screening	• Individuals 65 years of age and older; sooner if risk factors are present (daily steroid use, decreased exposure to estrogen from menopause prior to 45 years of age, or infrequent menses)
Visual impairment	• Routine screening	• Everyone 65 years of age or older

Note. From "Geriatric Screening and Preventative Care," by M. C. Spalding and S. C. Sebesta, 2008, *American Family Physician, 78*, pp. 206–215. Copyright 2008 by the American Academy of Family Physicians. Adapted with permission.

PISS TEST

problems (e.g., heart failure), osteoporosis, diabetes, prostate cancer, breast cancer, and thyroid disease. Several conditions common to the elderly can result in kidney or liver failure. Lab results may reveal reversible conditions that result in dementia symptoms (e.g., drug intoxication, electrolyte imbalance) or conditions that contribute to the disorder (e.g., thyroid disease, Vitamin B12 deficiency).

The relationship of the results of common lab tests to common disease processes in older adults is presented in Appendix 2A. When lab test results are provided, a "normal" range is typically reported. For some measures, the range that is considered normal varies with age. Depending on the specific test, results outside of the normal range may or may not be significant. For example, a high urine protein result might indicate several conditions, including urinary tract infection and kidney failure, while a low level of urine protein is considered normal.

Medication Assessment   Drugs : can cause affects.

As people age, they are likely to take more medications and possibly experience drug interactions and side effects. On average, older individuals take 4.5 medications daily (American Association of Retired Persons, 2004). Side effects often relate to the physical changes that accompany aging, which affect the way drugs are absorbed, distributed, metabolized, and eliminated from the body. For example, decreased cardiac output reduces the distribution of drugs to the kidneys and liver. Drugs that are excreted through kidneys are eliminated more slowly due to changes in renal functioning.

To avoid serious consequences, healthcare practitioners should be aware of the special risks that certain medications pose for elderly patients. The Beers Lists provide a resource that healthcare practitioners can consult to identify the risk level and potential side effects of medications (Fick et al., 2003). A list of medications that should be avoided when certain diseases or disorders are present is included in the Beers Lists and other pharmacologic guides. Of note, several medications may induce the common complex of anticholingeric side effects, which include effects ranging from dry mouth and constipation to increased heart rate and cognitive difficulties (e.g., delirium, confusion, memory problems).

Obviously, the benefit of the medication outweighs the risk in some cases; however, it is not uncommon for elderly people to take more than one medication that places them at risk. Curtis et al. (2004) reported that 21% of the elderly individuals they studied had been prescribed at least one medication on the Beers Lists, over 15% had been prescribed two drugs, and 4% had been prescribed three or more. Medication side effects and interactions can have a significant impact on several areas of concern to the speech-language pathologist (e.g., effects on cognitive functioning or swallowing).

To avoid problems related to side effects and interaction, each prescriber should regularly review all prescribed medications and doses. The older person should also be encouraged to use only one pharmacist, who can monitor the prescriptions and check for potential interactions. When new complaints arise, the healthcare practitioner should not assume that the problem is due to aging, but should determine if the medications might be a contributing factor.

Assessing Risk

Because people are living longer and are at risk for increased frailty and poor health, healthcare providers should pay particular attention to assessment of risks related to falls, failure to thrive, and elder abuse or neglect. All healthcare providers should be sensitive to these concerns. Frequently, it is not the primary care provider or nurse who first identifies a possible problem but instead other healthcare professionals who are working with the older persons to provide unrelated services.

Assessment for Fall Potential

Each year 1 in 3 Americans age 65 and older fall (Hausdorff, Rios, & Edelber, 2001; Hornbrook et al., 1994). Falls are the most common cause of nonfatal injuries and trauma-related hospital admission among older adults (CDC, 2008b). The risk of serious injury from falling increases as bones become more brittle with age (Stevens & Sogolow, 2005). The 1-year mortality rate estimates following a hip fracture vary between 12% and 32% (Schoen, 2006).

Because falls pose such a threat, all older adults who fall (whether or not they experience a fracture) should undergo an extensive assessment to understand the cause of the fall and any underlying intrinsic and extrinsic factors that contributed to it. A post-fall assessment should include a review of medications to identify potential side effects or pharmacological interactions that may be part of the problem. Gait and balance should also be tested, and visual status should be determined. If the fall was related to an environmental hazard at home, a home assessment by a qualified professional should be considered. Following a comprehensive post-fall assessment, the primary care provider should make appropriate referrals for treatment.

Recovery from a fall resulting in a fracture can be a stressful experience. Clients are often dealing with acute pain, immobility, and associated complications and depression. Depression may be related to acute loss of function and dependence on others for meeting the demands of daily living, including help with toileting, bathing, and dressing. Hospitalization can create disorientation. In addition to medical, surgical, and nursing care following a fall-related fracture, other potential resources for recovery may include the services of physical therapists, occupational therapists, counselors, and religious clergy. Long-term goals for recovery should focus on physical and mental well-being, including pain relief and independence in ADLs and IADLs. Finally, affected individuals should be provided with education and training to reduce risk of future falls. Internet resources can help both healthcare providers and consumers with training in fall prevention (http://www.stopfalls.org/).

Assessment for Failure to Thrive

Failure to thrive is a complex phenomenon more commonly discussed in the context of care for infants who fail to gain weight despite an absence of medical pathology. For older adults, failure to thrive is characterized by a refusal to eat or interact socially, and it may be caused by multiple factors, including cognitive impairment, depression, and limitations with physical function (including the ability to eat). Healthcare providers initially recognize failure to thrive through physical examinations and nutritional assessments. In long-term care facilities, mandated weighing of residents may be the first indication of this problem. Etiologic factors contributing to failure to thrive are often difficult to identify and treat. Treatment may require a change in a medication regimen, modification of the strategy used, or initiation of psychiatric care. Temporary nutritional support through parenteral or enteral tube feedings may be needed until effective treatment is in place, although care must be taken to be responsive to the wishes of the patient or those speaking on behalf of a patient who is not able (e.g., has end-stage dementia).

Assessment for Elder Abuse and Neglect

The incidence of elder abuse and neglect increases with age and increasing dependence on outside caregivers. Family members (usually spouses or adult children) account for approximately 90% of those who are abusing or neglecting an older person (Institute on Aging, 2009). These caregivers often experience escalating stress as demands increase in an environment that lacks adequate support. One consequence of increased demands and stress may be what is considered elder mistreatment. Examples of mistreatment include caregiver neglect, financial exploitation, psychological or emotional abuse, physical abuse, and sexual abuse. Elderly individuals may also demonstrate self-neglect, which may manifest as poor hygiene, malnutrition, fungal infections, and insect or rodent infestations in the home (Dowling-Castronova, Guadagno, & Fulmer, 2006). Healthcare providers have a unique responsibility to (a) recognize and report suspicious signs and symptoms of neglect or abuse and (b) ensure that dependent elders are receiving quality care in appropriate environments.

Aging Well Versus Aging Threats

At the beginning of this chapter (see Figure 2.1), it was suggested that aging individuals may be understood best by their placement on a continuum from those who exhibit optimal health and physical well-being to those who are most at risk. Both ends of this continuum warrant further discussion.

Promoting Healthy Aging

At the positive end of this continuum, the concept of aging well or healthy aging means different things to individual older adults and to healthcare professionals from different disciplines. For example, psychologists might focus on encouraging cognitive activity through mental challenges, and speech–language pathologists might emphasize enhanced opportunities for communication. Nursing professionals frequently use their understanding of physical aging to teach lifestyle changes in hopes of preventing common disorders or promoting daily functioning. What is common among disciplines, however, is the shared interest in maintaining quality of life through the various challenges that older adults may face.

Promoting Physical Health

In promoting healthy physical aging, some of the more common targets for behavioral change are nutrition, exercise, and sleep.

Nutrition. Recommended guidelines for maintaining health through appropriate nutrition tend to emphasize the following:

- maintenance of adequate caloric input to remain active and reduce risk of illness
- consumption of adequate amounts of protein (10% to 20% of calories)

- increased intake of high-fiber foods or supplements to reduce gastrointestinal problems like constipation and cardiovascular problems like heart disease and stroke
- increased intake of calcium and specific vitamins, such as D and B12
- intake of sufficient fluids for adequate hydration

The issue of maintaining appropriate hydration levels is a particularly important one for aging adults. Inadequate hydration can affect almost every aspect of daily functioning and can increase susceptibility to illness and even lead to death. Poor hydration is not always recognized by older individuals or their caregivers until a medical crisis occurs. It should not be assumed, however, that every elderly person needs, or can tolerate, equivalent amounts of water. Some health conditions, such as kidney disease, may increase the risk of hyponatremia (low blood sodium) if the elderly person drinks an excessive amount of water.

A variety of factors may affect hydration. Some of the medications taken more frequently by older adults have dehydration as a side effect; when two or more of these medications are being used, the risks to hydration increase dramatically. The elderly, particularly women, may be experiencing loss of bladder control and thus voluntarily limit fluid intake to avoid embarrassing episodes in public.

Physical Exercise. Exercise is critical throughout the lifespan. As we age, however, strength, balance, coordination, and endurance become even more important in maintaining ADLs and IADLs and in reducing risks. Each form of exercise has benefits in specific physical domains. For example, muscle-strengthening activities not only reduce joint stress and assist in fall prevention but also reduce bone loss associated with osteoporosis. Aerobic exercise is important for cardiovascular health.

In recent years, researchers and clinicians have begun to recognize that physical exercise also promotes healthy cognitive functioning (Geda et al., 2010; Lautenschlager et al., 2008). A series of simple tests can be used to assess an individual's current speed, strength, balance, and range of motion. It is important to note that people with health problems should receive clearance from their primary care provider before exercising and should ideally participate in programs run by professionals with specific training in exercise science.

Sleep. The importance of sleep is frequently underestimated in older adults. There is a common misperception that the elderly require less sleep, so problems created by inadequate sleep are frequently ignored. Adequate sleep is critical for maintaining alertness throughout the day, enhancing daily activity levels and independence, and reducing the risk of falls. Although there is no absolute number of required hours of sleep, night sleep of less than 7 hours or more than 8 hours is associated with higher rates of mortality (Hublin, Partinen, Koskenvuo, & Kaprio, 2007).

Promoting Psychosocial Health

Physical health cannot be separated from psychosocial health, since stress, depression, anxiety, and other products of psychosocial challenges directly affect physical elements such as the body's energy, alertness, and immune system. Generally, older adults should be encouraged to engage in their environment and participate in activities. When simple interventions fail to make a difference, older adults should be referred to clergy, a psychologist, or a psychiatrist for further professional help.

Promoting Spiritual Health

Finally, it is important to recognize the importance of spiritual health to some older adults. Their belief system may influence how they deal with the changes that take place in their life when they are confronted with disease, disability, and death. Because the topic is highly personal, healthcare providers often avoid discussing spirituality. If the older person approaches the topic, or indications of a belief system are evident, the healthcare provider's openness and acceptance can help the provider–patient relationship grow in strength, trust, and understanding. Conversely, if the older person expresses no interest in discussing spirituality, the healthcare provider should respect that choice as well.

Caregiver Health

Aging adults with health problems should not be the only target for promoting health. Because caregivers are also at high risk for declines in physical and mental health due to the stress and burden of caregiving, an assessment of the health and well-being of caregivers is an important part of the care of aging adults. When older adults live in the community, it is important to know with whom the client lives as well as the quality of the relationship. For those in assisted living or long-term-care facilities, family caregivers may still play an important role in the care of the older resident.

With aging and the loss of a significant other, clients may become more dependent on extended family members for caregiving. Increased dependency and role changes within families can lead to caregiver stress and the increased potential for abuse and neglect. Considering the constantly changing condition of many older adults, healthcare providers must continually assess and teach caregivers the skills necessary to ensure that they are properly equipped in dealing with the emotional and physical challenges they face.

Assistance with social support is important to caregivers and, ultimately, to older adults' quality of life. Social support can range from caregiver empathy to the promotion of respite services for caregivers. Caregivers must know that feelings such as frustration and hopelessness are very common among those caring for older adults. Healthcare providers should teach caregivers about support groups and other resources to aid in care. In addition, healthcare providers should link caregivers with social workers who can help them identify a range of other support services (e.g., respite) that can improve care quality and ultimately the physical, psychosocial, and spiritual well-being of the aging older adult.

The Environment as a Threat to Aging Well

The age-related changes to physical status described earlier in this chapter also jeopardize an aging person's ability to respond to and recover from illnesses. This fact becomes particularly important when the person is hospitalized for an acute medical crisis. It should not be surprising to learn that older persons are more likely than younger adults to be hospitalized. Typically, over a third of the elderly are admitted to the hospital each year, and more than 75% spend some time in a nursing home during their lifetime (Federal Interagency Forum on Aging-Related Statistics, 2008).

Hospitalized older adults are at greater risk for development of pneumonia and other infections that are unfortunately present in such an environment. In addition, hospitalization removes people from familiar surroundings, people, and routines and places them in an environment with limited sensory input. The individual is already sick enough to require hospitalization; now new medications are introduced. Additionally, a variety of confusing laboratory or imaging procedures may be performed with little explanation, and sleep is disrupted. Thus, for any individual, hospitals can create disorientation. For older persons, this disorientation may be compounded by the additional challenges noted above, plus older patients typically remain in hospitals longer than younger patients because of general frailty and compromised immune systems. A "perfect storm" of conditions may exist for undermining cognitive status. All too frequently, a cognitively functional elderly person, when hospitalized, will begin to show confusion, disorientation, even disruptive behavior, refusal to comply, or psychiatric phenomena such as apparent hallucinations.

These symptoms and behaviors are alarming to family and friends. Frequently, the older patient is described as displaying some form of dementia, even though dementia does not develop overnight or over the course of a few days. Instead, the reality is that the observed behaviors can be predictable reactions to the illness and to the changes being experienced. This cluster of behaviors, sometimes called *delirium*, may disappear fairly quickly once the patient leaves the hospital. In other instances, return to pre-morbid cognitive functioning levels may take longer.

Individuals experiencing some of these challenges during and after hospitalization are often at the high-risk end of the continuum illustrated in Figure 2.1. All healthcare professionals should recognize that hospitalization (or sometimes placement in long-term care) can affect mental functioning, but some of the observed changes are reversible. All too often, particularly with those individuals over age 80 or 85 years, professionals and caregivers assume that the older patient can no longer function independently, and what began as a physical threat alters the older person's quality of life in all domains. Responsibility for helping older adults age well physically should also include making certain that primary and secondary physical changes do not prematurely render the person totally dependent because of temporary changes in mental status due to illness and hospitalization.

Obstacles to Optimal Care

Some healthcare providers specialize in the treatment of older adults and provide services that meet the unique healthcare needs of older adults. Ideally, all older individuals would have a primary care provider with particular expertise in dealing with geriatric health issues. Unfortunately, despite awareness of the fact that the baby boomers will soon swell the ranks of the elderly, a shortage of such expertise continues to exist. Without more emphasis on meeting the special healthcare needs of older adults, the progression of this specialty through research and unique care practices may be constrained and ultimately weakened in quality.

Key Points

The future expected growth of the geriatric population, combined with an apparent lack of expertise, should inspire all healthcare providers to continue gaining geriatric expertise to promote health and prevent illness among this unique group of vulnerable individuals. Speech–language pathologists are particularly well-positioned to positively affect the process of healthy aging. Many secondary aging conditions interfere with speech, the ability to communicate, and therefore the ability to navigate the healthcare system. Major themes of this chapter on physical aging included the following:

- The provision of geriatric healthcare is a complex process that involves a variety of disciplines that come together to serve a population with unique, and sometimes complicated, needs. All healthcare providers must possess an appropriate level of education and skill to meet these challenges.
- Early changes consistent with secondary aging can be recognized at any time, at any place. Therefore, all healthcare providers must be able to recognize and differentiate these changes as primary or secondary aging.
- Healthcare providers should be aware of screening tests that help identify secondary changes that can threaten the health of older adults.
- For ongoing health, providers should be able to identify and encourage aspects of healthy lifestyles in promotion of healthy aging.

References

American Association of Retired Persons. (2004, December). *Prescription drug use among midlife and older Americans.* Washington, DC: Author.

Aminzadeh, B., Byszewski, A., Dalziel, W. B., Wilson, M., Deane, N., & Papahariss-Wright, S. (2005). Effectiveness of outpatient geriatric assessment programs: Exploring caregiver needs, goals, and outcomes. *Journal of Gerontological Nursing, 31,* 19–25.

Beers, M. H., & Berkow, R. (2000). Comprehensive geriatric assessment. In *The Merck manual of geriatrics* (sec. 1, chap 4). Retrieved July 7, 2009, from http://www.merck.com/mkgr/mmg/sec1/ch4/ch4b.jsp

Centers for Disease Control and Prevention. (2008a, November). *Chronic disease overview.* Retrieved July 8, 2009, from http://www.cdc.gov/NCCdphp/overview.htm

Centers for Disease Control and Prevention, National Center for Injury Prevention and Control. (2008b). *10 leading causes of nonfatal injury* [Data file]. Available from Web-based Injury Statistics Query and Reporting System (WISQARS), www.cdc.gov/ncipc/wisqars

Centers for Disease Control and Prevention and The Merck Company Foundation. (2007). *The state of aging and health in America 2007.* Whitehouse Station, NJ: The Merck Company Foundation.

Curtis, L. H., Osbye, T., Sendersky, V., Hutchison, S., Dans, P., Wright, A., et al. (2004). Inappropriate prescribing for elderly Americans in a large outpatient population. *Archives of Internal Medicine, 164,* 1621–1625.

Dowling-Castronova, A., Guadagno, L., & Fulmer, T. (2006). Violence and elder mistreatment. In P. Tabloski (Ed.), *Gerontological nursing* (pp. 271–291). New York: Prentice Hall.

Federal Interagency Forum on Aging-Related Statistics. (2008, March). *Older Americans 2008: Key indicators of well-being.* Washington, DC: U.S. Government Printing Office.

Fick, D. M., Cooper, J. W., Wade, W. E., Waller, J. L., Maclean, J. R., & Beers, M. H. (2003). Beers criteria for potentially inappropriate medications use in older adults. *Archives of Internal Medicine, 163,* 2716–2724.

Folstein, M. F., Folstein, S. E., & McHugh, P. R. (1975). "Mini-mental state": A practical method for grading the cognitive state of patients for the clinician. *Journal of Psychiatric Research, 12,* 189–198.

Geda, Y. E., Roberts, R. O., Knopman, D. S., Christianson, T. J. H., Pankratz, S., Ivnik, R. J., et al. (2010). Physical exercise, aging, and mild cognitive impairment. *Archives of Neurology, 67,* 80–86.

Hausdorff, J. M., Rios, D. A., & Edelber, H. K. (2001). Gait variability and fall risk in community-living older adults: A 1–year prospective study. *Archives of Physical Medicine and Rehabilitation, 82,* 1050–1056.

Healthcare Common Procedure Coding System. (n.d.). Retrieved July 7, 2009, from http://www.hcpcs.info/S_Codes/S0250.htm

Hornbrook, M. C., Stevens, V. J., Wingfield, D. J., Hollis, J. F., Greenlick, M. R., & Ory M. G. (1994). Preventing falls among community-dwelling older persons: Results from a randomized trial. *The Gerontologist, 34,* 16–23.

Hublin, C., Partinen, M., Koskenvuo, M., & Kaprio, J. (2007). Sleep and mortality: A population-based 22-year follow-up study. *Sleep, 30,* 1245–1253.

Institute on Aging. (2009). *Elder abuse prevention.* Retrieved July 28, 2009, from http://www.ioaging.org/services/elder_abuse/

Katz, S., Ford, A. B., Moskowitz, R. W., Jackson, B. A., & Jaffe, M. W. (1963). Studies of illness in the aged. The Index of ADL: A standardized measure of biological and psychosocial function. *Journal of the American Medical Association, 185,* 914–919.

Lautenschlager, N. T., Cox, K. L., Foster, J. K., van Bockxmeer, F. M., Xiao, J., et al. (2008). Effect of physical activity on cognitive function in older adults at risk for Alzheimer disease. *Journal of the American Medical Association, 300,* 1027–1037.

Lawton, M. P., & Brody, E. M. (1969). Assessment of older people: Self-maintaining and instrumental activities of daily living. *Gerontologist, 9,* 179–186.

Radloff, L. S. (1977). The CES-D scale: A self-report depression scale for research in the general population. *Applied Psychological Measurement, 1,* 385–401.

Schoen, D. C. (2006). Hip fractures. *Orthopaedic Nursing, 25,* 148–152.

Spalding, M. C., & Sebesta, S. C. (2008). Geriatric screening and preventative care. *American Family Physician, 78,* 206–215.

Stevens, J. A., & Sogolow, E. D. (2005). Gender differences for non-fatal unintentional fall related injuries among older adults. *Injury Prevention, 11,* 115–119.

Tinetti, M. E. (1986). Performance-oriented assessment of mobility problems in elderly patients. *Journal of the American Geriatrics Society, 34,* 119–126.

Yesavage, J. A., Brink, T. L., Rose, T. L., Lum, O., Huang, V., Adey, M. B., & Leirer, V. O. (1982–1983). Development and validation of a geriatric depression screening scale: A preliminary report. *Journal of Psychiatric Research 17,* 37–49.

The Relationship Between Lab Tests and Common Disease Processes in Older Adults

Comprehensive Metabolic Panel

Glucose	**High:** Diabetes **Low:** Hypoglycemia
Calcium	**High:** Hyperparathyroidism, cancer, hyperthyroidism, sarcoidosis **Low:** Malnutrition, renal failure, hypoparathyroidism, Vitamin D deficiency

Proteins

Albumin	**High:** Dehydration **Low:** Liver disease, kidney disease, malnutrition, inflammation
Total protein	**High:** chronic inflammation, viral hepatitis **Low:** Liver or kidney disorder, malnutrition, celiac disease

Electrolytes

Sodium	**High:** Dehydration **Low:** Diuretics, kidney disease, heart failure, kidney disease
Potassium	**High:** Kidney failure, diabetes, dehydration, infection **Low:** Dehydration, acetaminophen overdose
CO_2 (carbon dioxide, bicarbonate)	**High:** Vomiting, lung disease **Low:** Kidney disease, diabetic ketoacidosis, aspirin overdose

Kidney Tests

Blood urea nitrogen (BUN)	**High:** Acute/chronic renal disease **Low:** Low protein diet, severe liver damage, malabsorption
Creatinine	**High:** Early renal impairment **Low:** Muscle-wasting condition

Liver Tests

Alkaline phosphatase (ALP)	**High:** Hyperparathyroidism, neoplasm, hepatobiliary disease, chronic inflammatory bowel disease, thyrotoxicosis **Low:** May not be significant. May be low in hypothyroidism.

Liver Tests (continued)

Alanine aminotrans-ferase (ALT) Aspartate aminotrans-ferase (AST)	**High:** Necrosis of cells, including myocardial, skeletal muscles, liver **Low:** Not significant
Bilirubin	**High:** Liver damage, biliary tract blockage **Low:** May not be significant. May be seen in anemia.

Complete blood count (CBC)

White blood cell (WBC) count	**High:** Infection, inflammation, cancer, leukemia, steroid medications **Low:** Some medications (e.g., methotrexate), some auto-immune conditions, bone marrow failure
Red blood cell (RBC) count	**Low:** Anemia or fluid loss (due to diarrhea or dehydration)
Hemoglobin	
Hematocrit	
Platelet count	**High:** Bleeding, systemic lupus erythematosus, pernicious anemia, hypersplenism (spleen takes too many platelets out of circulation), leukemia, and chemotherapy
Mean corpuscular volume	**High:** B12 and folate deficiency **Low:** Iron deficiency and thalassemia
Mean corpuscular hemoglobin (MCH)	

Thyroid

Thyroid stimulating hormone (TSH)	**High:** Hypothyroidism **Low:** Hyperthyroidism
Thyronine (T3)	**High:** Hyperthyroidism
Thyroxine (T4)	**High:** Hyperthyroidism **Low:** Hypothyroidism

Prostate

Prostate-specific antigen	**High:** Indicative of prostate cancer

Diabetes

Fasting plasma glucose	**High:** Diabetes mellitus **Low:** Hypoglycemia

CHAPTER 3

Age-Related Hearing Loss

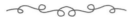

Michael B. Gluth, Colin L. W. Driscoll,
and Amy Hunter

GLUTH, DRISCOLL, AND HUNTER bring together perspectives from medicine and audiology to the discussion of age-related hearing loss. Much of the chapter is devoted to a description of presbycusis. Although presbycusis is viewed by many as a disorder, its prevalence in the elderly population is interpreted as a component of primary aging of the auditory system. Secondary disorders of hearing are introduced in this chapter, and the influence of tertiary aging on hearing in communicative contexts is described. The remainder of the chapter addresses evaluation, intervention, and prevention. Finally, obstacles to obtaining funding for services and hearing aids are presented.

The need to assess hearing loss in the aging population is such a common scenario that professionals working within the field of communicative science should consider it both an inevitable and a fundamental part of clinical practice. Indeed, hearing is a key element of communication for most individuals, with implications related to speech reception, speech production, and reception of environmental auditory cues. Accordingly, loss of hearing for an elderly individual may have major implications with respect to social well-being, professional competency, and overall quality of life. This chapter outlines the nature of age-related hearing loss and other pertinent diseases affecting the ear that are frequently seen in the aging population, with emphasis on clinical assessment, management, and associated global communicative implications.

Primary Aging

Primary aging of the hearing mechanism includes the typical spectrum of age-related changes that are known to commonly occur in the general population, without the additional effects of any other ear disease. Presbycusis is the term used to describe this natural age-related deterioration of hearing (Gates & Mills, 2005). Hearing is somewhat unique within the communicative sciences in that the "normal" hearing status for the elderly population consists of some degree of pathology and functional derangement. Accordingly, presbycusis is considered a part of primary aging. Given the progressive expansion of the elderly segment of the population, the impact of presbycusis on society will grow.

Understanding the nature of age-related hearing loss and other hearing disorders requires some knowledge of how we hear. The basic anatomy of the ear is depicted in Figure 3.1. It is beyond the scope of this chapter to provide a detailed description of hearing physiology, but a simplified version of the system follows. Sound waves travel down the ear canal, where they impact the eardrum, resulting in mechanical vibrations of the three ossicles within the middle-ear space. As the third bone (stapes) vibrates, sound pressure is transferred into the fluids within the inner ear (cochlea). Sound waves passing through the inner-ear fluids stimulate highly specialized sensory cells called *hair cells*. Hair cells are key elements of the inner-ear auditory sensory organs (organ of Corti) that are distributed upon a curled spiral partition called the *basilar membrane*. The physical properties of the basilar membrane and its attachments differentially direct stimulation to specifically located groups of inner-ear hair cells based on the pitch characteristics of the sound wave. In a process called *transduction*, the inner-ear auditory sensory organs then transform these mechanical fluid wave stimulations into electrical impulses within the adjacent auditory nerve fibers (also called the *cochlear nerve*). These impulses in turn travel up the central auditory pathway to the cortex of the brain, where sound is actually perceived.

Age-related hearing loss is primarily attributed to pathology involving the auditory sensory or neural elements of the inner ear. Most of the other anatomic structures comprising the hearing apparatus are relatively resistant to primary age-related changes. The ear canal, tympanic membrane (eardrum), and ossicles (middle-ear bones) do not undergo any clinically relevant degree of age-related functional loss. Therefore, in the clinical setting, presbycusis manifests as sensorineural or "inner-ear" hearing loss.

Large variations in the prevalence of presbycusis related to ethnicity or gender have not been definitively documented. Very rough estimated

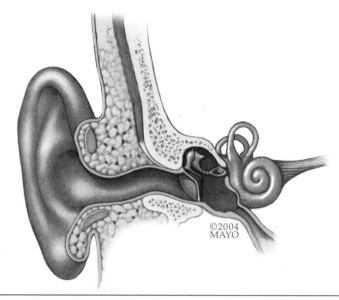

Figure 3.1. Anatomy of the ear. *Note.* From Mayo Clinic. (2004). *Cochlear Implants at Mayo Clinic*, (MC 5377). [Brochure]. Rochester, MN: Author. Copyrighted by and used with permission of Mayo Foundation for Medical Education and Research. All rights reserved.

rules of thumb suggest that in the United States, approximately 40% of individuals over age 65 have a significant hearing impairment with practical implications for daily function (Cruickshanks et al., 1998; Ries, 1994). The percentage of affected individuals in other societies may vary based on the degree of noise exposure (Goycoolea et al., 1986).

Typically, presbycusis consists of a symmetric bilateral high-frequency (4000–8000 Hz) hearing loss associated with deficits in speech discrimination. The negative impact of poor speech discrimination is perhaps the most commonly voiced complaint of hearing-impaired elderly adults. Pure-tone losses affect speech discrimination more severely if the major speech frequencies (500–4000 Hz) are also involved. When the speech discrimination capabilities are impaired, elderly individuals seem particularly prone to struggle in environments with background noise. This difficulty can be further aggravated by the presence of other cognitive and communication-related deficits. It should also be noted that impaired peripheral auditory signals may in turn affect central auditory processing with respect to specific parameters, such as temporal resolution, frequency resolution, loudness, and space localization (Williott, 1991).

Attempts have been made to correlate specific anatomic changes of the inner ear, particularly the stria vascularis, with the commonly recognized patterns of hearing loss associated with presbycusis (Nelson & Hinojosa, 2003; Schuknecht & Gacek, 1993). These efforts have resulted in the classification of four specific subtypes of presbycusis (see Table 3.1). The sensory subtype is most common. Much of the otopathology associated with sensory presbycusis is likely due to the accumulated effects of external toxic factors as opposed to strictly age-related change. Thus, age-related and acquired changes in anatomy and physiology are probably the result of both environmental insults (noise, ototoxic substance exposure, infection) and primary biological factors (genetic, metabolic) (Destefano, Gates, Heard-Costa, Myers, & Baldwin, 2003). In particular, mitochondrial DNA derangements are receiving attention for their role as relevant factors in age-related inner-ear degeneration (Fischel-Ghodsian et al., 1997).

Secondary Aging

Beyond presbycusis, there are a number of disease conditions and medical considerations common to the elderly population that should be familiar to clinicians dealing with communicative disorders. Despite having some typical characteristics, presbycusis is a diagnosis of exclusion; therefore, other potential causes of hearing loss must be considered. A brief discussion of the more common types of hearing loss and relevant related conditions with a focus on clinical aspects follows.

Conductive and Mixed Hearing Loss

The presence of a component of conductive hearing loss alone or in combination with underlying sensorineural hearing loss (thereby termed *mixed* hearing loss) definitively constitutes a condition that cannot be accounted for solely by age-related change. Conductive hearing loss results when sound waves are not properly "conducted" through the ear canal, eardrum, and middle-ear bones or middle-ear space; therefore, the sounds cannot be detected by the inner-ear sensory organs. Causes of conductive or mixed hearing loss common in the elderly population include cerumen (wax) impaction, eardrum perforation, impaired mobility of the eardrum, eustachian tube dysfunction, erosion of middle-ear bones, fluid within the middle-ear space (effusion), and otosclerosis (a disease that causes fixation of the stapes bone).

TABLE 3.1
Classification of Presbycusis

Type	Otopathology	Audiometric Findings
Sensory	Deterioration of cochlear sensory organs (organ of Corti); most prominent in basal turn of cochlea	Abrupt downsloping pure-tone loss in high frequencies; variable speech recognition; slowly progressive
Neural	Loss of auditory neural elements (spiral ganglion); equal distribution through-out cochlea	Relatively severe flat pure-tone loss in all frequencies; very poor speech recognition
Metabolic (strial)	Degeneration of stria vascularis	Relatively mild flat pure-tone loss in all frequencies; good speech recognition; earlier onset, slowly progressive
Mechanical (cochlear conductive)	Stiffening of basilar membrane; more severe in basal turn of cochlea	Gradual downsloping pure-tone loss in high frequencies; fair speech recognition

Sudden Sensorineural Hearing Loss

Sudden sensorineural hearing loss (SSNHL) refers to an abrupt drop of sensorineural hearing capacity that typically affects only one ear. Formally, this condition is defined as a drop of 30 decibels in three continuous frequencies over a period of less than 3 days, but less severe sudden losses certainly exist as well. Definitively determining the cause of SSNHL is usually not possible. The most common hypothesized causes include vascular compromise of the inner ear, unspecified viral infection affecting the inner ear or auditory nerve, and inflammation of the inner ear related to the host immune system (autoimmunity).

Asymmetric or Unilateral Sensorineural Hearing Loss

Because presbycusis is expected to be a process that occurs simultaneously in both ears at a similar rate, the presence of sensorineural hearing loss in only one ear or the presence of markedly asymmetric sensorineural hearing loss should alert the clinician to the possibility of a primary otologic or neurologic disease. In addition to the hypothesized factors that may be responsible for SSNHL, other conditions such as a tumor affecting the auditory nerve or otologic diseases such as autoimmune inner-ear disease (AIED) or Meniere's disease may be present. In particular, the presence of vertigo or other significant balance disturbances should alert the clinician to the possibility of one of these otologic disease conditions. Asymmetric noise exposure, such as firearm discharge or certain scenarios of occupational noise exposure, can also account for asymmetric sensorineural hearing loss.

Diabetes

Diabetes is a common disease condition encountered in the elderly population with a potential to cause sensorineural hearing loss (Kakarlapudi, Sawyer, & Staecker, 2003). Negative effects of diabetes include the potential for relevant related peripheral vascular disease and neuropathy. Such vascular disease can affect both the major blood vessel supply to the ear and the microscopic circulation within the inner ear. Furthermore, diabetic neuropathy has the potential to involve the auditory nerve.

Medications

Several medications commonly used in the elderly population also have the potential to cause temporary or permanent hearing loss. Examples include high-dose aspirin or other non-steroidal anti-inflammatory drugs (NSAIDs), loop diuretics (furosemide), certain chemotherapeutic agents, quinine derivatives, and certain antibiotics (aminoglycosides).

Tinnitus

Tinnitus is the perception of sound in the head or ears when no outside sound is actually present. It is often referred to as "ringing in the ears," but other forms of sound, such as roaring, hissing, chirping (crickets), whistling, swishing, or clicking noises, have also been described. Tinnitus, while not a cause of hearing loss, often accompanies presbycusis and frequently can be more bothersome to elderly individuals than hearing loss itself.

It is important to recognize that tinnitus is a symptom, not a specific disease condition. Tinnitus is felt to be a side effect of damage or wear within the inner ear or deranged hyperactivity within the central auditory pathway. In addition to sensorineural hearing loss, high blood pressure, noise exposure, specific medications, caffeine, alcohol, and a conductive hearing loss are all examples of factors that can result in or aggravate the symptom of tinnitus. Pulsatile tinnitus, which corresponds with an individual's heartbeat, may signal the presence of a serious vascular condition or tumor, indicating the need for a careful medical evaluation.

Tertiary Aging

Presbycusis can affect multiple facets of a person's life. For example, older individuals can be particularly dependent on hearing to compensate for other interrelated age-associated communicative disabilities, such as vision impairment, slowed cognition, age-related voice change, or diminished capacity for nonverbal communication. Furthermore, it has been hypothesized that decreased hearing may be a significant causative factor related to age-related decline in cognition (Wingfield, Tun, & McCoy, 2005). Common established psychosocial consequences of age-related hearing loss may include anxiety, low self-esteem, frustration, embarrassment, and social isolation (Erdman, Crowley, & Gillespie, 1984). There may also be concerns about or difficulty with understanding speech, responding appropriately, or appearing ignorant (Joensen & Saunders, 1984). These issues can lead to struggles or apprehension in the social and professional realms.

Despite the potential negative implications of age-related hearing loss, the average individual affected by a mild loss seems to adapt well and communicate without excessive perceived difficulty. This adaptation may be a result of the insidious onset of hearing loss that allows adults to make the needed adjustments (Garstecki & Erler, 1996). The ability to deal with communication deficits and related psychosocial implications may vary depending on an individual's environment, lifestyle, and personality.

Evaluation

Clinical evaluation of an elderly patient with hearing loss requires completion of a pertinent medical history, performance of a head and neck examination, and appropriate audiological testing. Details of the onset, nature, severity, and progression of hearing loss are obtained. Questioning about other associated symptoms such as tinnitus, vertigo, otalgia (pain), otorrhea (drainage), neurologic deficit, and facial nerve dysfunction is also required, as are queries regarding past or ongoing otologic disorders such as cerumen impaction, ear infection, eustachian tube dysfunction, or ear trauma. Other important points within the history include the nature of any past noise exposure, family history of hearing loss, prior otologic surgery, diabetes, ototoxic medication reception, and whether the patient has attempted use of an amplification device. Finally, knowledge of the relevant social or professional factors affected by hearing loss is needed to understand the impact on the individual patient.

After completion of the medical history, a head and neck examination is performed, with particular attention to the ears. Otoscopic examination allows for inspection of the pinna, ear canal, eardrum, ossicular landmarks, and middle-ear space. In doing so, medical professionals can note evidence of ear canal collapse, cerumen impaction, tympanic membrane perforation, or middle-ear effusion. A normal ear exam is expected in an elderly patient with presbycusis and no other ear pathology. Particular attention is also given to assessment of the cranial nerves, the voice, facial strength, and the eyes. Nystagmus, facial weakness, or cranial nerve deficits should raise concern for an underlying neurologic or neurotologic disorder and require a more in-depth evaluation.

The standard audiological evaluation will consist of pure-tone audiometry including air and bone conduction thresholds in both ears, speech audiometry to determine the speech reception threshold, and evaluation of suprathreshold word recognition. Other testing, such as tympanometry (dynamic measurement of ear canal volume that is indicative of the status of tympanic membrane integrity and compliance and the middle-ear pressure) or assessment of acoustic reflexes (the reflexive reactive contraction of the stapedius muscle in the middle ear when a loud noise is presented), may also be undertaken when clinically indicated.

While standard audiometric testing is helpful in characterizing a person's hearing loss, it is limited in terms of providing insight into how a person may function in "real world" conditions, which include factors such as background noise and multiple speakers. Other standardized word and speech recognition tests commonly used for evaluating cochlear implant patients (e.g., Hearing in Noise Test [HINT]; Nilsson, Soli, & Sullivan, 1994) can create a more realistic testing environment.

The functional decline in communication abilities due to decreased auditory performance is termed *hearing disability*; however, *hearing handicap* is the real-world, daily communication disadvantage that stems from such a disability. Attempts to measure and quantify hearing handicap have resulted in the development of specific tools. The American Medical Association/American Academy of Otolaryngology–Head & Neck Surgery (1979) has generated a formula to convert pure-tone threshold data into a percentage estimate of hearing handicap that is often utilized in legal matters related to worker's compensation:

Calculation of Hearing Handicap

Step 1: Calculate the pure-tone average (PTA) for each ear using pure-tone thresholds at 500 Hz, 1000 Hz, 2000 Hz, and 3000 Hz.

PTA = (500 Hz + 1000 Hz + 2000 Hz + 3000 Hz pure-tone thresholds) / 4

Step 2: Calculate the monaural percent impairment (MI) for each ear.

MI = 1.5 (PTA − 25)

Step 3: Calculate the percent hearing handicap (HH).

HH = [(5 × MI $_{better\,ear}$) + (MI $_{worse\,ear}$)] / 6

Asking the simple question "Do you have a hearing problem?" is a surprisingly sensitive way to screen for presbycusis (Gates, Murphy, Rees, & Fraher, 2003). Other self-assessment hearing handicap scales have also been validated for use as screening tools. Prominent among these are the Hearing Handicap Inventory for the Elderly–Screening Form (HHIE-S; Ventry & Weinstein, 1982) and the Self-Assessment of Communication (SAC; Schow & Nerbonne, 1982). Finally, other tools, such as the Communication Profile of the Hearing Impaired (CPHI; Demorest & Erdman, 1986) and Hearing Performance Inventory (HPI; Lamb, Owens, & Schubert, 1983), are useful in the assessment of the effects of hearing loss on overall communication and other more global consequences.

Prevention and Intervention

Noise Exposure

Although the prevention of presbycusis is not currently possible, mitigation of noise-induced hearing loss is achievable. The extent of injury due to noise is determined by two factors: loudness and duration of exposure. A permanent hearing loss may result from a single gunshot or accumulate more insidiously from repeated exposure to lower levels of noise encountered in many occupations. Some individuals are more susceptible to noise-induced hearing loss than are others. When presbycusis is already an issue, the additional damaging effects of noise exposure may be especially significant. Noise-induced hearing loss cannot be reversed but can be prevented. For that reason, it is critically important to counsel patients to protect their hearing by wearing ear plugs or protective ear muffs when in the presence of noise, even for brief exposures.

Behavioral or Listening Modifications

Any individual with hearing impairment struggling to communicate may misinterpret speech and provide inappropriate answers to questions. Ultimately, this struggle may compel him or her to disengage from conversations and social interaction. Several behavioral strategies can be used to help overcome such difficulties:

- Speakers should ensure that they have the listener's attention before speaking.
- Speakers and listeners should face each other while speaking and should make sure the lighting is appropriate.
- Listeners should wear glasses as needed.
- Speakers and listeners should be no more than 3 to 5 feet apart.
- Speakers should not cover their mouths or turn away from the intended speech recipient.
- Speakers should enunciate clearly and slowly and should refrain from shouting, as this can make understanding worse, given that loudness does not always mean clarity.
- Speakers should rephrase a misunderstood word or sentence instead of repeating the same phrase multiple times.
- Speakers and listeners should reduce background noise (e.g., turn off TV/radio, do not sit in the center of a loud restaurant, and do not sit by an open window).
- Listeners should sit with better ear toward speaker.
- Hearing-impaired listeners should repeat back what they perceive they have heard.
- Speakers might consider writing the topic of conversation or key points.
- Listeners should not nod or otherwise imply understanding when this is not the case.
- Speakers should ask hearing-impaired listeners what can be done to make conversation easier.

Hearing Aids

Adults with presbycusis can usually benefit from appropriately fit amplification. However, due to negative stigma associated with hearing aid usage, the average hearing-impaired adult may wait several years before seeking assistance for hearing loss. Over the last several years, the acceptance of hearing aids has increased due to more discreet devices, advanced device performance, better fitting techniques, and improved follow-up care.

Hearing aids consist of four basic parts. A *microphone* detects sound from the environment and changes it into an electrical signal. This signal is then transmitted to an *amplifier*. The amplifier increases the volume of the sound and then sends it to a *receiver*. The receiver transforms the electrical input back into sound and broadcasts it into the ear. The *battery* powers the device.

The majority of hearing aids dispensed today consist of digital technology, which affords advanced programming and processing capabilities that generally result in cleaner sound quality as compared to hearing aids with older, analog technology. The digital hearing aid utilizes a computer chip, which customizes the amplified sound according to an individual's particular hearing loss characteristics and the specific listening environment.

Several styles of hearing aids are available that may be classified by size and contour: completely in the canal (CIC), in the canal (ITC), in the ear (ITE), behind the ear (BTE), and open fit behind the ear. Each style has advantages and disadvantages. When counseling elderly patients regarding hearing aids, professionals should consider the presence of the patient's accompanying manual dexterity and vision problems, as these may affect his or her ability to manipulate the device and perform tasks such as aid insertion, aid removal, aid cleaning, and battery changing.

As a simple rule of thumb, when the average pure-tone hearing thresholds reach 40 dB, amplification is indicated (Gates & Mills, 2005). Despite the benefits that hearing aid use may potentially afford, only 20% of candidates for amplification actually purchase an aid (Popelka et al., 1998). This unfortunate phenomenon has been closely studied and noted to be multifactoral in origin. A complex mix of psychological and demographic factors, such as perceived stigma, financial status, social support, control-of-self attitudes, gender, and extent of perceived communication deficits, have been identified as key influences in the aging population with respect to hearing aid acquisition and utilization (Garstecki & Erler, 1998).

Assistive Listening Devices

Assistive listening devices may also be appropriate for individuals with presbycusis. One such device is the pocket amplifier, which can be worn like a portable music player. This device contains a headset with earphones that are connected to a box comprising a microphone and volume control switch. When communicating with an individual using a pocket amplifier, the speaker directs sounds toward the microphone, and those sounds are then amplified into the headset.

Another assistive listening device that can be coupled to a hearing aid is the FM system. This is a coupled device that includes one component connected to a behind-the-ear hearing aid and another component that consists of a microphone and transmitter. The signal from the microphone/transmitter is conveyed directly to the receiver through a wireless FM signal, thereby allowing one-way communication without significant interference from environmental sounds.

Finally, nonauditory alerting devices may be used to promote both safety and independence. Examples include a flashing light that is activated when someone is ringing the doorbell or when a telephone is ringing. Similarly, modified smoke detectors can be equipped with a strobe light to better alert hearing-impaired individuals.

Cochlear Implants

Cochlear implants are an option for individuals with hearing loss who receive limited benefit from conventional hearing aids. The cochlear implant effectually bypasses the damaged parts of the inner ear by transmitting electrical sound signals directly to the auditory nerve. As shown in Figure 3.2, the cochlear implant consists of an externally worn component (appears similar to a hearing aid) and a surgically implanted internal component. The external component is composed of a microphone, a speech processor, and a transmitter. The microphone receives sound and sends it to the speech processor, where it is converted into a digital code. The transmitter then broadcasts this digital signal across the skin into the implanted internal component that consists of a receiver and an electrode array. Receipt and conversion of this signal controls the rate and pattern of electric impulses, which are fired throughout the electrode array coiled within the cochlea, thereby directly stimulating the fibers of the auditory nerve. With time and rehabilitation, the cochlear implant recipient can learn to clearly interpret these electrical signals into meaningful sounds and speech. Cochlear implants are becoming more common in the aging population as candidacy criteria continue to evolve.

Cerumen

Impacted cerumen (earwax) is a common problem in the elderly population. Cerumen normally migrates toward the opening of the ear canal and is generally removed easily with normal washing. However, plugging does occur at times due to the presence of a narrow ear canal, excessive or overly

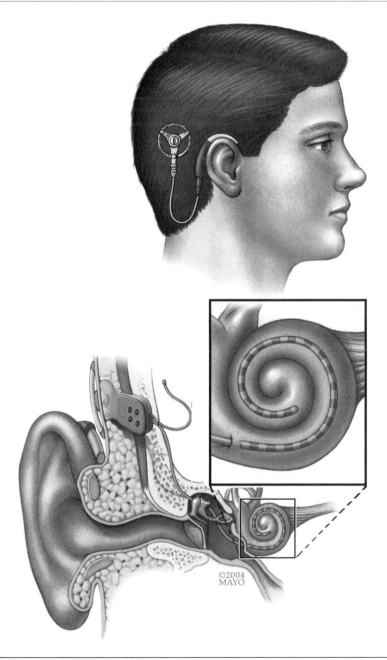

Figure 3.2. Cochlear implant. *Note.* From Mayo Clinic. (2004). *Cochlear Implants at Mayo Clinic*, (MC 5377). [Brochure]. Rochester, MN: Author. Copyrighted by and used with permission of Mayo Foundation for Medical Education and Research. All rights reserved.

aggressive use of cotton swabs (which can push cerumen farther into the ear canal toward the eardrum), or other unknown factors. When blockage occurs to an excessive degree, affected individuals may notice a decrease in hearing or experience a plugged sensation. Hearing aid users may also report that their aids are no longer working properly. Impacted cerumen can be cleared in a number of ways, including irrigation, use of cerumen-removal ear drops, or curettage performed by a healthcare professional.

Reimbursement

While most audiology services do not require physician supervision, the procedures must be ordered by a physician to qualify for reimbursement from most insurance companies and Medicare. Audiologists use codes that correspond to a wide range of procedures, including audiological assessment procedures, hearing aid assessment and fitting, vestibular and balance system assessment, cochlear implant services, and auditory habilitation and rehabilitation. Audiologists may also bill for cerumen management. With few exceptions, charges for audiology services are based on the procedures performed during a contact, not on the time spent with a client during that contact.

Auditory assessment procedures are described by Current Procedural Terminology (CPT) codes that specify individual procedures or by comprehensive codes that describe a combination of procedures (American Medical Association [AMA], 2009a). If a comprehensive code is billed, the codes for the individual procedures should not be reported. One example of a CPT code that describes a combination of procedures is the one used to designate a comprehensive audiometry threshold and speech recognition evaluation. This code indicates that air and bone conduction have been performed and that speech audiometry thresholds and recognition have been tested. If those procedures are not completed on the same day, CPT codes representing each individual procedure should be billed. Although a specific code applies to removal of cerumen, that procedure is assumed to be part of the audiometric test and cannot be billed as a separate procedure.

Another comprehensive code applies to acoustic immittance testing. That code includes tympanometry, acoustic reflex threshold testing, and acoustic reflex decay testing; however, individual codes apply if all procedures are not completed in one contact. Similarly, the basic vestibular evaluation code includes spontaneous nystagmus testing, positional nystagmus testing, optokinetic nystagmus testing, and oscillating tracking testing. Individual codes apply if all four procedures are not performed.

Certain distinct procedures can be performed on the same day, with each CPT being reported. Performance of distinct procedures requires addition of a numeric modifier. For example, tinnitus assessment can be billed on the same day as a loudness balance test. Modifiers are also used to identify reduced procedures, such as audiometric testing of only one ear.

Hearing aid assessment and fitting procedures are described by both CPT codes and the Healthcare Common Procedure Code System (HCPCS; AMA, 2009b). Medicare does not cover routine hearing examinations; however, a percentage of the expense of diagnostic hearing examinations is covered by Medicare Part B. Private insurance companies vary in the hearing services covered, but most standard health insurance plans do not provide coverage for hearing aids. An older person may be able to obtain coverage by paying an additional fee or by purchasing supplemental insurance, but these funding limitations may reduce an older person's access to appropriate testing and intervention.

Evaluation for auditory rehabilitation may be provided by audiologists or speech–language pathologists. Although a code exists for auditory rehabilitation for postlingual hearing loss, the code is not covered for audiologists; speech–language pathologists use the procedure code that applies to rehabilitation of speech, language, voice, and auditory processing.

Key Points

The medical and audiological perspectives on hearing in the elderly were presented in this chapter. Primary points of information included the following:

- Age-related hearing loss (presbycusis) is a common condition that is caused by multifactoral deterioration of the sensory and neural elements of the inner ear.
- The pattern of hearing loss associated with presbycusis most commonly consists of a bilateral, symmetric, down-sloping sensorineural loss involving the higher frequencies (4000–8000 Hz) and diminished speech discrimination.
- Elderly individuals with hearing loss sufficient to affect speech recognition encounter particular difficulty in environments with background noise.

- Because presbycusis is a diagnosis of exclusion, careful assessment of other possible causes of hearing loss or underlying ear disease is important.
- The management approach to presbycusis consists of a combination of protection against acoustic trauma, modification of behavioral listening techniques, and usage of mechanical devices such as assistive listening devices, hearing aids, or cochlear implants.
- Current limits on funding for hearing evaluations and hearing aids may restrict an older person's access to appropriate services and interventions.

References

American Medical Association. (2009a). *Current procedural terminology (CPT) 2010*. Chicago: Author.

American Medical Association. (2009b). *Healthcare common procedure coding system 2010: Level II*. Chicago: Author.

American Medical Association/American Academy of Otolaryngology. (1979). Guide for the evaluation of hearing handicap. *Journal of the American Medical Association, 241*, 2055–2059.

Cruickshanks, K. J., Wiley, T. L., Tweed, T. S., Klein, B. E. K., Klein, R., Mares-Perlman, J. A., et al. (1998). Prevalence of hearing loss in older adults in Beaver Dam, Wisconsin: The epidemiology of hearing loss study. *American Journal of Epidemiology, 148*, 879–886.

Demorest, M. E., & Erdman, S. A. (1986). Scale composition and item analysis of the Communication Profile for the Hearing Impaired. *Journal of Hearing and Speech Research, 29*, 515–535.

Destefano, A. L, Gates, G. A., Heard-Costa, N., Myers, R. H., & Baldwin, C. T. (2003). Genome-wide linkage analysis to presbycusis in the Framingham Heart study. *Archives of Otolaryngology–Head & Neck Surgery, 129*, 285–289.

Erdman, S. A., Crowley, J. M., & Gillespie, G. G. (1984). Considerations in counseling the hearing impaired. *Hearing Instruments, 35*, 50–58.

Fischel-Ghodsian, N., Bykovskaya, Y., Taylor, K., Kahen, T., Cantor, R., Ehrenman, K., et al. (1997). Temporal bone analysis of patients with presbycusis reveals high frequency of mitochondrial mutations. *Hearing Research, 110*, 147–154.

Garstecki, D. C., & Erler, S. F. (1996). Older adult performance on the Communication Profile for the Hearing Impaired. *Journal of Speech, Language, and Hearing Research, 39*, 28–42.

Garstecki, D. C., & Erler, S. F. (1998). Hearing loss, control, and demographic factors influencing hearing aid use among older adults. *Journal of Speech, Language, and Hearing Research, 41*, 527–538.

Gates, G. A., & Mills, J. H. (2005). Presbycusis. *Lancet, 366*, 1111–1120.

Gates, G. A., Murphy, M., Rees, T. S., & Fraher, A. (2003). Screening for handicapping hearing loss in the elderly. *Journal of Family Practice, 52*, 56–62.

Goycoolea, M. V., Goycoolea, H. G., Farfan, C. R., Rodriguez, L. G., Martinez, G. C., & Vidal, R. (1986). Effect of life in industrialized societies on hearing in natives of Easter Island. *Laryngoscope, 96,* 1391–1396.

Joensen, J. P., & Saunders, D. J. (1984). Psychological correlates of geriatric hearing loss: Understanding the emotional and behavioral consequences of impaired hearing. *The Hearing Journal, 45,* 47–54.

Kakarlapudi, V., Sawyer, R., & Staecker H. (2003). The effect of diabetes on sensorineural hearing loss. *Otology & Neurotology 24,* 382–386.

Lamb, S. H., Owens, E., & Schubert, E. D. (1983). The revised form of the Hearing Performance Inventory. *Ear and Hearing, 4,*152–159.

Mayo Clinic. (2004). *Cochlear implants at Mayo Clinic* (MC 5377). [Brochure]. Rochester, MN: Author.

Nelson, E. G., & Hinojosa, R. (2003). Presbycusis: A human temporal bone study of individuals with flat audiometric patterns of hearing loss using a new method to quantify stria vascularis volume. *Laryngoscope, 113,* 1672–1686.

Nilsson, M., Soli, S., & Sullivan, J. (1994). Development of the Hearing in Noise Test for the measurement of speech reception thresholds in quiet and noise. *Journal of the Acoustical Society of America, 95,* 1085–1099.

Popelka, M. M., Cruickshanks, K. J., Wiley, T. L., Tweed, T. S., Klein, B. E., & Klein, R. (1998). Low prevalence of hearing aid use among older adults with hearing loss: The epidemiology of hearing loss study. *Journal of the American Geriatrics Society, 46,* 1075–1078.

Ries, P. W. (1994). Prevalence and characteristics of persons with hearing trouble: United States, 1990–1991. *Vital Health Statistics, 188,* 1–75.

Schow, R. L., & Nerbonne, M. A. (1982). Communication screening profile: Use with elderly clients. *Ear and Hearing, 3,* 135–147.

Schuknecht, H. F., & Gacek, H. R. (1993). Cochlear pathology in presbycusis. *Annals of Otology Rhinology and Laryngology, 102,* 1–16.

Ventry, I., & Weinstein, B. (1982). The hearing handicap inventory for the elderly: A new tool. *Ear and Hearing, 3,* 128–134.

Williott, J. F. (1991). *Aging and the auditory system: Anatomy, physiology, and psychophysics.* San Diego, CA: Singular.

Wingfield, A., Tun, P. A., & McCoy, S. L. (2005). Hearing loss in older adulthood: What it is and how it interacts with cognitive performance. *Current Directions in Psychological Science, 14,* 144–148.

CHAPTER 4

Voice Disorders in the Aging Patient: A Physician's Viewpoint

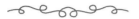

Michael B. Gluth and C. Blake Simpson

GLUTH AND SIMPSON PRESENT a medical perspective on primary, secondary, and tertiary aging of the laryngeal system. In discussing normal and pathological changes in laryngeal structures and functions, the authors highlight the challenge of determining when an "old-sounding" voice (often called *presbyphonia*) may be considered problematic by the aging individual. In the secondary aging section, laryngeal pathologies are described. Methods of evaluation are then introduced, followed by a discussion of how voice disorders might be prevented or treated.

A clinician evaluating speech and voice abnormalities in an elderly patient is presented with a distinct set of challenges that requires both an understanding of the relevant potential pathologic processes as well as the usual age-related changes involved. While some degree of anatomic and physiologic change in vocal function is expected with senescence, it is the onus of the clinician to determine when these processes have passed beyond the realm of normal aging and into the disordered range. It is also necessary to possess a working knowledge of the most common disease processes and other medical considerations that are intrinsic to the larynx itself as well as those affecting other related body systems in the elderly population. With careful, systematic clinical assessment and analysis, medical professionals can develop and execute appropriate plans for management and treatment with a multidisciplinary approach in order to maximize successful communication.

One important component of multidisciplinary assessment and intervention is understanding the differing perspectives of each professional discipline. To meet this need, two chapters on speech and voice disorders have been provided in this book. This chapter, the first of the two, reflects the views of two otolaryngologists and emphasizes anatomic changes and laryngeal pathology. Chapter 5 provides the perspective of two speech–language pathologists and focuses on vocal functions that cause or perpetuate voice problems. That chapter also includes more comprehensive discussions of other speech processes and disorders.

Primary Aging

Primary aging of speech and voice refers to the changes that fall within the expected range for what one would generally consider "normal aging." Relevant structural and physiologic alterations within the speech and vocal apparatus are described, with some anatomic changes highlighted, in Table 4.1. Despite the reality of these changes, it should be noted at the outset of this section that the majority of active elderly adults maintain a level of speech and voice quality that is satisfactory for communication needs.

Documented trends suggest that these collective alterations in structure tend to correlate with perceptible changes in function with age. However, it is important to note that there can be considerable variation within the aging population with respect to the degree and consequences of these changes. It is particularly important to realize that the biological process of aging can significantly vary from one individual to another, having poor correlation with chronologic age. In general, the healthy older person adapts to anatomic and physiologic changes in the vocal tract without experiencing a significant deterioration of speech functioning unless the system is stressed by physical or environmental factors (Hooper & Cralidis, 2009). Thus, significant changes in the intelligibility of an elderly person's speech should alert the physician to a potential disease process.

In contrast to other aspects of speech, age-related anatomic alterations seem to bear more recognizable consequences with respect to voice. In fact, the ability to ascertain variations in phonation between young and elderly individuals is generally inherent even for untrained listeners. These changes generally consist of increased degrees of coarseness, pitch change, tremulousness, and breathiness. A summary discussion of normative vocal acoustic parameters within the aging population is undertaken in Chapter 5. Nevertheless a few correlates between elderly anatomy and physiology are worth further limited discussion—most notably the topics of cricoarytenoid joint degeneration and age-related vocal cord transformation.

TABLE 4.1

Age-Related Anatomic Changes of the Oral Cavity and Larynx

Location	Anatomic changes
Oral cavity	• Thinned mucosa • Loss of dentition • Minor salivary gland degeneration • Tongue and pharyngeal muscle atrophy • Sensory and motor neuronal degeneration
Laryngeal framework	• Laryngeal cartilage ossification • Minor salivary gland degeneration • Extrinsic laryngeal muscular atrophy • Sensory and motor neuronal degeneration • Cricoarytenoid joint erosion
Glottis	• Thinned mucosa • Vocalis muscle atrophy/replacement with collagen • Vocal ligament stiffening and degeneration • Edema (females) or thinning (males) of lamina propria • Diminished, thickened mucous coating

Laryngeal cartilage ossification is a progressive process that begins during the middle decades and continues well into the later stages of life. Although males seem to begin this process roughly one decade earlier than female counterparts (usually within the third decade in males), both sexes may eventually be affected by its consequences. Some clinicians contend that the degree of laryngeal cartilage ossification is a rough marker of laryngeal biologic age, but it remains unclear whether the rates of other anatomic or physiologic changes exactly correlate with this indicator. As aging and ossification progress, the structure and orientation of the laryngeal cartilages and cricoarytenoid joints can be altered, resulting in diminished range of motion. This change, in combination with other degenerative changes such as joint fibrosis, ultimately can impair glottal closure and cause an increased degree of breathiness.

Over time, the vocal cord also undergoes distinct changes in structure. Atrophy of the vocalis and other intrinsic laryngeal muscles is a common finding in the aging larynx that may be related to social isolation, long periods of relative nonvocalization, and resultant vocal deconditioning. This atrophy can result in diminished vocal cord bulk and altered shape, with a tendency toward thinning and bowing. The contour of the glottis and degree of closure can be thereby affected, also potentially contributing to breathiness.

Changes in the lamina propria of the vocal fold occur with aging, and the effects seem to be more evident in males. In the superficial layer of the lamina propria, elastin becomes irregular and disorganized, while the corresponding deep layer of the lamina propria shows similar changes with collagen fibers. The combination of these senescent changes leads to a loss of the layered structure and reduction in viscoelasticity and thickness of the vocal folds. In contrast, females tend to develop edema of the superficial lamina propria (possibly due to the hormonal effects of reduced estrogen production) and a thickening of the vibratory tissues.

Laryngeal muscle atrophy, in combination with changes in the lamina propria, as well as thickening and reduction of overlying mucous secretions, can adversely affect the vibratory characteristics. In general, studies show a trend toward an increase in pitch in elderly males and decrease in pitch in elderly females—again, the latter is likely due to increased vocal cord edema. Age-related vocal cord transformation in combination with a decrease in neuromuscular control can also affect vocal tremulousness, coarseness, and the ability to sustain phonation.

Secondary Aging

While laryngeal structures and functioning may be affected, a significant change in speech functioning is not associated with normal aging and may signal a health problem. In the elderly, disease processes that affect speech are often neurological, with a wide range of static and progressive conditions being possible. Specific characteristics of the person's speech may help identify the etiology or site of lesion, and in some cases, speech problems may be the first symptom reported. It is beyond the scope of this book to present a medical perspective on the numerous neurological disorders associated with speech disorders. Information relevant to specific motor speech problems is contained in Chapter 5. Cognitive–linguistic disorders are discussed in Chapters 8 and 10.

In many cases, medical interventions for conditions that underlie an older person's articulation and fluency problems do not have significant benefits for the person's communication. This is less true of voice disorders, where the treatments offered by the physician are likely to have a direct impact on the person's communication.

As outlined, the changes associated with primary aging generally do not constitute a pathologic process in most individuals. However, the art of clinical medicine involves the application of a customized set of standards for each individual patient in order to determine when these changes have breached the threshold of normalcy into the realm of a primary age-related voice disorder. Such standards may be based on a combination of social aspects, psychological factors, and professional demands unique to each individual. For example, the perceived desirability of an "old-sounding" voice may vary between two individuals. Furthermore, the consequences of a relatively breathy, weak, or coarse voice differ depending on specific lifestyle demands.

In the clinical realm, the term often used to describe a primary age-related voice disorder is *presbyphonia* (although there is some debate about whether this label implies pathology). The subjective finding of a coarse, breathy voice along with the physical finding of vocal fold atrophy and "bowing" is commonly used to make the clinical diagnosis of presbyphonia (Pontes, Brasolotto, & Behlau, 2005). Figure 4.1 illustrates the vocal fold thinning and "bowing" that characterize presbylaryngis. However, each clinician must understand that a diagnosis of presbyphonia is largely subjective and can be reached by the determination that (a) a specific vocal parameter has undergone an unacceptable degree of age-related change or (b) common subtle alterations are unsuitable for a particular patient's quality of life.

Beyond presbyphonia, there is also a set of common disease conditions intrinsic to the larynx that may be encountered in the aging population.

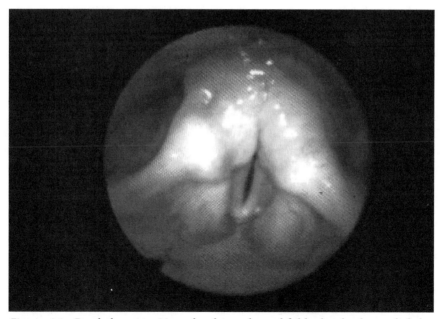

Figure 4.1. Presbylaryngis. Note the thinned vocal folds that lead to a slightly concave contour and incomplete closure during phonation.

Clinicians must be knowledgeable of these conditions because most elderly patients who present for laryngologic evaluation with voice complaints suffer primarily from conditions other than presbyphonia (Woo, Casper, Colton, & Brewer, 1992). Although this section is not intended to be an encyclopedic discussion of laryngeal pathology, it offers a brief outline of some of these pathologies, with emphasis on elements unique to the aging population.

Vocal Cord Paralysis

Paralysis (complete weakness) or *paresis* (partial weakness) of the vocal fold is generally the result of underlying damage or dysfunction of the recurrent laryngeal nerves. The recurrent laryngeal nerve innervates all of the intrinsic laryngeal musculature, with the exception of the cricothyroid muscle. This condition is most often unilateral and generally results in signs and symptoms of glottic insufficiency, including a weak or breathy voice, excessively effortful phonation, dysphagia, cough, or aspiration that is most prominent with ingestion of thin liquids. In most instances, a distinct point of onset is evident. In the elderly population, this condition can be caused by inadvertent damage during a surgical procedure involving the thyroid, cervical spine, or chest. Long-term or traumatic endotracheal intubation, blunt neck or chest trauma, viral infection, tumor (skull base, thyroid, chest), and stroke are other common identifiable causes.

Superior Laryngeal Nerve Palsy

The superior laryngeal nerve is responsible for motor innervation of the cricothyroid muscle and sensory innervation of the supraglottic larynx. Injury to this nerve can occur as a result of surgery to the neck (carotid artery, cervical spine, and thyroid). Other cases may be related to viral infection or stroke. Signs and symptoms of superior laryngeal nerve palsy are usually more subtle than those observed with vocal cord paralysis. Most often this condition is associated with a normal conversational voice that is impaired in the upper pitch range, with a tendency toward early fatigue. The patient may also complain of dysphagia or coughing, especially with thin liquids.

Chronic Laryngitis and Benign Vocal Cord Lesions

Chronic laryngitis is a nonspecific clinical term used to describe a state of chronic laryngeal irritation. In most cases, chronic laryngitis is a multifactoral condition resulting from a combination of cigarette smoke, laryngo-pharyngeal reflux, vocal abuse, inhaled irritant exposure, laryngitis sicca, and allergic sequellae. Generally, this is a noninfectious condition. Symptoms of chronic laryngitis may include a coarse voice, early vocal fatigue, throat discomfort, cough, excessive throat mucus, or foreign body sensation (globus pharyngeus). Chronic laryngeal irritation can also result in the secondary development of related benign or malignant laryngeal neoplasms.

Vocal cord nodules are discreet masses that form in the superficial layer of the vibratory edge of the vocal cords in a manner similar to a callous. Vocal abuse is thought to be the overwhelming contributing factor in the development of most nodules, although chronic laryngitis may lead to an increased risk of developing nodules (or perhaps more sizable nodules). Although generally uncommon in the aging population, nodules may be encountered in elderly singers or other individuals with heavy vocal usage. Symptoms of vocal nodules may include hoarseness, vocal fatigue, restricted vocal range, or breathiness, and those symptoms vary depending on bulk and extent.

A *vocal polyp* is a reactive inflammatory neoplasm that is also derived from within the superficial layer of the vocal cord and is usually found on one side only. In addition to being a potential consequence of chronic laryngitis, some vocal polyps may originate from a vocal fold hemorrhage or vocal misuse. Depending on size or location, polyps can result in hoarseness, breathiness, or even stridor with inspiration.

A *granuloma* is an inflammatory vocal cord lesion that usually forms in the posterior glottis adjacent to the vocal process of the arytenoid cartilage. Often these lesions form as a consequence of traumatic contact with an endotracheal tube; however, uncontrolled laryngopharyngeal reflux or vocal abuse (such as chronic cough and throat clearing) can also result in granuloma formation. If they are bulky, these lesions can result in breathiness due to obstructed glottic closure, hoarseness, cough, or mild discomfort with phonation; however, they are often asymptomatic.

Reinke's Edema (Polypoid Corditis)

Reinke's edema is a condition seen predominantly in middle-age and elderly females who smoke cigarettes. Figure 4.2 provides a view of the effects of this condition on the vocal folds. Although Reinke's edema can rarely be caused by hypothyroidism or other sources of laryngeal irritation, it is properly considered a smoker's disease that results in the abnormal accumulation of gelatinous fluid within the superficial layer of the vocal cord. As a result, patients experience signs and symptoms that result from having

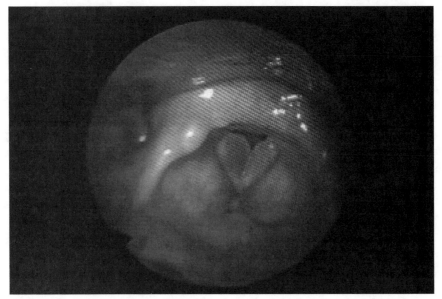

Figure 4.2. Reinke's edema. Note the convex contour of the vocal folds due to deposition of subcutaneous polypoid tissue and edema.

bulky, engorged vocal cords, such as a coarse voice with lowered pitch and, in some cases, dyspnea or stridor with inspiration.

Laryngitis Sicca

Laryngitis sicca is a term used to describe a vocal cord irritation that results from drying and insufficient hydration. It is common in the aging population. A healthy voice is dependent on vocal cords that are kept continually moist and lubricated with thin watery mucus. Without adequate mucus, normal vocal cord vibratory function is adversely affected, resulting in inflammation and an increased workload required to generate normal phonation. This inflammation can result in a voice that is coarse, decreased in pitch, and easily fatigued. Causes of laryngitis sicca include excessive alcoholic or caffeinated beverage intake, inadequate intake of water, chronic mouth breathing, dry air exposure, and certain medications (e.g., diuretics, antihistamines, some anti-anxiety medications).

Laryngopharyngeal Reflux

Laryngopharyngeal reflux (LPR) is a common condition that results from abnormal regurgitation of stomach contents up through the esophagus into the pharynx and larynx. Common symptoms of LPR include hoarseness, frequent throat clearing, pain or irritation in the throat, feeling of lump in throat (globus pharyngeus), dysphagia, a foul or bitter taste in the mouth, cough, asthma-like symptoms, and excessive throat mucous. It is critical to understand that heartburn may or may not be present with LPR, thereby rendering some patients with this condition surprised or even skeptical to learn their diagnosis.

Laryngeal Cancer

Cancer of the larynx is most prominent in males over the age of 55, although females and younger patients can certainly be affected as well. By far the most significant risk factor for developing laryngeal cancer is cigarette smoking. Other notable risk factors include heavy alcoholic beverage use, inhalant exposure to certain occupational hazards (e.g., nickel, sulfuric acid, and asbestos), history of other throat or lung cancer, and severe uncontrolled laryngopharyngeal reflux. Specifically, laryngeal cancer is almost always squamous cell carcinoma that develops from the outer soft tissue covering of the upper aerodigestive tract. This cancer most often results in hoarseness, especially in lesions that derive from the vocal cord itself. More advanced bulky lesions can also result in hemoptysis, dysphagia, odynophagia, shortness of breath, or even sequelae of vocal cord paralysis if laryngeal nerves are invaded.

Muscle Tension Dysphonia

Excessive tension in the muscles of the supraglottic larynx is a frequently encountered scenario that may result in a voice that is strained, pitch-locked, and easily fatigued. Most cases of muscle tension dysphonia are the result of attempted compensation for underlying glottic insufficiency that is due to age-related vocal fold atrophy or vocal fold paralysis or paresis. Other factors may contribute to the development of this condition, including laryngeal irritation (LPR, vocal overuse, and smoking), psychological stress, and related strain in the neck and shoulder musculature. An acute variant of muscle tension dysphonia is also recognized in patients who overuse their voice in the midst of a bout of acute infectious laryngitis.

Non-Laryngologic Illnesses

A number of other general health issues may potentially play a role in speech and voice production in the elderly population (Sataloff, Rosen, Hawkshaw, & Spiegel, 1997). Notably, the effects of chronic pulmonary diseases such as emphysema, asthma, or restrictive lung disease on voice production can be detrimental. By reducing airflow through the vocal tract during attempted phonation, pulmonary disease can affect the resultant volume as well as heighten the effort required to phonate. Additionally, steroid-containing inhalers commonly used to treat chronic pulmonary disease can cause fungal laryngitis.

Neurologic disorders in the elderly can also have adverse consequences relative to communication. Foremost, stroke can result in derangements in neuromuscular coordination, motor deficits, and sensory deficits throughout the upper aerodigestive tract that diminish the quality and efficiency of speech, breathing, swallowing, and voice. Other notable neurologic disorders with speech and vocal consequences more prominent in the aging population include Parkinson's disease, essential tremor, and drug-induced tremor. A number of these are addressed in Chapter 5.

Finally, age-related hearing loss (presbycusis) is an extremely common and frequently untreated condition that can have significant effects on voice production. Deficient hearing may result in compensatory vocal abuse, and the loss of auditory feedback can render both the control and matching of pitch quite difficult.

Tertiary Aging

In the context of speech and voice disorders, *tertiary aging* refers to the more global consequences of age-related dysfunction. In specific, speech and voice disorders can result in disability or handicap, and can have a measurable effect on quality of life (Verdonck-de Leeuw & Mahieu, 2004). Dysphonia may affect an individual's ability to perform activities of daily living, to socialize, or to meet professional demands—all of which can have a negative bearing on emotional well-being and self-sufficiency. In general, quality-of-life studies involving patients with voice disorders have demonstrated decreased scores similar to those involving other common chronic diseases.

Evaluation

Clinical evaluation of an elderly patient with a speech or voice complaint requires acquisition of a detailed medical history and performance of a thorough relevant physical examination. First, a clear understanding of the primary complaint with respect to onset, severity, timing, progression, attempted treatments, and associated symptoms is obtained. Second, an inquiry is made regarding pertinent voice performance requirements, usage habits, and related expectations. This inquiry should include an understanding of relevant social or professional voice requirements and singing habits.

In taking a history from an elderly patient with a vocal disorder, a physician must be aware that the general medical and surgical history may be particularly relevant. It is specifically important to review the presence of any pulmonary, allergic, neurologic, rhinologic, or otologic conditions. Several progressive neurologic disorders may be associated with dysphonia in the elderly (e.g., Parkinson's disease, amyotrophic lateral sclerosis, essential tremor). In some instances, the presenting complaint for these disease states is dysphonia or dysphagia. When taking a surgical history, the clinician should take particular notice of any procedures performed in the neck or chest, or other interventions that may have required an extended period of endotracheal intubation. A social history should include a review of tobacco, caffeine, and alcoholic beverage usage in addition to an inquiry regarding the nature of the patient's living conditions and social support. Finally, the medication list should be surveyed for agents that might have an influence on vocal health, such as corticosteroids, antihistamines, diuretics, hormones, or psychotropic medications.

After the medical history is reviewed, a complete ear, nose, and throat examination is required. Table 4.2 outlines the particularly important elements of a physical examination for an elderly patient with a voice disorder. Laryngeal examination, at a minimum, requires indirect mirror laryngoscopy. However, the examiner is ideally afforded the benefits of modern laryngoscopy utilizing either a flexible or rigid laryngeal scope. Currently available laryngeal imaging techniques can provide improved visibility, increased magnification, video replay capabilities, and stroboscopic assessment of vocal fold motion.

Table 4.3 outlines the typical laryngeal exam findings for common voice disorders encountered in the aging population. Despite the presence of such laryngeal findings, it should be stressed that in many instances, a careful assessment of the voice itself is most helpful in diagnosis and in subsequent treatment planning.

Prevention and Intervention

A comprehensive discussion of the management of each laryngeal disease mentioned thus far is beyond the intended scope of this text. However,

TABLE 4.2
Key Elements of Physical Examination
in an Elderly Patient with a Voice Complaint

System	Foremost aspects of exam
General	Assess for malnutrition, obesity, and abnormal emotional state.
Ears	Assess outer and middle ears for pathology resulting in conductive hearing loss. At a minimum, perform a gross hearing screen.
Nose	Assess for stigmata of allergic rhinitis, chronic nasal airway obstruction resulting in mouth breathing, and evidence of chronic sinusitis.
Oral cavity	Assess extent of mucosal hydration, tongue mobility, and presence of fasciculation. Inspect dentition.
Oropharynx	Assess for signs of infection (exudate or fungal element), signs of chronic irritation, and evidence of tonsillar disease.
Speech	Assess articulation, rate, and fluency.
Voice	Assess for hoarseness, breathiness, tremor, pitch abnormality, and abnormal vocal fatigue. Consider formal acoustic measurements if indicated.
Neurologic	Assess for cranial nerve dysfunction, gross focal motor deficits, and tremor.
Neck	Palpate larynx, thyroid, and cervical musculature. Assess for pathologic lymphadenopathy. Grossly evaluate cervical range of motion.
Breathing	Assess airflow and respiratory effort. Consider lung auscultation and spirometry if indicated.
Hypopharynx	Assess for signs of infection (exudate or fungal element), signs of chronic irritation, presence of pooled secretions, and presence of neoplasm.
Larynx	Assess for signs of infection (exudate or fungal element), signs of chronic irritation, signs of presbylarynx, presence of neoplasm, abnormal vocal cord mobility, abnormal glottic closure, abnormal mucosal wave (amplitude, phase, symmetry), and abnormal pattern of muscle contraction.

specific recommendations related to the management of presbyphonia, as well as a general paradigm for dealing with most vocal disorders, are outlined. Management of presbyphonia and other vocal disorders commonly encountered in the aging population ideally involves a multidisciplinary approach that may include elements of appropriate vocal hygiene, speech or voice therapy, medical therapy, or surgery.

TABLE 4.3
Typical Laryngeal Exam Findings for
Common Voice Disorders Affecting Elderly Patients

Condition	Exam findings
Presbylarynx	Thinned/bowed true vocal folds, quiver or tremor with arytenoid motion, incomplete glottic closure
Vocal cord paralysis/paresis	Immobility or partial mobility of arytenoid and vocal fold, incomplete glottic closure, bowed or fixed vocal fold, increase in vibratory amplitude or mucosal wave, or "chasing" mucosal wave
Superior laryngeal nerve palsy	Vocal fold on affected side shortened and bowed, posterior glottis rotated to affected side, asymmetric supraglottic sensory function, "scissoring" of vocal folds during glottic closure
Chronic laryngitis	Red, thickened, edematous mucosa, bulky vocal folds with injected vasculature, and thick laryngeal mucous
Vocal nodules	Small, rounded bilateral white nodular lesions located at junction of anterior 1/3 of true vocal fold, "hourglass"-shaped glottis
Vocal polyp	Sessile or pedunculated rounded unilateral vocal fold lesion, may have prominent feeding vasculature, prominent inflammatory changes, may result in reactive vocal fold lesion on the contralateral vocal fold, possible incomplete glottic closure
Granuloma	Inflammatory hypervascular lesion located at posterior glottis, unilateral or bilateral, possible incomplete glottic closure
Reinke's edema	Bulky, rounded, "polypoid" vocal folds
Laryngitis sicca	Thick, tenacious vocal fold mucous banding
Laryngopharyngeal reflux	Red, thickened, edematous mucosa—most prominent at posterior glottis, interarytenoid regions, and the infraglottis (often referred to as pseudosulcus); "cobblestoned" pharyngeal wall; possible associated neoplasm
Laryngeal cancer	Irregular ulcerative plaque, diminished or absent mucosal wave, possible vocal cord paralysis if bulky
Muscle tension dysphonia	Anterior–posterior compression of the supraglottic larynx and excessive lateral compression of the false vocal folds, both leading to an inability to obtain a complete view of the vocal folds during phonation

Vocal Hygiene

Vocal hygiene is a term that refers to a set of general voice care guidelines aimed at promoting laryngeal health, optimizing vocal performance, reducing sources of chronic laryngeal irritation, and preventing laryngeal disorders. General vocal hygiene guidelines are as follows:

- *Assure sufficient laryngeal hydration.* In general, intake of at least 2 quarts (64 oz) of plain water per day is recommended (unless contraindicated due to cardiac or renal conditions). Caffeinated and alcoholic beverages tend to have a dehydrating effect on the larynx and should be taken in smaller quantities, while compensating with added quantities of water. Dry air can also result in dehydration. Such dehydration is often encountered on airplanes, near a heating furnace, or in locations with low humidity. Use of an air humidifier may be helpful in these conditions.
- *Avoid excessive throat clearing.* Excessive throat clearing causes a collision of vocal cords, with resultant trauma and irritation. It can become a habitual condition that may be difficult to cease. Education regarding less traumatic throat-clearing techniques and treatment of potential contributing factors such as chronic bronchitis, allergic rhinitis, chronic sinusitis, and laryngopharyngeal reflux may be helpful.
- *Avoid vocal strain.* Phonating too loudly, for too long, or while fatigued can strain the voice. Heavy vocal demands may be particularly damaging in the midst of a bout of laryngitis or a common cold. It is recommended that individuals avoid forceful vocalization or whispering for long periods of time, eliminate excessive speech in noisy environments, and phonate with a soft glottal onset to minimize trauma. It is also recommended that hearing loss be properly addressed because it can result in excessively loud speech.
- *Minimize tobacco smoke exposure.* Cancer-causing chemicals and tar in tobacco cause inflammation of the vocal cords and dry out the vocal tract. It is not realistic to expect a normal voice in a smoker. Smoking cessation and avoidance of smoke-filled environments are recommended for optimal vocal health.
- *Take measures to minimize laryngopharyngeal reflux.* Surges in reflux activity generally take place 30 to 60 minutes after meals during the daytime, but nighttime reflux can occur as

well. Meals should be at least 2 hours before bed, tight-fitting clothing should be avoided, and the head of the bed may be raised 4 to 6 inches. Spicy foods, mint, chocolate, to-bacco, and caffeine exacerbate gastroesophageal reflux and should be avoided. Weight loss is advocated because excess body weight can also strongly promote laryngopharyngeal reflux.

- *Avoid prolonged exposure to polluted air.* Environments with excessive dust, mold, or chemical elements can adversely af-fect the health of the larynx. Use of a facemask when per-forming yard work, woodshop tasks, and housecleaning may be helpful.

Speech Therapy

Speech therapy is the cornerstone of most treatment strategies needed to deal with speech and voice disorders encountered within the aging popula-tion. In particular, vocal exercises can be highly effective in dealing with or preventing the sequelae of presbyphonia and improving quality of life (Berg, Hapner, Klein, & Johns, 2008). Details regarding speech therapy are covered in Chapter 5.

Medical Therapy

Usage of expectorants may be of variable benefit in thinning secretions and reducing throat-clearing triggers. Guaifenesin, the most widely used expectorant, should be dosed appropriately high to achieve clinical ef-fectiveness. Uncontrolled laryngopharyngeal reflux is ideally treated with long-acting acid suppressant medications, the proton pump inhibitor sub-class being the most effective. Proper twice-daily dosing is often needed to achieve clinical efficacy. Occasionally, antibiotics are needed to cover the usual upper respiratory pathogens associated with a prolonged upper respiratory tract infection. Antibiotics are generally not needed over long periods of time and should be used judiciously. Medical therapy to treat conditions affecting the voice, such as allergy or pulmonary disease, may be necessary as well.

Surgery

When speech therapy and vocal exercises fail to adequately overcome the manifestations of presbyphonia, surgical intervention may play a role in management. Specifically, vocal cord injection with fat or other biocompatible materials has been used successfully to add bulk to thinned vocal folds and thereby improve glottic closure while positively influencing pitch and vocal projection. Data available on surgical results associated with this procedure suggest generally favorable outcomes with acceptably low complication rates (Ford, 2004).

Benign vocal cord lesions that fail to resolve sufficiently with noninvasive measures such as vocal hygiene, medications, and speech therapy may require microsurgical phonosurgery. Although only a minority of benign vocal cord lesions eventually require removal, properly executed newer microsurgical techniques have the potential to eliminate these lesions with minimized negative impact and subsequent improved vocal performance. Vocal cord paralysis may also be managed surgically with a high rate of success using one of a variety of procedures aimed at medialization of the affected vocal cord and elimination of the manifestations of glottic insufficiency.

Reimbursement

When assessing the vocal tract, physicians and speech–language pathologists and physicians may perform the same procedure for different reasons. If the same procedure is performed by two different professionals on the same day, only one will be eligible for reimbursement. Both the physician and the speech–language pathologist may perform indirect laryngoscopy, flexible or rigid laryngoscopy, or stroboscopy. Although the procedures used by the two professions overlap, some codes are considered physician codes and must be billed by the physician or by a physician-directed setting, even when performed by the speech–language pathologist. A discussion of reimbursement issues related to the speech–language pathologist's procedures for assessing and remediating speech disorders is presented in Chapter 5.

Key Points

The physician's perspective on aging and speech is presented, with an emphasis on changes in the peripheral speech structures and the medical interventions that may have a direct impact on speech. Key points are as follows:

- The larynx undergoes structural changes with biologic aging that may affect speech and vocal function. Despite these changes, most healthy elderly individuals maintain sufficient speech and vocal quality to effectively communicate without concern or significant disorder.

- Presbyphonia is addressed when associated vocal function is inadequate to meet individualized social or professional patient needs.
- Most elderly patients presenting for clinical assessment with voice disorders have contributing disease entities beyond age-related change to account for their symptom complaints.
- Clinical assessment must involve an understanding of each patient's specific vocal demands and expectations in addition to a complete review of possible contributing age-related general medical factors alongside a careful physical examination.
- Treatment of speech and voice disorders in the aging population ideally involves a customized multidisciplinary approach including disorder-specific appropriate elements of vocal hygiene, medical therapy, surgery, and speech therapy.

References

Berg, E., Hapner, E., Klein, A., & Johns, M. (2008). Voice therapy improves quality of life in age-related dysphonia: A case-control study. *Journal of Voice, 22,* 70–74.

Ford, C. (2004). Voice restoration in presbyphonia. *Archives of Otolaryngology–Head & Neck Surgery, 130,* 1117.

Hooper, C. R., & Cralidis, A. (2009). Normal changes in the speech of older adults: You've still got what it takes; it just takes a little longer. *Perspectives on Gerontology, 14,* 47–56.

Pontes, P., Brasolotto, A., & Behlau, M. (2005). Glottic characteristics and voice complaint in the elderly. *Journal of Voice, 19,* 84–94.

Sataloff, R. T., Rosen, C. D., Hawkshaw, M., & Spiegel, J. R. (1997). The aging adult voice. *Journal of Voice, 11,* 156–160.

Verdonck-de Leeuw, I., & Mahieu, H. (2004). Vocal aging and the impact on daily life: A longitudinal study. *Journal of Voice, 18,* 193–202.

Woo, P., Casper, J., Colton, R., & Brewer, D. (1992). Dysphonia in the aging: Physiology versus disease. *The Laryngoscope, 102,* 139–144.

CHAPTER 5

Aging Speech:
Voice, Resonance, and Articulation

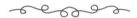

Leah Skladany and Mary Ann Toner

IN CONTRAST TO THE emphasis on anatomic changes in Chapter 4, this chapter provides an overview of the effects of primary aging on the respiratory, phonatory, and articulatory systems from a perceptual perspective. The section on secondary aging further clarifies the differing roles of the speech–language pathologist and otolaryngologist by describing the vocal functions and habits that contribute to or perpetuate laryngeal pathologies. The speech disorder discussion is expanded to include dysarthria and apraxia. In the evaluation portion of this chapter, readers are provided with an outline of basic assessment procedures and significant results, with tables and appendices containing additional procedures and norms. Treatment addresses each of the component systems and includes discussion of issues surrounding the potential use of augmentative and alternative communication devices. The authors clarify conditions surrounding when a speech–language pathologist may or may not be reimbursed for a procedure.

The aging process differs among individuals of the same chronological age. Some individuals are more successful in "aging well" than others, and this may be reflected in their speech. In preparation for differentially diagnosing and managing pathology, it is crucial that the practicing clinician understand the changes in speech associated with the normal aging process.

The basic speech subsystems include respiration, phonation, resonation, articulation, and prosody. The functions of these systems are coordinated to produce the final speech product. Changes in voice may be the aspect of speech production that is most associated with "sounding old." The voice is also subject to several pathologies that are seen with greater frequency in the elderly. For that reason, voice will be addressed as a part of the general speech process and as a separate category of pathologies.

Primary Aging

While some changes in speech production take place as a result of aging, they do not usually result in a significant disruption of communication; in many cases, the person is relatively unaware of any change. To identify normal versus abnormal change, it is important to assess each of the speech subsystems. Although the subsystems will be discussed separately, it should be remembered that these processes interact to produce speech, and a disruption in one system can result in changes in one or all of the others.

Speech–language pathologists do not diagnose or treat respiratory disorders, but they do deal with respiration as it functions to provide the power source for speech. Respiration supports both voiced and voiceless speech sounds and is adjusted to vary the characteristics of our voice and prosody. Lung volumes are reduced as an effect of primary aging, but healthy older people adjust naturally by saying fewer syllables per breath. Most will not be aware of this adjustment; however, singers and others who continue to use their voices professionally are likely to recognize the effect.

Phonation serves as the sound source for voiced sounds and is described by the pitch, loudness, and quality of the voice. Research by Woo, Casper, Colton, and Brewer (1992) has suggested that the onset of age-related voice changes is between the seventh and ninth decades of life. Pitch drops in women after menopause, while elderly men have been shown to demonstrate a rise in pitch. Conversational loudness may increase, with intensity being more variable. Both pitch and dynamic (loudness) ranges decrease. Vocal roughness also increases and is reflected in higher perturbation measures (e.g., jitter and shimmer). These changes vary greatly from person to person, with some continuing to demonstrate young voice traits into their 80s.

Resonation shapes the sound as it is transferred through the vocal tract. It is a primary factor in production of vowels and the nasal consonants. As noted in Chapter 4, the vocal tract undergoes several age-related anatomic changes. Lengthening of the vocal tract, atrophy of tongue and pharyngeal muscle, and declines in sensory-motor functioning appear to be associated with changes in formant frequencies and a tendency toward centralizing production of vowels and some consonants (Linville & Rens, 2001).

Articulation involves production of the speech phonemes and the rapid movements required to blend those sounds into a cohesive speech unit. A convenient model for understanding the role that each of the subsystems plays in consonant articulation is provided by the traditional descriptors: manner, place, and voicing. Manner involves the way in which the airflow is restricted and released (e.g., frication, stopping, nasalization), place is described by the point in the vocal tract where the primary restriction of the airflow occurs (e.g., bilabial, linguadental, velar), and voicing is determined by the presence or lack of vocal fold vibration. Vowel sounds do not vary in voicing or manner, but are described by characteristics such as position of the tongue (e.g., high/low, front/back), degree of lip rounding, and tension—factors that affect the resonance characteristics of the vocal tract.

A listener's perception of voice quality is based primarily on vowel characteristics, while the intelligibility of speech relies heavily on adequate production of consonant phonemes. In primary aging, articulatory precision is slightly reduced, with voice onset time for plosives becoming more variable (Linville & Rens, 2001; Torre & Barlow, 2009). Perhaps the most consistent finding is the variability demonstrated by older speakers, with both intrasubject and intersubject variability significantly exceeding that found for younger subjects.

Prosody also illustrates the interaction of the speech subsystems. It is defined by factors such as the rate, intonation, and inflectional characteristics of speech. Rate and rhythm influence the listener's perception of the speaker's fluency. Older individuals tend to show increased intonation in conversational speech and a reduction in speech rate (Amerman & Parnell, 1992). Although there is some disagreement about the effect of aging on speech fluency, even speakers of very advanced age maintain normal fluency levels (Searl, Gabel, & Fulks, 2002). However, the smooth flow of an older person's speech is more likely to display interjections, revisions, and word repetitions. These changes may be due to changes in cognitive-linguistic as well as neuromuscular functioning. Cognitive–linguistic effects on fluency are described in greater detail in Chapter 9.

Secondary Aging

Advancing age increases the risk of multiple diagnoses contributing to speech and voice disorders. Diagnostic categories frequently noted in an aging population include laryngeal disorders, neurologic disorders, pulmonary illnesses, medication effects, Alzheimer's disease and related dementias, cardiovascular disease, rheumatoid arthritis, and endocrine dysfunctions (particularly thyroid). While all of these etiologies may have an effect on communication, individuals with neurological disorders are most likely to require speech–language services to achieve or maintain functional communication. Because of the impact of motor speech disorders on communication in the aging population, the characteristics of those disorders will be discussed.

Motor Speech Disorders

Central or peripheral nervous system damage may result in the motor speech disorders classified as dysarthria and apraxia. In the dysarthrias, the direct and/or indirect activation pathways may be disrupted. The direct pathways facilitate voluntary, skilled movement, while the indirect pathways regulate characteristics such as posture and tone that support the skilled movements and inhibit activities that may interfere with them. The dysarthrias impair the speed, range, precision, and accuracy of speech and may substantially limit functional communication. The five physiological speech subsystems (respiration, phonation, articulation, resonance, and prosody) are affected to varying degrees. Symptoms depend on the site and degree of nervous system damage.

The second category of motor speech disorders, apraxia, is characterized by disrupted central programming of the motor elements to execute precise voluntary movements in the absence of substantial muscle weakness. Most frequently, apraxia disrupts articulation and prosody of speech without significantly impairing voice, resonance, or respiration. In severe cases, however, patients may be unable to vocalize voluntarily, leaving them essentially mute.

The specific nature of symptoms encountered with dysarthria or apraxia depends on the site and degree of nervous system damage. The etiology of the damage and the neuromuscular conditions observed during an oral mechanism examination will provide information about the type of motor speech disorder that might be present; however, the perceptual characteristics are of primary importance to the speech–language pathologist's diagnosis. Perceptual characteristics associated with flaccid, spastic, ataxic, hyperkinetic, hypokinetic, and mixed dysarthria were described in the classic work by Darley, Aronson, and Brown (1975). *Upper motor neuron dysarthria* and *undetermined* are categories that were described later (Duffy, 2005). It is beyond the scope of this text to provide a detailed discussion of motor speech disorders; therefore, only a brief summary of the primary types is provided. Table 5.1 presents an overview of six basic forms of dysarthria plus apraxia of speech.

TABLE 5.1
Overview of Motor Speech Disorders

Motor speech disorder	Site of lesion	Physical characteristics	Distinctive speech symptoms	Possible etiologies
Flaccid dysarthria	Peripheral nerve, particularly CN V, VII, IX, X, XII	Flaccid paralysis/weakness, fibrillation, fasciculation then atrophy, hypotonicity, loss of reflexes	Breathiness, audible inspiration, hypernasality with nasal emission.	Surgery (neurological, chest, thyroid), bulbar ALS, multiple systems atrophy, myasthenia gravis, tumor, brainstem stroke, Guillain-Barre, radiation
Spastic dysarthria	Bilateral damage in the corticobulbar tract, direct and indirect activation pathways	Spastic paralysis, hypertonicity, pathologic reflexes, drooling, pseudobulbar affect	Strained-strangled voice, slow but regular AMR	Primary lateral sclerosis, bilateral cortical strokes, corticovascular disease, traumatic brain injury
Unilateral upper motor neuron dysarthria	Unilateral damage in the corticobulbar tract, direct and indirect activation pathways	Unilateral symptoms, increased tone, unilateral lower facial weakness, unilateral tongue weakness	Mild in severity, imprecise articulation, irregular AMR, harsh voice	Unilateral CVA, tumor, neurosurgery
Ataxic dysarthria	Cerebellar control circuit	Incoordination, dysmetria, dysdiadochokinesis, intention tremor	Irregular articulatory breakdowns, distorted vowels and prolonged phonemes, excess and equal stress	Cerebellar degeneration, multiple sclerosis, cerebellar stroke, alcohol or drug toxicity, traumatic brain injury

(continues)

TABLE 5.1 (continued)

Motor speech disorder	Site of lesion	Physical characteristics	Distinctive speech symptoms	Possible etiologies
Hypokinetic dysarthria	Basal ganglia control circuit	Resting tremor, rigidity, decreased movement, masked facies, "freezing"	Rushes of speech, reduced stress, monopitch, monoloudness, stuttering-like repetitions	Parkinson's, cerebral hypoxia, drug toxicity
Hyperkinetic dysarthria	Basal ganglia control circuit	Abnormal movement (rhythmic or regular, rapid or slow), dystonia	Vary widely—depending on type of dyskinesia or dystonia present and speech system(s) affected	Essential tremor, orofacial dyskinesia/dystonia/tremor, drug toxicity, spasmodic dysphonia, Huntington's Chorea, Tourette's, torticollis
Apraxia of speech	Left cerebral hemisphere	May be none. Unilateral UMN symptoms common	Volitional speech more disrupted than automatic, distortion/substitution of sounds, attempts to self-correct, groping	Left-hemisphere stroke, dementia, neurosurgery, tumor

Flaccid dysarthria is unique in that damage is in the peripheral nervous system. The damage may be located anywhere from the origin of the motor nerve in the brainstem to the muscle being innervated. Unlike other types of dysarthria, flaccid symptoms may occur in one isolated muscle group or may encompass all five physiological speech subsystems. Weakness and hypotonia are prominent characteristics of flaccid dysarthria. Speech effects vary according to the peripheral nerves that are damaged. Damage to the recurrent laryngeal nerve (RLN) or superior laryngeal nerve (SLN) is associated with both voice and swallowing difficulties. Those disorders are discussed under the laryngeal pathologies section of this chapter.

Spastic dysarthria and unilateral upper motor neuron dysarthria both involve damage to the upper motor neuron tract anywhere along the continuum from cortex to the brainstem. Spastic dysarthria results from bilateral damage, while unilateral upper motor neuron dysarthria (UUMND) results from a unilateral lesion. UUMND typically results in an impairment that is relatively mild in comparison to spastic dysarthria. These categories of dysarthria often coexist with aphasia and apraxia as the result of focal frontal lobe damage; thus, substantial language production deficits and motor programming deficits may overlay the dysarthria.

Hypokinetic dysarthria results from damage in the basal ganglia circuit, a complex circuit that regulates muscle tone, goal-directed muscular activity, postural adjustments, and new motor learning. This is the dysarthria associated with Parkinson's disease, a progressive movement disorder with a typical onset in the 50s and 60s. Tremor, a festinating gait, a mask-like facial expression, and rigidity are common physiological symptoms. This dysarthria is unique in that it is associated with a rapid rate of speech.

Hyperkinetic dysarthrias are also associated with damage to the basal ganglia control circuit and occasionally the cerebellum. Their hallmark is involuntary movements that overlay and disrupt the voluntary. All, some, or only one level of speech production may be compromised. Clinical symptoms include dyskinesia, myoclonus, tics, chorea, athetosis, dystonia, spasm, and tremor. Speech characteristics vary widely, depending on the type of involuntary movement present and the level(s) of the speech system affected. Spasmodic dysphonia and essential voice tremor are classified under this category, but those disorders will be discussed under the laryngeal pathologies section of this chapter.

Ataxic dysarthria results from cerebellar damage. The cerebellum refines and coordinates motor movements. Cerebellar damage commonly results in abnormalities in the range of movements, with both undershooting and overshooting of targets. The lack of coordination of movements is also seen in the performance of alternate motion rate (AMR) tasks. These neuromuscular characteristics disrupt the articulatory and prosodic elements of speech. Cerebellar strokes and tumors, traumatic brain injury (TBI), or chronic alcohol abuse may produce this category of dysarthria.

Mixed dysarthria is very common, with observed symptoms depending on the sites of nervous system involvement. Degenerative neurological diseases, such as amyotrophic lateral sclerosis (ALS) and progressive supranuclear palsy (PSP), and demyelinating diseases, such as multiple sclerosis (MS), are associated with mixed dysarthria. The complexity of this category stems from multiple and simultaneously occurring neurologic conditions disrupting more than one aspect of the nervous system.

Acquired apraxia of speech typically coexists with aphasia. Volitional movement is impaired, while reflexive or spontaneous motor movements remain intact. Apraxia of speech is usually associated with the articulation subsystem, but it may appear as a vocal apraxia. Patients with a vocal apraxia may be unable to initiate voice voluntarily and may have difficulty inhaling and exhaling upon command. The more commonly seen speech apraxia is characterized by inconsistent articulation errors, substitution, omission, reversals, additions, trial-and-error articulatory movements, and numerous filled or unfilled pauses.

Laryngeal Pathologies

Voice disorders are often classified as *functional* or *organic*, but voice clinicians are aware that these terms describe a continuum more than distinct categories. Similarly, the terms *hyperfunctional* and *hypofunctional* are used to categorize voice disorders; however, a hyperfunctional behavior may result in a hypofunctional voice. Rather than classify disorders using those terms, this section will discuss voice disorders in terms of their physiological bases.

The aging process predisposes the elderly to several types of voice disorders, and they are at higher risk for health and environmental influences that precipitate and perpetuate the problems. The otolaryngologist is responsible for examining the condition of the laryngeal apparatus and for diagnosing laryngeal pathology. Laryngeal changes and disorders associated with secondary aging are discussed in Chapter 4. Speech–language pathologists are responsible for identifying abnormal parameters of voice production and the behaviors that might contribute to both the perceptual characteristics of the voice and the underlying pathology.

Dysphonia refers to an abnormal-sounding voice irrespective of age. The voice of an elderly individual may be termed presbyphonia or "old voice." The larynx of presbyphonia exhibits a bowed configuration, reduced intrinsic muscle mass, and a persistent glottic space during the closed phase of vibration. While often considered a primary aging process, these laryngeal changes may result in dysfunction or pathology that can vary among affected individuals, with a resulting voice that is often weak, breathy, and limited in range.

Voice disorders resulting from damage to the recurrent laryngeal nerve or the superior laryngeal nerve are technically a flaccid dysarthria, although they are often not discussed in that category. Paralysis of the laryngeal adductor secondary to RLN damage results in a breathy, weak voice. In contrast, SLN damage affecting the laryngeal tensor reduces the flexibility and range of the voice. In both cases, aspiration is a concern. Similarly, spasmodic dysphonia and essential tremor fall into the category of dysarthria but are often described as voice disorders. Spasmodic dysphonia may affect the laryngeal adductors or abductors, with the strained-strangled sound of the adductor type being most familiar. An improved voice may be observed during singing, falsetto voice, or emotionally charged speech. The quavering voice of essential tremor is often mistakenly associated with old age, although the resulting voice may be quite different from that of presbyphonia. The vocal tremor is frequently accompanied by tremor in other parts of the body, but may affect the voice alone. Essential voice tremor is a periodic, 4-7 Hz vibration that is more pronounced during sustained vowels. The tremor may be temporarily relieved by alcohol. Speech–language pathologists play a role in discriminating spasmodic dysphonia and essential tremor from other dysphonias, such as muscle tension dysphonia.

Many laryngeal pathologies result in a change in the mass of the vocal folds. The resulting dysphonias have similar perceptual characteristics. For example, any mass on the medial edge of vocal folds (nodules, polyps, cancer) or a condition associated with edema (reflux, chronic laryngitis) tends to result in lower pitch, increased breathiness, and hoarseness. Several of these voice disorders also share underlying factors that predispose a person to the disorder, precipitate the dysphonia, and perpetuate the pathology. For example, an upper respiratory infection may lead to frequent throat clearing, which can contribute to nodules, polyps, or laryngitis.

Dysphonia may result from increased effort needed to speak in an adverse environment or to compensate for a system weakened by illness. For example, it is not uncommon for patients to report the onset of vocal fatigue or demonstrate muscle tension dysphonia following a respiratory infection or influenza. The continued struggle to speak and the reaction of listeners may result in the older person limiting communication situations.

While the elderly are commonly aware of experiencing voice changes beyond hoarseness, they tend to attribute even pathological changes to the aging process and do not seek medical evaluation or voice intervention (Turley & Cohen, 2009). Because of the awareness of the relationship between hoarseness and cancer, adult patients in every age group are more likely to seek medical evaluation for unexplained hoarseness than other voice symptoms; however, they frequently do not follow up with voice therapy once they are reassured that their condition is not malignant.

Tertiary Aging Factors in Speech

Quality of life is often compromised by advancing age and illness; however, older individuals who maintain a healthy lifestyle, exercise regularly, and have regular opportunities to communicate are more likely to delay or avoid the appearance of "old" speech or voice characteristics. Those who "start out strong" also benefit; for example, older individuals who are trained singers demonstrate fewer age-related voice symptoms. Unfortunately, many elderly individuals are exposed to multiple factors that can increase the risk of aging affecting speech and voice. Bereavement, loss of independence, loss of control and support, reduced income, anxiety, depression, disability, and social and environmental isolation are all inextricably linked to diminished life satisfaction in the aged. Communication is often limited by environmental noise, peers that are hard-of-hearing, and/or uninterested family members or facility staff. Being home-bound or confined to a nursing facility limits communication opportunities and almost guarantees feelings of isolation and reduced self-worth. Individuals with voice and speech issues face additional challenges. Communication now requires speaker effort and listener patience; communication is frustrating because of the need to repeat; and communication anxiety may exist, particularly with authority figures and/or caregivers.

Evaluation

The clinical evaluation of the aged with speech and voice disorders is ideally interdisciplinary. Evaluation of speech and voice is based on a thorough review of all speech production subsystems. Both subjective and objective (instrument based) methods may be used to determine the nature and consequence of speech and voice disorders. It is important that any communication disorder also be viewed in the context of its impact on quality of life.

Review of Medical History

Review of medical reports prior to the patient interview is important to preparation. Medical reports provide information about diagnoses, surgeries, current medications, prior assessments and results, current findings, and prior recommendations. This information is crucial when evaluating the elderly, who are often chronically ill, medically fragile, and present with multisystem pathology. Numerous medications may also impact speech and voice performance.

Patient Interview

The information provided in the interview is important when making diagnostic and therapeutic decisions. Enhancing communication begins by establishing a good rapport. Asking brief, direct questions, clarifying, and finally verifying information through restating is encouraged. Due to mobility issues, memory problems, supportive needs, or preference, the elderly patient is often accompanied to an evaluation by a spouse, family member, friend, or caregiver. If appropriate, those accompanying the patient may be included in the interview; but it is important that most questions continue to be directed toward the patient. Actively engaging elderly individuals in the interview may improve the quality of the information communicated and enhance the quality of their care.

When interviewing the elderly patient, past and current medical diagnoses, surgical history, and current medications should be reviewed. Habits and lifestyle factors that may predispose a person to a disorder or perpetuate the problem should be assessed, including smoking and alcohol history, daily communication demands, vocal abuses (extended talking, loud speech), singing, occupational risks, and throat clearing. A description of the onset and progression of the problems should be obtained, as well as the patient's description of the effects of the problem on communication and any variability experienced. It is important not to assume that communication demands no longer exist as one ages. Professional voice use may continue to be profitable and enjoyable throughout one's lifespan.

Subjective/Perceptual Evaluation of Speech and Voice

To assess the structural-functional basis for speech, the oral mechanism is assessed at rest, during sustained postures, and during both nonspeech and speech movements. While the tasks may vary from clinician to clinician, a thorough evaluation allows observation and clinical judgment of all speech subsystems. Instruments such as the *Frenchay Dysarthria Assessment–Second Edition* (FDA-2; Enderby & Palmer, 2008) or *Dworkin-Culatta Oral Mechanism Exam and Treatment System* (D-COME-T; Dworkin & Culatta, 1996) are available to help clinicians organize their procedures and observations.

Observation of the face, lips, tongue and velum at rest or in sustained movements can be helpful in identifying the site of a neurological lesion. When observing the facial muscles at rest, it is important to remember that the strong (normal) side should be wrinkled on an older person; the paralyzed side often lacks normal facial lines and appears smooth. Drooping of the entire side of one face versus weakness of only the lower portion of one side may help discriminate peripheral from central lesions. Impression of muscle tone and observations of any abnormal or extraneous movements are noted. Tremors or muscle tics may indicate a lesion of the extrapyramidal system, while fasciculations suggest a peripheral nerve lesion. Scarring or other structural deviations should be observed. Strength and steadiness can be assessed when the person attempts to hold a structure in a sustained position. Reflexes may be assessed to determine if pathological reflexes are present, such as the rooting, biting, or snouting reflexes.

To assess the speech structures in nonspeech movements, patients may be asked to open and close their mouth; protrude, elevate, lateralize, and retract the tongue; smile and pucker their lips; and puff their cheeks. During these tasks, the range, speed, symmetry, accuracy, strength, and coordination of movement can be assessed. Deviation of a structure when a voluntary movement is attempted helps identify laterality of a problem. For example, a protruded tongue may deviate to the weak side. Weakness may also be demonstrated by a limited range and slow rate of movement. Poorly coordinated voluntary movements or inaccurate movements may suggest a cerebellar problem.

Perceptual judgments made during performance of a variety of speech tasks provide information central to identifying speech disorders and planning remediation. The choice of speech tasks presented may vary based on the symptoms observed. If it is apparent that only one subsystem is compromised, tasks can be chosen to target that process. At a minimum, most evaluations will include assessment of maximum phonation duration, alternate motion rate (AMR), sequential motion rate (SMR), and a connected speech sample, for example, reading of a standard passage. These tasks provide a means of identifying disruptions in any or all subsystems. Additional tasks can be chosen to further examine the subsystem(s) that appear to be disordered during performance of those tasks.

Respiration

Respiration underlies the other speech processes; therefore, it is difficult to distinguish respiratory contributions from symptoms due to impairments in other subsystems. The maximum phonation duration task, which involves the patient taking a deep breath and sustaining /a/, provides some information about respiratory support for phonation. While this measure alone cannot differentiate a pulmonary problem from a phonatory insufficiency, it provides a gross estimate of a potential respiratory–phonatory issue (Kent, Kent, & Rosenbeck, 1987). Determination of the number of speech syllables produced per breath in oral reading or conversation also provides information about breath support for speech. In middle life, both men and women begin to experience speech breathing changes that continue into later years and result in fewer syllables per breath. (See Appendix 5A for normative data.)

Phonation

Observation of pitch, loudness, roughness or hoarseness, breathiness, strain, effort, and onset characteristics during maximum phonation duration (MPD) tasks, connected speech, and pitch range tasks provides information about the integrity and functioning of the phonatory subsystem. Onset of voicing and coordination of voicing with other processes can be evaluated during alternate motion rate (AMR) and sequential motion rate (SMR) tasks as well as connected speech. Additional tasks that discriminate between specific phonation disorders may include reading sentences or paragraphs loaded with voiced or voiceless consonants. These tasks help the clinician discriminate between disorders such as spasmodic dysphonia, essential tremor, and muscle tension dysphonia (Roy, Mauszycki, Merrill, Gouse, & Smith, 2007). The clinician may also palpate the circumlaryngeal area to assess the position of the larynx, tension in the muscles, and points of pain.

Experienced clinicians often use their own methods of rating to provide descriptions of the problem; however, there are protocols available that promote consistency in documenting these perceptions. One of these protocols, the Consensus Auditory Perceptual Evaluation–Voice (CAPE-V) was designed by a group representing the American Speech-Language-Hearing Association (ASHA) Voice and Voice Disorders Special Interest Division (ASHA, 2003). Using this protocol, the clinician rates the overall severity, roughness, breathiness, strain, pitch, and loudness using a visual analog scale. Another protocol, the Grade, Roughness, Breathiness, Aesthenia, Strain Scale (GRBAS; Hirano, 1981), provides equal-appearing-interval (EAI) ratings of vocal characteristics. Both of these scales have been reported to provide reliable clinician ratings (Karnell et al., 2007).

It is also important that the patient's perception of the voice disorder be considered. The Voice-Related Quality of Life (V-RQOL; Hogikyan & Sethuraman, 1999) asks patients to rate their responses to 10 statements that are designed to measure the impact of dysphonia on specific aspects of daily life. The Voice Handicap Index (VHI; Jacobson et al., 1997) asks the patient to rate the functional, physical, and emotional impact of the voice disorder. Both of these protocols use an EAI scaling method. Pre- and post-therapy administration of protocols such as these can provide information about the overall success of intervention programs beyond that available from the clinician's assessment of the voice parameters.

No longer the sole domain of the physician, laryngoscopy is within the speech–language pathologist's scope of practice. Visualization of the vocal folds using a rigid oral or flexible fiberoptic nasal endoscope provides information on the anatomy and physiology of the larynx. Stroboscopy also involves endoscopy, but it employs an intermittent light source synchronized with the fundamental frequency of the voice. It provides an optical illusion of "slow motion" vibration of the vocal folds and permits observation of the vibratory characteristics of the mucosal wave, duration of the open versus the closed phase, and the glottic configuration. This technology is crucial to the diagnosis of subtle pathology, vocal fold scarring, and adynamic vocal fold segments not otherwise visible using laryngoscopy alone.

Resonance

Nasality characteristics are judged during the MPD and connected speech tasks, but hypernasality and nasal emission may be most prominent during the production of AMR and SMR tasks performed using the voiceless plosives. Comparing SMR performance using the standard stimuli (pʌtʌkʌ) with performance using the syllables in "monica" can help discriminate resonance problems from those due to other processes. Additional tasks performed to clarify the contribution of a resonance deviation to the overall speech problem might include alternately squeezing and releasing the nares during production of a sustained /i/ or production of high-pressure consonants (e.g., plosives, affricates, fricatives) in a variety of speech contexts. Function of the velopharyngeal mechanism can also be observed and judged during nasoendoscopy.

Articulation

Articulatory deviations may be observed if a standard, phonetically balanced paragraph is used to obtain a sample of connected speech. Additional testing may be performed with standard articulation tests, and intelligibility of speech may be assessed using an instrument such as the Assessment of Intelligibility of Dysarthric Speech (Yorkston & Beukelman, 1981). If a neurological etiology is present, an apraxia assessment may be required. Verbal apraxia is usually assessed by eliciting speech samples that progress from simple, rote speech to propositional speech that varies in phonetic requirements. The co-occurrence of aphasia or dysarthria often confounds the identification of apraxia. However, the presence of speech apraxia may be evidenced in the contrast between "overlearned" tasks performed in the typical manner with performance in the reverse order, such as counting from 1 to 20 versus 20 to 1 or saying the days of the week and then reversing the order. Speech apraxia is indicated if no errors are noted when the tasks are performed in the typical sequence but errors are noted when the sequence is reversed. Additional speech tasks that vary in length, complexity, and propositionality can be used to further delineate the characteristics of the apraxia.

Prosody

Deviations in prosody are usually apparent in the tasks performed to assess other speech subsystems. Assessing the prosodic elements of speech involves evaluating the perceptual and visual characteristics of speech naturalness, particularly during conversational speech. Clinicians may evaluate a variety of characteristics, including rate, rhythm, intonation, and stress patterns. Facial expression and gestures are also important aspects of naturalness that may influence the perception of prosody.

Objective/Instrumental Evaluation of Speech and Voice

While nothing can replace a listener's perception to determine the impact of a speech or voice disorder on communication, objective measures can provide valuable information about the physiological integrity of each subsystem and allow an unbiased means of tracking progress. Instrumentation is not influenced by the comparison of one client with another, personal expectations of or experience with the client, or listener fatigue. Not all clinicians have access to instrumentation, but computer technology is making these measures increasingly available. Sample normative data are provided in Appendix 5A; however, it should be remembered that normative data vary with the instrumentation used and the test sample measured.

Respiration

Aerodynamic analysis provides a quantitative assessment of general respiratory function in terms of lung volumes and capacities, air pressure, airflow, and durational measures. Normal aging results in a decrease in lung volumes and capacities, and pathologic aging and a sedentary lifestyle cause further reductions to occur. Respiratory insufficiency is important diagnostically since it may negatively affect both voice and speech in advancing age.

Phonation

Acoustic analysis provides a supplement to the clinician's perceptions. The following parameters are typically measured: speaking fundamental frequency, maximum phonational frequency range (MPFR), pitch sigma, cycle-to-cycle variation in period (jitter), intensity instability (shimmer), habitual loudness, intensity dynamic range, and noise-to-harmonic ratio. Frequency of vocal tremor may also be identified.

Resonance

Although not as widely used as respiratory or acoustic measures, nasalance can be used to provide an objective estimate of nasality. Measures of nasalance may be calculated as the patient reads a standard passage. Higher nasalance percentage scores are related to greater nasality; however, the passage read affects the level of nasalance measured. For example, when comparing two commonly used reading passages, the Zoo Passage is associated with lower percentages than is the Rainbow Passage.

Articulation

It is difficult to separate articulation from the other subsystems. For example, voice onset time may be an important feature that distinguishes voiced from voiceless consonants, but this feature relies on the integrity of the phonatory system. Identification of areas of spectral energy and formant transitions may be helpful in clarifying articulatory deviations, but the interpretation of those spectral features is relatively subjective. The Iowa Oral Performance Instrument (IOPI) can also be used to provide a measure of tongue or lip strength; however, it should be remembered that a strong relationship between maximum strength and intelligible speech has not been established. In fact, Neel, Palmer, Sprouls, and Morrison (2006) found that individuals with reduced tongue strength did not show significant loss of articulatory accuracy or speech intelligibility.

Prosody

Objective assessment of prosodic factors may include measures of frequency and intensity variability across a speech signal and an objective count of the rate of speech. In general, however, prosodic assessment relies heavily on the listener's subjective assessment of the appropriateness of characteristics such as intonation and word stress in connected speech. The multiple features that influence prosody of speech and the wide range of acceptability of those features make it difficult to objectively assess the impact of any one feature on the final speech product.

Remediation

Clinicians should not assume that speech and voice changes experienced after retirement do not have a significant impact on quality of life or that therapy will not have a significant positive effect. In women over the age of 50, quality of life was reported as substantially reduced when communication was judged as being unsatisfactory (Kerr, Engle, Schlesinger-Raab, Sauer, & Holzel, 2003). Significant quality-of-life improvement following voice therapy was reported in dysphonic individuals over the age of 60 (Berg, Hapner, Klein, & Johns, 2008). In every age group, however, compliance of the patient may be an issue. Lack of insight into the diagnosis and the need for intervention may be a primary factor in the lack of compliance, but the elderly are likely to face additional obstacles to therapy. Older people are often highly motivated to improve their communication to maintain their lifestyle and are aware that they must be actively involved in their rehabilitation. However, mobility issues, transportation issues, and limited financial resources may result in failure to obtain services or missed appointments. The elderly patient may benefit from more extensive education, a more flexible appointment schedule, a positive supportive environment, and a written appointment schedule and assignments to facilitate needed attendance and compliance.

Patient education may be even more important with the elderly population than it is with other age groups. As will be discussed in Chapter 7, older people are more likely to attend and respond if the rationale for treatment is clear to them and the results are made relevant to their life. It may be necessary to explain the basic anatomy and physiology of speech and voice production and the effect the diagnosed disorder has on those functions. It is essential that patients are aware of treatment options, the anticipated outcomes, and the expectations for their involvement. They must understand that they are learning a new behavior and practice is needed.

The goal of intervention for dysarthria and apraxia is typically to regain intelligible speech that is as natural as possible. The goal of intervention for most voice therapy is to achieve the best voice possible using healthy phonation patterns. Many intervention strategies are designed to target a specific subsystem or change a specific behavior; however, the speech subsystems are highly interactive. As a result, most speech and voice interventions will affect all of the basic subsystems to some degree. Additionally, if the most basic subsystem's problems are remediated, deviations in other subsystems may be reduced without being directly targeted in therapy. It is also important that intervention strategies not require excessive effort or concentration and that the resulting speech sound and look as natural as possible.

Respiration

Although it is not within the speech–language pathologist's scope of practice to treat respiratory illnesses, respiratory behaviors that support speech can be addressed. Strategies that improve breath support for speech also address one or more of the other subsystems. To provide adequate airflow for phonation, the patient may be placed in a posture that promotes diaphragmatic breathing and deeper inhalation. Pausing more often to replenish available air or producing fewer words on a breath also compensate for weak respiratory support. If adequate respiratory support for audible speech cannot be achieved, some form of abdominal support or a respiratory paddle may help increase the expiratory force, or a personal amplification device might be used.

Phonation

Appropriate vocal hygiene is important for all patients. Intervention involves more than just reducing vocally abusive behaviors, such as throat clearing. It includes instruction in basic habits that affect overall health (e.g., appropriate hydration) and strategies that enhance the communication setting (e.g., not talking over noise, increasing proximity to the listener). Equal emphasis on all aspects of a vocal hygiene program may reduce the likelihood of compliance. If patients are asked to change too many aspects of their life, they may change none. Compliance may be improved if one or two factors that have the greatest impact on the voice are identified and targeted specifically. (See the vocal hygiene handout provided in Appendix 5B.)

If the voice is strained or strangled, strategies that reduce laryngeal effort and tension are indicated. These strategies might include easy onset, yawn-sigh, chewing, or forward/facial focus techniques. If the voice is weak and breathy, therapy might include maximum effort tasks, such as hard glottal onsets or performance of sustained phoneme and pitch range tasks. Numerous approaches may be used to remediate phonatory problems seen in the elderly. Five of these approaches are described in this section. Each of the selected strategies addresses the physiology of vocal fold function and is appropriate for use with a variety of voice disorders.

- *Vocal function exercises.* This is a therapeutic program encompassing systematic strengthening and rebalancing of respiration, phonation, and resonance. Exercises include maximum prolongation of the vowel /i/ followed by pitch glides from lowest to highest then highest to lowest while saying "knoll" or "whoop." A forward voice focus is encouraged. This exercise may be followed by a power exercise that involves prolongation of the musical notes C-D-E-F-G using the syllable "ol" as in "old" (Stemple, 1993).
- *Confidential voice.* In this technique, individuals are taught to speak using lower volume, a gentle sound, and easy onset. This approach reduces forceful vocal fold closure. It may be an initial strategy used to reduce abuse. A cue for its implementation may be, "If you cannot touch a person, don't talk to them." Close proximity reinforces the need for confidential voice. This technique appears most beneficial for laryngeal lesions that are secondary to vocal abuse and misuse, such as nodules, polyps, contact granuloma, Reinke's edema, and postsurgical voice cases.
- *Resonant voice therapy (RVT).* Voice-focusing strategies such as RVT (Verdolini, 2000) employ the concept of easy, relaxed, effortless phonation through optimizing voice focus and laryngeal relaxation. This technique begins with production of nasal consonant–vowel combinations, first as a sigh, then at varying rates and intensities. RVT progresses to monotonic chanting of nasal-loaded sentences, to similar tasks that alternate the nasal-loaded stimuli with stimuli containing a voiceless plosive. This exercise is followed by

inflected speech that gradually increases in length as cues to phrasing are removed.

- *Manual laryngeal musculoskeletal reduction.* Hyperfunctional disorders are often characterized by excessive tension in the extralaryngeal muscles. While many of these voice problems are easily remediated using facilitation techniques such as chewing, yawn-sigh, or focusing, some are characterized by a long-standing dysphonia that is very resistant to change. In those cases, physical manipulation of the larynx may result in fairly dramatic and rapid improvement. As described by Aronson (1990) and Roy (1993), anterior-to-posterior massage is provided on the hyoid then moved to the thyrohyoid space. Massage should then progress down the posterior border of the thyroid lamina. An elevated larynx can then be moved down. Circumlaryngeal massage and laryngeal repositioning are techniques that disrupt patterns of abnormal extralaryngeal muscle tension, allowing clients to become more aware of tension patterns and gain control over their voice.

- *Lee Silverman Voice Treatment® (LSVT).* LSVT is a therapeutic approach that was initially designed for the management of the hypokinetic dysarthria of Parkinson's disease and has recently been extended to vocal fold paralysis and other forms of dysarthria. Extensive research has firmly established the efficacy of this approach (Pinto et al., 2004; Spielman, Ramig, Mahler, Halpern, & Gavin, 2007; Yorkston, Spencer, & Duffy, 2003). LSVT targets increased vocal loudness but results in overall improvement in the effort and coordination of all of the speech production subsystems. The traditional program is a short-term, intensive program (4 sessions per week for 4 weeks) that requires the patient to learn to use increased phonatory and respiratory effort when sustaining vowels, performing pitch range exercises, and producing progressively longer speech stimuli. The patients are taught to breathe more deeply, increase their effort, expel air more forcefully, and "think shout." The availability of LSVT has been increased by development of an extended program, called LSVT X (Spielman, Ramig, Mahler, Halpern, & Gavin, 2007), which requires 2 sessions per week for 8 weeks. For patients who cannot be seen in a clinical setting, LSVT®eLOUD provides the program via a webcam. A "virtual therapist" LSVT computer program has also been created (Yan, 2008).

For some voice disorders, medical interventions provide good outcomes. These interventions include vocal fold medialization procedures for a paralyzed vocal fold and Botox treatments for spasmodic dysphonia. Still, people who undergo these procedures may benefit from voice therapy. For example, it has been demonstrated that voice therapy helps patients extend the time between Botox treatments (Murry & Woodson, 1995).

Resonance

Resonance characteristics may show improvement with the physiological voice therapies described earlier. Use of an exaggerated mouth opening and light contacts assist airflow through the mouth and help reduce nasality by reducing oral resistance. Slow rate with precise articulatory contacts reduces the perceived effects of hypernsality. Tasks that strengthen or increase the tension of other muscles (e.g., pushing or pulling tasks) may improve the vegetative movement of the velar muscles. Use of a continuous positive airway pressure (CPAP) during performance of specially designed speech tasks has also been reported to improve velar muscle functioning (Kuehn, 1997). The use of most nonspeech oral–motor exercises (e.g., sucking, cheek puffing, blowing against resistance) has not been found to have a significant effect on speech (McCauley, Strand, Lof, Schooling, & Frymark, 2009; Powers & Starr, 1974). It appears that speech resonance improvement requires speech tasks. If hypernasality interferes significantly with the intelligibility of speech and cannot be remediated with behavioral strategies, a palatal lift prosthesis or an obturator may be needed. Not all hypernasal clients are good candidates for these prostheses or will benefit from them, so the recommendation should be made cautiously.

Articulation

Some interventions for articulation disorders include strategies to address basic muscle functions such as strength, tone, and range of movement; however, the benefit of oral strengthening exercises for dysarthric speech is not clearly supported by research. Articulation disorders experienced by most elderly adults are better remediated using reduced speech rate, exaggeration of consonant production, syllable-by-syllable attack, and explicit instruction on phonetic placements for speech targets. To obtain intelligible speech, it is often necessary for the dysarthric patient to learn a compensatory articulatory strategy. If articulation compensations are required, designing a compensation that maintains the manner of the target phoneme usually provides the best auditory cues and promotes intelligibility. It is also helpful if the compensation "looks" like the target sound; therefore, approximating the place of articulation as closely as possible can provide visual cues and promote naturalness of speech. If lingual strength and range of movement are severely limited, a palatal drop may allow articulatory contacts by reducing the distance between the tongue and the hard palate.

Most intervention methods for acquired apraxia of speech involve systematic movement and intensive drill using a carefully designed hierarchy of speech stimuli. Efficacy has been reported for several approaches. One approach with a relatively strong evidence base is sound production treatment (SPT; Wambaugh, 2004). This approach targets speech sounds and works from imitation of a target word in a minimal pair contrast (e.g., *pay–bay*), progressing to imitation of the target sound in isolation, and then moving to the next target sound. It shares many of the features of other apraxia programs, such as repetition, modeling, placement cues, and integral stimulation. Although this approach and others have been effective in remediating verbal apraxia, all approaches may be confounded by the presence of aphasia.

Prosody

Use of a slower rate is basic to treatment of almost every speech disorder experienced by the elderly. Rate reduction provides opportunities for more conscious planning and use of newly learned behaviors. In addition, listener understanding is facilitated if distinct word boundaries are present. Contrastive stress practice also promotes a more natural prosody.

Augmentative and Alternative Communication Devices

When intelligible or audible speech cannot be achieved, augmentative and alternative communication (AAC) devices can provide a means of communication for many elderly patients. These devices may be the only means of communication or they may provide a supplement to disordered speech. Available devices range from high-technology, speech-generating devices to simple picture or letter boards. Adults of all ages often resist use of these devices, or at least the more technologically sophisticated ones. This resistance may be due to the desire to regain speech as the primary means of communication. If a motor speech disorder is accompanied by aphasia, the language problems created by the aphasia may interfere with understanding and using symbols on AAC systems. Careful assessment and use of devices on a trial basis may ensure more successful AAC outcomes.

Reimbursement

Speech–language pathology services are frequently covered by Medicare, Medicaid, private healthcare payers, and managed healthcare plans. A physician referral and a pre-authorization are typically needed for speech–language pathology services. Many insurance plans limit reimbursement for acquired speech or voice disorders if the therapy is not considered to be a medical necessity. For example, voice therapy for a polyp may not be reimbursed because it is addressing the consequence of a "behavior," while therapy following surgical injury to the vocal cords would be authorized. The speech–language pathologist should clearly document that the therapy provided is recognized as effective, perhaps providing references that demonstrate the efficacy of the procedures.

Intervention for speech, language, voice, communication, or auditory processing is described by a single Current Procedural Terminology (CPT) code (American Medical Association [AMA], 2009a). Evaluation of speech, language, voice, communication, or auditory processing is also described by a general code; however, special evaluation procedures may be conducted and billed using individual codes. These individual procedures include codes for laryngeal function studies (i.e., aerodynamics and acoustics), laryngeal videostroboscopy, and evaluation for and fitting of a voice prosthesis.

The stroboscopy code is considered a physician's code; therefore, a physician must be on the premises when the speech–language pathologist performs the procedure. The speech–language pathologist cannot bill for a stroboscopy if a physician also performed a flexible fiberoptic examination on that day. Stroboscopy, a speech–language evaluation, and laryngeal function studies may be performed and billed on the same day; however, it is typically necessary to include a qualifier that indicates the procedures were distinct. The separate and distinct nature of the procedures should be supported in the documentation. If a clinician performs acoustic analysis but does not complete an aerodynamic assessment, a modifier should be included that indicates a reduced service for the laryngeal function study procedure.

Healthcare Common Procedure Coding System (HCPCS; AMA, 2009b) codes address devices and equipment not covered in the CPT codes. Speech-generating devices are often identified by these codes, as are speech amplifiers (see Chapter 10). HCPCS codes also cover devices and supplies used with laryngectomy and tracheostomy patients.

Key Points

The major themes of this chapter are the unique challenges the aging individual may present to the speech–language pathologist. The major discussion points included the following:

- Primary aging of the speech subsystems is usually not consequential enough to result in perceived deviance, disability, or handicap.
- The elderly are at increased risk for multiple health conditions that contribute to speech and voice disorders, with neurological disorders being prevalent.
- Tertiary aging factors increase the risk for voice abuse and increase the communication challenges for elderly individuals who demonstrate speech or voice disorders.
- Speech evaluation involves the inclusion of all five speech subsystems and both subjective/perceptual and objective/instrumental assessments.
- Efficacy has been established for several intervention approaches, but a return to "normal" may be an unrealistic expectation for the elderly patient. Intelligible speech is the primary goal for most dysarthric patients and optimal, healthy voice for most elderly voice patients.
- Speech–language pathology services are typically reimbursable if medical necessity can be established and efficacy of procedures is documented.

References

American Medical Association. (2009a). *Current procedural terminology (CPT) 2010*. Chicago: Author.

American Medical Association. (2009b). *Healthcare common procedure coding system 2010: Level II*. Chicago: Author.

American Speech-Language-Hearing Association Special Interest Division 3. (2003). *Voice disorders: Consensus auditory-perceptual evaluation of voice (CAPE-V)*. Retrieved March 30, 2008, from http://www.asha.org/

Amerman, J., & Parnell, M., (1992). Speech timing strategies in elderly adults. *Journal of Phonetics, 20,* 65–76.

Aronson, A. (1990). *Clinical voice disorders* (3rd ed.). New York: Thieme Medical Publishers, Inc.

Berg, E., Hapner, E., Klein, A. & Johns, M. (2008). Voice therapy improves quality of life in age-related dysphonia. *Journal of Voice, 22,* 70–74.

Brown, W., Morris, R., Hicks, D., & Howell, E. (1993). Phonational profiles of female professional singers and nonsingers. *Journal of Voice, 7,* 219–226.

Darley, F., Aronson, A., & Brown, J. (1975). *Motor speech disorders.* Philadelphia: Saunders.

Duffy, J. (2005). *Motor speech disorders: Substrates, differential diagnosis, and management* (2nd ed.). St. Louis, MO: Elsevier Mosby.

Dworkin, J., & Culatta, R. (1996). *Dworkin-Culata oral mechanism exam and treatment system.* Farmington Hills, MI: Edgewood Press.

Enderby, P., & Palmer, R. (2008). *Frenchay dysarthria assessment* (2nd ed.). Austin, TX: PRO-ED.

Hirano, M. (1981). *Clinical examination of voice.* New York: Springer-Verlag.

Hogikyan, N., & Sethuraman, G. (1999). Validation of an instrument to measure voice-related quality of life (V-RQOL). *Journal of Voice, 13,* 557–569.

Hoit, J., & Hixon, T. (1987). Age and speech breathing. *Journal of Speech and Hearing Research, 30,* 351–366.

Hoit, J., Hixon, T., Altman, M., & Morgan, W. (1989). Speech breathing in women. *Journal of Speech and Hearing Research, 32,* 353–365.

Hollien, H., & Shipp, T. (1972). Speaking fundamental and advancing age in males. *Journal of Speech and Hearing Research, 15,* 155–159.

Karnell, M., Melton, S., Childes, J., Coleman, T., Dailey, S., & Hoffman, H. (2007). Reliability of clinician-based (GRBAS and CAPE-V) and patient-based (V-RQOL and IPVI) documentation of voice disorders. *Journal of Voice, 21,* 576–590.

Kelley, A. (1977). *Fundamental frequency measurements of female voices from twenty to ninety years of age.* Unpublished manuscript, University of North Carolina at Greensboro.

Kent, R., Kent, J., & Rosenbeck, J. (1987). Maximum performance tests of speech production. *Journal of Speech and Hearing Disorders, 52,* 367–387.

Kerr, J., Engle, J., Schlesinger-Raab, A., Sauer, H., & Holzel, D. (2003). Communication, quality of life and age: Results of a 5-year prospective study. *Annals of Oncology, 14,* 421–427.

Kuehn, D. (1997). The development of a new technique for treating hypernasality: CPAP. *American Journal of Speech–Language Pathology, 6,* 5–8.

Jacobson, B., Johnson, A., Grywalski, C., Silbergleit, A., Jacobson, G., Benninger, M. S., et al. (1997). The voice handicap index (VIT): Development and validation. *American Journal of Speech–Language Pathology, 6,* 66–70.

Linville, S. E., & Rens, J. (2001). Vocal tract resonance analysis of aging voice using long-term average spectra. *Journal of Voice, 15,* 323–330.

Manning, L. A., Gluth, M.B., & Toner, M. A. (n.d.). *Caring for your voice* [Brochure]. Springdale, AR: Author.

McCauley, R. J., Strand, E., Lof, G. L., Schooling, T., & Frymark, T. (2009). Evidence-based systematic review: Effects of nonspeech oral motor exercises on speech. *American Journal of Speech–Language Pathology, 18,* 343–360.

Morris, R., Brown, W. S., Jr., Hicks, D. M., & Howell, E. (1995). Phonational profiles of male trained singers and nonsingers. *Journal of Voice, 9,* 142–148.

Murry T., & Woodson, G. (1995). Combined-modality treatment of adductor spasmodic dysphonia with botulinum toxin and voice therapy. *Journal of Voice, 9,* 460–465.

Mysak, E. (1959). Pitch and duration characteristics of older males. *Journal of Speech and Hearing Research, 2,* 46–54.

Neel, A., Palmer, P., Sprouls, G., & Morrison, L. (2006). Tongue strength and speech intelligibility in oculopharyngeal muscular dystrophy. *Journal of Medical Speech–Language Pathology, 14,* 273–277.

Pinto, S., Ozsancak, C., Tripoliti, E., Thobois, S., Limousin-Dowsey, P., & Auzou, P. (2004). Treatments for dysarthria in Parkinson's disease. *The Lancet, 3,* 547–556.

Powers, G. L., & Starr, C. D. (1974). The effects of muscle exercises on velopharyngeal gap and nasality. *Cleft Palate Journal, 11,* 28–35.

Ptacek, P., Sander, E., Maloney, W., & Jackson, C. (1966). Phonatory and other changes in advancing age. *Journal of Speech and Hearing Research, 9,* 353–360.

Roy, N. (1993). Effects of the manual laryngeal musculoskeletal tension reduction technique as a treatment for functional voice disorders: Perceptual and acoustic measures. *Journal of Voice, 7*(3), 242–249.

Roy, N., Mauszycki S., Merrill, R., Gouse M., & Smith, M. (2007). Toward improved differential diagnosis of adductor spasmodic dysphonia and muscle tension dysphonia. *Folia Phoniatrica et Logopaedica, 59,* 83–90.

Searl, J. P., Gabel, R. M., & Fulks, J. S. (2002). Speech dysfluency in centenarians. *Journal of Communication Disorders, 35,* 383–392.

Spielman, J., Ramig, L., Mahler, L., Halpern, A., & Gavin, W. (2007). Effects of an extended version of the Lee Silverman Voice Treatment on voice and speech in Parkinson's disease. *American Journal of Speech–Language Pathology, 16,* 95–107.

Stemple, J. (1993). *Voice therapy: Clinical studies.* St. Louis, MO: Mosby.

Stoicheff, M. (1981). Speaking fundamental frequency characteristics of non-smoking female adults. *Journal of Speech and Hearing Research, 24,* 437–441.

Torre, P., & Barlow, J. A. (2009). Age-related changes in acoustic characteristics of adult speech. *Journal of Communication Disorders, 42,* 324–333.

Turley, R & Cohen S. (2009). Impact of voice and swallowing problems in the elderly. *Otolaryngology–Head and Neck Surgery, 140,* 33–36.

Verdolini, K. (2000). Resonant voice therapy. In J. C. Stemple (Ed.), *Voice therapy: Clinical studies,* (2nd ed., pp. 46–62). San Diego, CA: Singular.

Wambaugh, J. (2004). Stimulus generalization effects of sound production treatment for apraxia of speech. *Journal of Medical Speech–Language Pathology, 12,* 77–97.

Woo, P., Casper, J., Colton, R., & Brewer, D. (1992). Dysphonia in the aging: Physiology versus disease. *Laryngoscope, 102,* 139–144.

Yan, J. (2008). A 3-D pedagogical agent enhanced virtual therapy system for people with idiopathic Parkinson disease. *The International Journal of Virtual Reality, 7,* 59–61.

Yorkston, K., & Beukelman, D. (1981). Communication efficiency of dysarthric speakers as measured by sentence intelligibility and speaking rate, *Journal of Speech and Hearing Disorders, 46,* 296–301.

Yorkston, K., Spencer, K., & Duffy, J. (2003). Behavioral management of respiratory/phonatory dysfunction from dysarthria: A systematic review of the evidence. *Journal of Medical Speech–Language Pathology, 11,* 12–38.

Sample Normative Data for Speech and Voice

Respiratory support measures

	Age 50	Age 75
Total lung capacity in liters—Mean (SD)		
Men[a]	7.07 (1.07)	6.63 (.66)
Women[b]	5.31 (.66)	4.86 (.66)
Vital capacity—Mean (SD)		
Men[a]	5.09 (.80)	4.47 (.67)
Women[b]	3.60 (.39)	2.94 (.39)
Speech rate in syllables/breath		
Men[a]	18	12.5
Women[b]	19	17

Phonation measures

Habitual pitch—Fundamental frequency in Hertz

	Age 50–59	Age 60–69	Age 65–79	Age 80+
Men	118[c]	112[c]	119.3[d]	146[c]
Women	214[e]	209[e]	196[f]	199.8[f]

Maximum frequency range in semitones

	Non singers age 65+	Singers age 65+
Men	29.7[g]	36.4–36.5[g]
Women	33[h]	35–38[h]

Articulation measures

AMR/SMR rates for ages 65+ in syllables/second (SD)

	pʌ	tʌ	kʌ	pʌ tʌ kʌ
Men[i]	5.4 (1.2)	5.3 (1.0)	4.9 (1.0)	4.4 (1.3)
Women[i]	5.0 (1.1)	4.8 (1.1)	4.4 (1.1)	3.6 (1.3)

Note. AMR = alternate motion rate; SMR = sequential motion rate. [a]Hoit & Hixon, 1987. [b]Hoit, Hixon, Altman, & Morgan, 1989. [c]Hollien & Shipp, 1972. [d]Mysak, 1959. [e]Kelley, 1977. [f]Stoicheff, 1981. [g]Morris, Brown, Hicks, & Howell, 1995. [h]Brown, Morris, Hicks, & Howell, 1993. [i]Ptacek, Sander, Maloney, & Jackson, 1966.

101

Caring for Your Voice

Introduction

Do you take your voice for granted? Is the quality of your voice important to you? Has your voice ever sounded raspy, hoarse, or felt like it was going to "give out" on you? These voice symptoms may indicate that you are misusing your voice or that you are experiencing irritation of the voice box (larynx). Repeated overuse or misuse of your voice is often called "vocal abuse." Vocal abuse is one of several factors that can cause significant irritation of the vocal cords and may cause your voice to have less agility, range, and quality. Prolonged irritation of the voice box may even result in physical damage such as swelling, callous formation, or scarring. In some cases, non-cancerous or cancerous growths can form on the vocal cords after long periods of irritation. The following information is intended to help you become aware of good vocal health in order to avoid the factors that cause deterioration of voice quality and poor health in the throat and voice box.

Symptoms of Vocal Irritation

The following symptoms signal vocal problems:

- Hoarseness
- Raspiness
- Severe dryness of the throat
- Fullness or "lump" in the throat
- Excess or excessively thick mucus in the throat
- Voice fatigue after a period of voice use
- Throat irritation or soreness
- Loss of vocal range (especially the higher notes)
- Coughing up blood
- Difficulty with swallowing

Note. From "Caring for Your Voice," by Lance A. Manning, Michael B. Gluth, and M. A. Toner. Copyright by the Ear, Noise, and Throat Center of the Ozarks. Reprinted with permission.

Causes of Vocal Irritation and Recommended Voice Care

By identifying specific causes of voice abuse and targeting treatments at each particular cause, voice quality can by optimized. The following are the most common causes of vocal abuse and irritation.

Throat Dehydration

A healthy voice is *very* dependent on vocal cords that are kept continually moist with watery mucus. Thin, watery mucus in the throat is normal and necessary. It allows the vocal cords to slip easily past each other during voice production. Without adequate mucus, the vocal cords must work harder to produce sound, which leads to inflammation or swelling of the vocal cord tissues.

In general, it is recommended that you drink at least 2 quarts (64 oz.) of plain water per day (unless advised otherwise by another physician due to heart or kidney problems). In general, generous amounts of water, fruit juice, and other decaffeinated beverages are preferred for optimal voice hygiene. Caffeinated and alcoholic beverages actually pull water out of the tissues in your voice box. Even though they are liquids, these substances can work in this manner to cause dehydration of the throat and voice box. Small amounts of caffeinated and alcoholic beverages are acceptable, but only if counteracted by added quantities of water.

Dry air can also result in dehydration. This is often encountered on airplanes, near a heating furnace, or in locations with low humidity. Consider using an air humidifier at your bedside at night if dry air is commonly encountered.

Although there is no substitution for proper intake of water, the following recipe can be used to relieve symptoms of dry throat:

> Mix 1/2 tsp. of salt, 1/2 tsp. of baking soda, 1/2 tsp. of clear corn syrup, and 6 oz. of warmed, distilled water.
> Gargle quietly and gently for 2 minutes.
> Do not rinse and use as often as necessary.

Laryngopharyngeal Reflux

Reflux of stomach contents into the esophagus and throat is an extremely common condition that results in irritation and poor voice. Symptoms of this condition may include one or many of the following: throat fullness/tightness, excessive throat mucous, frequent sore throat, frequent belching, hoarseness, frequent sour contents in the mouth, or heartburn. It is important to know that many people with this condition rarely experience heartburn.

Most often, surges in reflux activity will take place 30–60 minutes after meals during the daytime, yet nighttime reflux can occur as well. Although reflux can be exacerbated by lying down flat after meals, it will still occur even if awake and standing or sitting upright.

Suggestions to deal with laryngopharyngeal reflux include: plan meals at least 2 hours before lying down for sleep, elevate the head of your bed at least 4–6 inches, and wear loose fitting clothing. Spicy foods, mint, chocolate, tobacco, and caffeine often make this condition worse. Excess body weight can strongly promote laryngopharyngeal reflux. If you are overweight, consulting with your primary care physician to formulate an appropriate weight loss program is advised. Medications may be prescribed by your physician that suppress stomach acid production and thereby reduce irritation to your throat and voice box.

Throat Clearing

There is a correct and incorrect way to clear your throat. When done incorrectly, a person produces a sound like a car trying to start and not catching. This bangs the vocal cords together and causes irritation. Clearing your throat correctly keeps the vocal cords from colliding.

Tips on Throat Clearing
- First, become aware. Ask someone to help you. Pick a time during the day when they can point out every time you clear your throat. If you feel the urge to clear your throat, try these behaviors instead:
  - Take a drink of water and don't speak for a few seconds.
  - Swallow *hard*.
  - Sniff, then swallow hard.
  - Yawn to relax your throat.
  - Do a "silent cough"—inhale deeply then exhale with a strong "hhh" sound.
- If you *must* clear your throat, clear quietly and gently.

It may help to start small. Choose one hour each day and do not clear your throat during that hour. Each day, add some minutes to that hour. The more you clear your throat, the more you will feel the need to clear your throat. The less you clear your throat, the less you will feel the need to clear your throat.

Conditions that affect the nose, throat, and lungs such as chronic bronchitis/COPD, asthma, allergies, chronic rhinitis/sinusitis, and laryngopharyngeal reflux may have the potential to result in throat mucous that is excessive in thickness or quantity. Proper treatment of these conditions may be needed to alleviate excess wear on the voice box related to throat clearing.

Voice Strain

Talking too loudly, for too long, or when you are tired can strain your voice. If you experience vocal strain, limit the use of your voice and sharply reduce any excessive demands such as singing, long conversations, or shouting.

- Do not force your voice or whisper. Forcing your voice and whispering places more tension on your vocal cords.
- Avoid excessive speech in noisy environments.
- Speak at the same tone you say "umm-hmm."
- Don't do all the talking!
- Lower your pitch slightly if you sing.
- Try not to raise your voice volume or pitch when you get excited.
- Don't shout across a room or talk over loud background noise. Move closer to your listener when speaking.
- Properly address hearing loss (if possible), as this can result in excessively loud volume of speech.
- Practice relaxation techniques and deep breathing.
- If needed, learn to use your voice more efficiently with less stress by having regular sessions with a speech therapist.

Smoking

Cancer-causing chemicals and tar in tobacco cause inflammation of the vocal cords and dry out the vocal area. It is not realistic to expect a good voice if you smoke. The lining tissue of the vocal cords eventually thickens and swells, and a lesion or growth may form. If you smoke, stop. Research shows that most people who develop cancer of the throat have a history of smoking.

Drinking

Alcohol irritates the swallowing system and robs the throat of its much needed water content. Caffeinated coffee, tea, or soft drinks also dehydrate the throat. Minimize alcohol and caffeinated beverages for optimal vocal cord health.

Medications

Certain common mediations can have effects on the throat and voice. These include antihistamine medications for allergies, diuretics (water pills), and progesterone-dominant contraceptive pills—among others. Anesthetic throat sprays can also adversely affect vocal performance (like playing the piano wearing gloves).

Polluted Air

Avoid prolonged exposure to polluted air. Environments with excessive dust, mold, and/or chemical elements can adversely affect the health of the throat and voice box. Consider use of a facemask when performing tasks such as yard work, woodshop tasks, house cleaning, etc. A high-quality air purifier/filter might be helpful in certain circumstances.

Infection

The voice box can be involved with viral, bacterial, and fungal infections. Most cases of "laryngitis" are viral infections that also affect other parts of the upper respiratory tract (nose, throat, wind pipe). Viral infections usually last anywhere from 5–10 days and will not respond to antibiotics. The best policy to deal with viral laryngitis is to rest the voice, to assure good hydration (warm liquids), and to be patient. Vigilant hand-washing and appropriate usage of antiseptic hand cleansing lotions are key in preventing viral infections.

Fungal infections of the voice box may be particularly common in persons with diabetes or when steroid inhaler medications and/or antibiotic medications have been used over an extended period of time.

Surgical Therapy

Usually, a lesion forms on the vocal cords after months or years of vocal irritation. Most lesions occur from a combination of a recent event, such as respiratory infection, and a chronic condition irritating the voice box. An example of this is continuation of singing when you have viral laryngitis. Most conditions affecting the vocal cords improve over time with good vocal hygiene and removal of irritation. However, permanent lesions or growths may require surgical removal. Although surgery often results in voice improvement, it will always temporarily interfere with the normal function of the voice box. Recovery of voice after surgery requires time and rest. Some people continue to have problems with hoarseness, irritation, scarring, or re-growth of abnormal lesions following surgery.

Conclusion

The best way to treat vocal irritation is to prevent it. Pay close attention to the care of your voice and maintain good vocal hygiene before significant physical damage to the voice box occurs. By recognizing the earliest symptoms of vocal irritation and by caring for your voice, you may avoid or eliminate voice problems.

CHAPTER 6

Aging and Swallowing

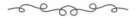

Mary Ann Toner

TONER DISCUSSES PRIMARY, SECONDARY, and tertiary aging factors as they affect swallowing, noting that many elderly persons assume that swallowing problems are a part of the normal aging process. The discussion of primary aging includes sensory and motor changes, reduced saliva, nutritional requirements, and common adaptations made by older adults. For secondary aging, medical conditions often associated with dysphagia are identified. Toner highlights the importance of tertiary factors in eating and swallowing. Evaluation and intervention sections emphasize the speech–language perspective but also include some medically related procedures. A discussion of the reimbursement requirements for assessment and intervention procedures concludes the chapter.

The ability to eat is basic to maintaining physical and psychological health in the geriatric population. Regardless of age, swallowing remains safe and efficient as long as health is maintained; however, changes do take place as part of the normal aging process. The swallowing characteristics associated with normal aging are known as *presbyphagia*. Although the swallowing patterns associated with aging are not considered a disorder (i.e., dysphagia), they do increase the risk of a significant swallowing problem if another negative health factor is introduced.

The elderly obviously experience more health problems than the younger population; therefore, the prevalence of dysphagia is expected to be high, particularly in institutionalized elderly. Even in the noninstitutionalized elderly, approximately one third self-report a current swallowing problem (Roy, Stemple, Merrill, & Thomas, 2007). Although many elderly are aware of voice or swallowing problems, they often do not seek treatment, either because they attribute the problems to normal aging or because they are not aware of treatment options (Turley & Cohen, 2009). Particularly in the older population, delays in seeking appropriate intervention for dysphagia can lead to additional health complications and a poorer prognosis even with treatment.

Optimal services for an elderly patient with swallowing problems include the perspectives of a variety of healthcare professionals, caregivers, and, most importantly, the patient. The primary concern of those involved may vary from threat to health to enjoyment of eating to financial issues. All perspectives are important, and all should be considered in designing appropriate assessment and intervention.

Primary Aging

To understand the significance of the effects of aging, it is necessary to be aware of the swallowing characteristics of younger adults. Swallowing begins once the food is delivered to the mouth and includes oral, pharyngeal, and esophageal stages. In the oral stage, the food is prepared for the swallow by chewing it if necessary, mixing it with saliva, forming a bolus, and propelling it to the pharynx. The pharyngeal stage involves movement of the bolus toward the epiglottis, where it splits into two parts that pass through the lateral channels and pyriform sinuses, reuniting to pass through the upper esophageal segment (UES). To accomplish this stage efficiently, the velum is raised, the larynx is elevated, the airway is closed, and the tongue base contacts the posterior pharyngeal wall to propel the bolus downward. The elevation of the larynx helps open a relaxed UES, creating a negative pressure "under the bolus." A positive pressure above the bolus is created by closure of the velopharyngeal port, pressure from the tongue base, and laryngeal elevation. This pressure differential helps move the bolus rapidly through the pharynx and into the esophagus. Movement of the food through the esophagus to the stomach comprises the esophageal stage.

All elderly individuals experience changes in motor and sensory functions, saliva production, and nutritional requirements. These effects appear gradually, allowing the healthy older person to adapt. Similar swallowing characteristics and adaptations might signal a disorder in a younger person but should not be identified as such in the elderly. Inappropriate identification of normal changes as symptoms of a disorder can result in unnecessary restrictions in eating and swallowing habits. While such restrictions might be seen as preventative, they can have significant physical and psychological repercussions. It is essential, therefore, that healthcare providers be able to discriminate presbyphagia from dysphagia.

Motor Functioning

The swallowing pattern associated with aging is characterized by decreases in the strength and tension of the lips, tongue, maxillo-mandibular area, pharynx, and larynx. These effects result in several alterations of the oral stage, including slower oral manipulation and transit, extra tongue effort and motion, reduced biting force, and reduced tongue force. The pharyngeal stage is similarly affected, with delayed onset of the pharyngeal swallow, frequent penetration, filling of the valleculae prior to the onset of laryngeal elevation, and stasis in the valleculae or pyriform sinuses after the swallow without awareness or significant aspiration. Butler, Stuart, Markley, and Rees (2009) reported observing inconsistent silent trace aspiration in some healthy elderly subjects' swallows.

The condition of the UES plays a primary role in the efficiency of the oropharyngeal swallow. In the elderly, UES relaxation is often incomplete, resulting in slower transit times and less tongue driving force. Incomplete UES relaxation interferes with development of the pressure differential necessary to move the bolus efficiently through the system.

Aging also affects the esophageal stage of swallowing. Changes in esophageal musculature result in weaker primary esophageal peristalsis (triggered by the swallow) and reduced secondary peristalsis (resulting from distention of the esophagus). Clinically, these changes in peristalsis are sometimes referred to as *presbyesophagus*. Slower esophageal emptying makes reflux and indigestion more common. Diminished muscle tone and function can also cause a slowing of waste movement through the lower intestine and contribute to constipation.

Sensory Functions

Sensory experience of food is basic to maintaining a healthy appetite. Enjoyment of the taste and smell of foods early in the meal increases further intake of food. By enhancing the sensory experience of eating, individuals reduce their risk for malnutrition and weight loss. Some variations in the sensory experiences basic to eating are expected in the elderly and should be considered when preparing meals.

Taste

The number of taste buds decreases as we age, causing elevation of taste detection and recognition thresholds. Older people are more likely to experience a "background" taste in their mouths and have more food complaints. Declines in other senses (particularly smell) have a major influence on taste perception.

Smell

Changes in the olfactory membranes, the endocrine system, the olfactory nerve, and the brain result in elevated detection and recognition thresholds for olfactory stimuli. A more concentrated odor is needed for an elderly person to become aware of it.

Other Senses

The visual appeal, temperature, consistency, weight, volume, and "sound" of the food can affect overall perception of the taste of food. These factors may become more important as taste and smell decline. The volume, temperature, and viscosity of the bolus affect the response of the oropharyngeal swallowing mechanism.

Reduction of Saliva Secretion

A reduction in saliva can affect both sensory and motor functions. Less saliva mixed with the food requires more effort for oral manipulation of the bolus. If the bolus is not mixed with an adequate amount of saliva, it is difficult to spread the bolus across the taste buds or form a cohesive bolus. It is also more difficult to move the bolus out of the oral cavity, and the likelihood of residue remaining in the mouth increases.

Nutritional Requirements

The risk of nutritional deficiencies is often increased by the activity level, lifestyle, health, dentition, economic situation, and social environment of the elderly person. These factors can affect nutritional needs and influence choice of food. For example, reduction in outdoor activity may result in Vitamin D deficiency. To prevent nutritional deficiencies, the elderly should maintain a diet that includes adequate protein, calcium, and fiber. Protein-rich foods, such as salmon and tuna, are also a good source of Vitamin B12. High-fiber foods help elderly people reduce cholesterol and maintain regularity. Specific nutrition guidelines for the elderly are provided in the Modified MyPyramid for Older Adults (Lichtenstein, Rasmussen, Yu, Epstein, & Russell, 2008). See Chapter 2 for additional discussion of nutrition guidelines.

Decreased muscle mass and activity levels lower calorie requirements and often result in some weight loss. The elderly are likely to demonstrate an intolerance of large amounts of fat due to decreased pancreatic lipase. Pathological effects of these changes may be avoided through frequent small meals, eating high-calorie foods early in the meal, and daily multivitamin supplements. Some healthy elderly people choose to drink nutritional supplements to maintain their weight. These supplements may reduce the demands for planning and preparing well-balanced meals, but they should not become a replacement for nutritious foods.

Common Adaptations

People often joke that they must be getting old if they are eating in a restaurant during the "early bird specials." Eating at those times may actually show adaptation to several aging effects. There is usually better lighting early in the day, so they can see the menu more easily. It is quieter, so they can hear the person waiting on them without difficulty. They can eat in a calm environment with no pressure to eat quickly to make room for others. It may also improve the social eating experience when they are not eating with younger people, who may finish their meals rapidly and indicate impatience with the older person's slow rate and eating behaviors.

Despite declines in motor and sensory functioning, the healthy elderly maintain a safe, efficient swallow by adapting. Some of the common adaptations include taking smaller bites and using more chewing strokes, which leads to slower eating and longer meals. Older individuals also make new flavor and food choices, preferring those with stronger smells and tastes while avoiding foods that are hard to chew, irritate their esophagus, or are hard to digest. The elderly often adjust to the reduction in taste sensation by adding more salt and sugar to foods.

These adaptations are illustrations of reserve capacity. Reserve capacity allows the elderly person to alter function to cope with age-related declines. In some cases, the person's use of reserve capacity resources may mask early signs of disease or injury. As reserve capacity declines with physiological aging, the ability to cope also declines. This decline leads to increased risk of disorder due to injury or disease and decreased ability to adapt to the consequences of aging.

Secondary Aging

The changes associated with primary aging increase the risk for developing swallowing problems secondary to almost any condition that weakens an elderly person. Furthermore, the elderly are more likely to have multiple health problems that contribute to swallowing problems. Many of the chronic problems experienced by the elderly can contribute to an age-related form of anorexia.

To provide a complete and appropriate assessment of feeding and swallowing and to design effective interventions, the swallowing therapist must be aware of any existing medical conditions that may cause or exacerbate the problem. The elderly frequently demonstrate dysphagia secondary to neurological conditions. When pathology involves the cerebral cortex, cognitive impairment or loss of voluntary control of the oral structures may result in feeding apraxia or problems in oral manipulation and transit. Conditions that affect lower cerebral centers (e.g., basal ganglia) might result in abnormal movements, such as tremor or repetitive uncoordinated movements of the tongue. Disorders affecting the brainstem or peripheral nerves are likely to affect the pharyngeal stage, resulting in a delayed or absent swallowing reflex.

It is also common for the elderly to experience dysphagia due to chronic health conditions, surgery, or other medical procedures used to treat health problems. These factors can obviously reduce the overall functioning of the elderly person in dramatic ways, resulting in generalized weakness of the swallow. Treatments such as radiation for head and neck cancer reduce flow and alter the viscosity of saliva, resulting in xerostomia (dry mouth). The lack of saliva affects the ability to mix food with saliva, stimulate taste, form a cohesive swallow, and clear the oral cavity. Structural abnormalities can also result in stasis of the food.

The digestive system is interactive; therefore, a disorder in one part of the system often affects functioning in another part. For example, disorders that obstruct the esophagus or reduce its motility can result in pharyngeal stasis. It is important, therefore, that the swallowing clinician be aware of disorders affecting any aspect of the swallowing sequence. Examples of medical conditions that are commonly associated with dysphagia in the older population are shown in Table 6.1.

Feeding and swallowing problems in the elderly frequently result in additional, serious health complications. Pneumonia, dehydration, malnutrition, abnormal weight loss, and change in bone condition are among the most prominent. Not only can these conditions be a consequence of dysphagia, but they also may further contribute to the swallowing disorder.

Polypharmacy is common in the elderly, with increases in both prescription and over-the-counter medications. Medications used to treat common health problems can be a primary factor in the appearance or exacerbation of dysphagia symptoms. For example, medications prescribed to treat pain, high cholesterol, cardiac conditions, diabetes, osteoporosis, and neuromuscular disorders add to the primary aging effects of reduced saliva, diminished sensory functioning, reduced gastrointestinal (GI) motility, and slowed responses. Medications that affect functioning of the

TABLE 6.1
Common Causes of Dysphagia in the Elderly

Category	Examples
Static neurological disorders	• Cerebral vascular accidents (stroke) • Peripheral nerve damage (e.g., superior laryngeal nerve palsy)
Progressive neurological disorders	
Neuromotor	• Amyotrophic lateral sclerosis—motor • Neuron disease • Parkinson's disease • Myasthenia gravis
Cognitive	• Alzheimer's disease • Lewy-body dementia • Multi-infarct dementia
Cancer	• Surgical effects • Radiation effects • Chemotherapy
Pharyngeal/cricopharyngeal disorders	• Cricopharyngeal achalasia • Cervical osteophytes • Neoplasm • Postcricoid web • Zenker's diverticulum
Gastroesophageal disorders	• Barrett's esophagus • Hiatal hernia
Esophageal obstruction	• Lower esophageal/Schatzki ring • Cervical spine disease • Esophageal stricture • Esophageal web • Neoplasms
Esophageal motility disorder	• Esophageal achalasia • Diffuse esophageal spasm
Dental conditions	• Dentures • Periodontal disease
Chronic conditions	• Diabetes • Chronic obstructive pulmonary disease • Thyroid disease • Rheumatologic conditions • Kidney disease • Cushing's disease

central nervous system may alter muscle function or impair cognition. Several common medications can damage the membranes of the mouth, pharynx, or esophagus, resulting in dysphagia. The risk of medication damaging the tissues of the older person is increased by the natural decrease in saliva and the slower movement of the bolus. Examples of medications that may contribute to the development of a swallowing problem are provided in Appendix 6A.

While not typically considered to be a direct cause of dysphagia, medications that alter the taste and smell of food or contribute to constipation should be considered relevant. In elderly people who have multiple health problems or cognitive impairment, the reduction in taste and smell may result in difficulty triggering a swallow or a lack of awareness of the presence of the bolus. Even in healthier people, these sensory alterations may result in changes in preferred foods, reduction of appetite, and reduction of food intake. Common examples of medications that have the potential to alter perception of taste and smell include angiotensin-converting enzyme (ACE) inhibitors, antibiotics, beta blockers, muscle relaxants, and the statin class of cholesterol-lowering agents. Frequent constipation also has a significant effect on the older person's appetite and willingness to eat. Anticholinergics, opioids, and bisphosphonates are medication classes that can cause constipation. Dementia patients in particular may not be able to describe the reason for their discomfort and refusal to eat, so it is important that the caregiver be aware of the potential effect of these drugs.

Tertiary Aging

Tertiary aspects of aging can both contribute to swallowing problems and be a consequence of those problems. The elderly experience social, economic, and psychological conditions that have an effect on their swallowing efficiency and motivation to eat. Roy, Stemple, Merrill, and Thomas (2007) found that swallowing problems had a significant impact on the quality of life of the noninstitutionalized elderly, with limitations on activities, taking longer to eat, greater effort required when eating, and embarrassment being reported among the socioeconomic effects. Factors that diminish an elderly person's motivation or enjoyment of eating increase the potential for swallowing problems and malnutrition. In addition, if elderly individuals begin to experience swallowing problems, they may avoid social contacts.

The social network of the elderly is often altered by retirement, the death of a spouse or friends, change of residence, and a loss of mobility. Financial problems may make it difficult to buy the foods needed to maintain nutrition. Physical limitations may prevent preparation of nutritious foods or adequate meals. It is not surprising, therefore, that depression is common in this population. Depression results in loss of appetite, rejection of foods, reduction in activity level, agitation, and lack of motivation. Depression may also be associated with odynophagia (pain when swallowing), globus pharyngeus ("lump in the throat" feeling), and fatigue.

Evaluation

The availability of dysphagia evaluation procedures is influenced by the elderly person's living arrangements and the healthcare setting. For independent-living seniors, healthcare providers often rely on the patient, family members, or primary healthcare providers to identify signs of dysphagia. At-risk patients in acute care settings should be systematically screened to identify potential swallowing problems. In a long-term-care center, patients may be unable to self-report problems; therefore, it is important that the caregivers and healthcare providers are alert to early signs of dysphagia.

Medical Evaluation

Elderly people may misinterpret abnormal swallowing characteristics as part of the normal aging process and consequently may not report the problems to healthcare providers. It is important, therefore, for the primary care provider to regularly assess risk for swallowing disorders when conducting an examination. Table 4.2 in Chapter 4 describes the elements of the physical examination for elderly patients with voice complaints. Those procedures and observations are also appropriate for assessing elderly patients with swallowing problems.

When dysphagia is suspected, more attention is paid to complaints of eating or swallowing difficulties, including loss of appetite. The patient should be questioned regarding the types of food or liquid that cause problems, the frequency and consistency of the problem, sensations of food sticking in the mouth or throat, trouble chewing, globus sensation, odynophagia, coughing during or after eating, drooling, nasal regurgitation, weight loss, heartburn, and recurrent pneumonia. The patient's medical history should be reviewed for potential etiologies of dysphagia, including reflux, chronic obstructive pulmonary disease (COPD), stroke, neuromuscular disease, diabetes, thyroid disease, dementia, and cancer. In particular, a prominent history of tobacco use or alcoholic beverage intake should heighten suspicion for an underlying malignancy involving the aerodigestive tract. Medications should be reviewed to identify those that might affect swallowing, appetite, and gastrointestinal functioning. It may also be necessary to review the patient's nutritional supplements and vitamins.

Some observations made during the physical examination are particularly important to identifying potential swallowing problems. The presence of halitosis (bad breath), dysarthria, a "wet" vocal quality, general weakness, or signs of malnutrition are significant if the older person is at risk for a swallowing problem. During the examination of the oral cavity, clinicians should look for glossitis, stomatitis, and gingivitis. These conditions may indicate essential vitamin or mineral deficiency. Lung auscultation should be performed to identify crackles, wheezing, or rhonchi (coarse rattling). Cranial nerve function should be checked (particularly V, VII, IX, X, and XII), and the patient's cognitive status should be assessed. The neck should also be inspected for evidence of past surgical procedures.

Speech–Language Pathology and Evaluation

The speech–language pathologist should use the medical diagnosis to guide choice of both diagnostic procedures and intervention strategies. Not all patients with a swallowing disorder will be identified through medical examination and referral. Many patients are initially identified through screening of at-risk patients.

Dysphagia Screening

Systematic screening of at-risk patients has been shown to improve early identification of swallowing problems and lead to a reduction in related health complications (Hinchey et al., 2005). For the general population, "at-risk" might include those who experience an unexpected weight loss, report difficulty swallowing, or demonstrate a physical condition or disease that might cause a swallowing problem. In the elderly population, "at-risk" is expanded to include any older person who is in a weakened condition.

Dysphagia screening procedures are used to determine if a potential swallowing problem may exist and, if so, the type of diagnostic procedure that should be recommended. Some screening procedures involve questionnaires or patient observations, without the introduction of food substances. Other screenings involve presentation of a variety of substances and monitoring of the patient's swallow with manual palpation or auscultation. Still others include an observation of the patient during meals. Many screening procedures reveal difficulty in getting food to the mouth and oral-stage swallowing problems. Procedures designed to obtain information about the pharyngeal stage typically attempt to evaluate the ability to initiate a swallow and the presence of aspiration. Perhaps the biggest challenge in effective screening is identification of possible silent aspiration.

The choice of screening procedure should be based on the patient's characteristics and needs. Examples of screening procedures that may be implemented by trained professionals include the following:

- *Toronto Bedside Swallowing Screening Test* (TOR-BSST). As described by Martino et al. (2009), this instrument is appropriate for use with stroke patients in both acute and rehabilitative settings. It can be administered by trained healthcare personnel in less than 10 minutes. Patients are evaluated on the basis of tongue movement, performance on a 50-ml water swallow test (administered in 5-ml amounts), and voice at the beginning and end of the screening.

- *Gugging Swallowing Screen* (GUSS). This instrument is designed to assess risk for aspiration in stroke patients. As described by Trapl et al. (2007), the GUSS includes an indirect assessment composed of yes–no responses regarding observations of patient alertness, cough or throat clear, and saliva management. The direct assessment includes presentation of liquid, semisolid, and solid substances. The actual swallow is scored on a 3-point scale indicating *no swallow, delayed swallow,* or *successful swallow.* Scores are also given for a cough, drooling, or voice change. A total score for both the indirect and direct assessments is calculated.

- *Cough response.* Using a nebulizer, the patient is asked to orally inhale a mist of citric acid–physiologic saline for 1 minute. The number of coughs during that minute is observed, with more than 5 being considered a normal response (Wakasugi et al., 2008).

- *Water swallow tests.* A variety of screening tests involve swallowing of different amounts of water. Examples of these protocols include the following:

  - *100-ml water test* (Nathadwarawala, McGroary, & Wiles, 1994). The patient is given 100 ml of distilled water and asked to drink all of the water as rapidly as possible. Drinking is stopped if the patient coughs before finishing the water. If the patient is able to finish the water, he or she is observed for at least 1 minute after the swallow to determine if he or she coughs or demonstrates a change in voice quality. Speed of drinking is also assessed, with

10ml/s being considered abnormal. This water test may be accompanied by auscultation or pulse oximetry.

- *Modified water test* (Tohara, Saitoh, Mays, Kuhlemeier, & Palmer, 2003). The patient is given 3 ml of cold water and instructed to swallow. If the patient is able to swallow without apparent difficulty, he or she is asked to perform two dry swallows. If the patient can complete both dry swallows, the whole process is performed two additional times. Scoring is based on the patient's ability to perform a swallow, any difficulty breathing after the swallow, or a completed swallow followed by coughing or voice changes. If the patient attempts the dry swallows, the score is based on the ability to perform one or both dry swallows.
- *Oxygen desaturation with 50-ml water swallow* (Lim et al., 2001). The patient is given 50 ml of water and monitored for coughing or choking during drinking or a voice change after drinking. After 10 minutes, oxygen saturation levels are checked. An abnormal water swallow or an oxygen saturation drop of more than 2% is considered significant.

- *The McGill Ingestive Skills Assessment* (MISA; Lambert, Abrahamowicz, Groher, Wood-Dauphinee, & Gisel, 2005). The MISA is an assessment of mealtime functioning and ingestive skills. Positioning, self-feeding skills, oral-motor skills, and overall safety are evaluated during a mealtime observation. It includes a 3-point rating of 42 items. The MISA scores are predictive of pulmonary infection and time to death in an elderly population with neurogenic dysphagia in long-term-care settings.
- *Mayo Dysphagia Questionnaire* (MDQ; Grudell et al., 2007). The MDQ is a 26-item questionnaire designed to identify esophageal dysphagia. Items include determination of presence, onset, frequency, and severity of dysphagia, heartburn, and acid regurgitation. It also assesses the effects of different foods on dysphagia.

In addition to identifying potential swallowing problems in the elderly, the healthcare provider must be alert to signs of poor nutritional status. Wilson and Morley (2004) described the SCALES as a sensitive screening tool that can be used in a variety of clinical settings to detect undernutrition in the elderly. The SCALES assesses nutritional risk based on Sadness, Cholesterol level, Albumin level, Loss of weight, Eating problems, and Shopping/cooking ability.

Diagnostic Procedures

The symptoms identified by the physician, speech–language pathologist, or other healthcare provider can be used to select the diagnostic procedures that will be most likely to reveal the patient's problem. The procedures vary in the aspects of the swallow assessed, the settings in which they can be performed, and their usefulness in identifying factors that improve the swallow.

Barium Esophagram

The barium esophagram or air contrast esophagram may be recommended when a structural esophageal problem is suspected. Patients who report problems with solids but not with liquids are often referred for an esophagram. The barium esophagram requires the patient to drink a cup of liquid barium, and then the bolus is tracked to the stomach using a fluoroscope. A more detailed view of the anatomy can be obtained using an air contrast esophagram, in which air is introduced into the esophagus before the barium is swallowed. Speech–language pathologists are not typically involved in the barium swallow procedure or treatment of esophageal disorders. However, some patients with an esophageal abnormality report symptoms typically associated with oropharyngeal dysphagia (e.g., food sticking in the throat). For that reason, speech–language pathologists should consider the results of the esophagram when evaluating a patient's swallow.

Videofluoroscopic Evaluation of Swallowing

The videofluoroscopic evaluation of swallowing (VFS) remains the most used procedure for diagnosing swallowing disorders. This procedure is also known as a *modified* barium swallow. This evaluation requires the patient to consume foods of various consistencies that have been mixed with barium. As the patient swallows, the dynamics of all stages can be viewed and recorded using the videofluoroscope. The swallow can be visualized in a lateral view to identify aspiration and in an anterior–posterior view to assess laterality of the swallow. The effectiveness of strategies that might facilitate a safe swallow can be examined. Unfortunately, not all elderly patients have access to VFS or are able to cooperate with the procedure. Problems with vocal fold closure, secretion management, and penetration may not be revealed during a VFS study. Additionally, barium can cause coating of the tongue and suggest a more severe problem than would be evidenced with unaltered foods in people with reduced tongue strength (Steele & Lieshout, 2005).

Flexible Endoscopic Evaluation of Swallowing

Flexible endoscopic evaluation of swallowing (FEES) and fiberoptic endoscopic evaluation of swallowing with sensory testing (FEESST) are used increasingly in a variety of settings. FEES involves insertion of a flexible fiberoptic scope through the nose to directly view the patient swallowing solids and liquids. This process provides a view of the structures and functions involved in the pharyngeal swallow. If pharyngeal or laryngeal sensory impairment is suspected, FEESST may be indicated. A specially equipped fiberoptic scope is used to direct pulses of air toward areas of the larynx to determine if an airway protection response is present. It is important that both FEES and FEESST be performed without application of topical anesthetic agents to the pharyngeal or laryngeal mucosa. These procedures may be performed simultaneously with VFS in some settings. Fiberoptic procedures are more portable than VFS, do not expose the patient to radiation, and allow use of unaltered foods (with the exception of blue or green coloring). FEES may also be more revealing of secretion management problems and penetration than VFS. Additionally, patients who have difficulty with barium adhering to the tongue might be better evaluated with FEES. As in VFS, compensatory strategies can be attempted and evaluated. Unfortunately, some patients who might benefit most from the FEES or FEESST technique object to placement of the scope

Manometry

Although used less frequently than VFS or FEES, manometry can be particularly useful in evaluating an elderly person's swallow when an abnormality in UES function is suspected. Manometry may be done in conjunction with either VFS or FEES. It involves placement of sensors in the upper pharynx, lower pharynx, upper esophageal sphincter, and esophagus. This placement allows assessment of the pressures and timing that take place during the swallow, providing insight into the underlying problem.

Scintigraphy

Scintigraphy also has some particular benefits for the elderly. This procedure requires the patient to swallow a radioactive substance. The movement of the bolus is tracked with a gamma camera. It is a powerful tool for identifying silent aspiration of secretions and for quantifying the amount of a bolus that is aspirated. It also allows identification and quantification of gastroesophageal reflux.

SWAL-QOL and SWAL-CARE

The patient's perception of the effects of the swallowing problem and the care received are important factors to consider for optimal outcome. McHorney, Martin-Harris, Robbins, and Rosenbeck (2006) reported that measureable improvements in swallowing function do not correlate strongly with patients' ratings of quality of life and satisfaction with care. The SWAL-QOL and SWAL-CARE are designed to assess these domains. The SWAL-QOL consists of 44 items that assess quality of life in terms of burden, eating duration, eating desire, symptoms experienced, food selection, communication, fear of eating or swallowing, fatigue, social effects of the problem, and mental health. Sleep is also assessed. The SWAL-CARE assesses quality of care provided, including advice on foods and liquids to eat or avoid, treatment options, swallowing strategies, emergency strategies, goals of therapy, and patient satisfaction with the care provided.

A problem that can occur with all instrumental assessments is that the patient's swallowing in the formal test conditions often does not reflect the swallow demonstrated during a regular meal. Comparison of instrumental study results with SWAL-QOL, SWAL-CARE, or MISA results may reveal that the person experiences significant problems during meals but compensates for the problems when instructed to swallow test substances. It may be harder to document dysphagia in these patients, but the possibility that a disorder exists should be considered when a patient or caregiver insists that a problem is present.

Prevention and Intervention

A team of professionals should be involved in the care of dysphagic patients. These professionals might include the primary care physician, radiologist, otolaryngologist, gastroenterologist, neurologist, occupational therapist, physical therapist, dietician, speech–language pathologist, and nurses.

Medical Interventions

Gastroesophageal reflux disease (GERD) is very common in the elderly, and many take prescription or over-the-counter medications to control the symptoms. For control of mild-to-moderate GERD, histamine receptor antagonists (e.g., Zantac, Pepcid) may be recommended. These medications reduce but do not completely block acid production in the stomach. Unfortunately, some patients develop resistance to the effects of histamine receptor antagonists. For more severe cases, proton pump inhibitors may be recommended (e.g., Nexium, Prevacid). These highly effective medications disable the acid pumping mechanisms in the stomach. GERD may also be treated by tightening or thickening the gastroesophageal juncture. A Nissen fundoplication reduces GERD by wrapping the top of the stomach around the bottom of the esophagus. Other evolving innovative techniques involve a variety of interventions aimed at augmenting the function of either the upper or lower esophageal sphincter by means of controlled scarring or the placement of implantable devices. For example, one treatment method currently being studied is the LINX™ Reflux Management System, which involves use of a device made of magnetic beads that is placed around the lower esophageal sphincter (*USC News*, 2009). The force of the magnets helps keep the sphincter closed to prevent reflux, while still allowing it to open for food to enter the stomach.

A lack of UES relaxation (cricopharyngeal achalsia) is frequently a contributing factor in the dysphagia experienced by the elderly. This problem may require invasive treatment approaches, such as a cricopharyngeal myotomy or dilation. Both of these procedures are intended to promote better passage of the bolus into the esophagus by reducing the UES tension. Patients should be informed that these procedures are not without risk and may not have a permanent effect. It should also be noted that the rate of success varies for different types of patients; for example, a relatively low success rate has been reported for cricopharyngeal myotomy in patients who have undergone head and neck radiation (Jacobs et al., 1999). Another condition that may require an invasive procedure is Zenker's diverticulum. Some people who have a diverticulum do not experience serious problems; however, when symptoms are excessive, these outpouchings of the upper esophagus can be treated endoscopically with a high rate of success and a reasonably low complication rate (Scher & Richtsmeier, 1998).

When a safe swallow cannot be achieved or adequate nutrition and hydration cannot be maintained through oral feeding, the person may require an alternate means of nutrition. For short-term needs, a nasogastric (NG) tube might be recommended. For long-term needs, a percutaneous endoscopic gastrostomy (PEG) or a jejuneostomy (J-tube) might be indicated. If the digestive system is not functioning or there is a blockage in the intestinal tract, it may be necessary to temporarily resort to total parenteral nutrition (TPN). In cases where a swallowing disorder is accompanied by severe chronic aspiration that is not responsive to other treatment measures (often seen with neuromuscular disorders), insertion of a tracheostomy tube may be indicated. The tracheostomy tube does not eliminate aspiration, as at least part of the bolus can leak around a cuffed tube, but it does facilitate suctioning and clearing of secretions and mucus from the airways.

Again, these interventions are not without risk or complication, and they rarely solve all swallowing and nutritional issues. Even when they are not eating orally, patients need to be aware of the importance of oral care to reduce complications such as periodontal disease and aspiration of bacteria in their oral secretions. Placement of a feeding tube does not eliminate the risk of aspirate pneumonia, particularly in the bedridden or frail patient (Nakajoh et al., 2001). It should be noted that placement of a feeding tube does not prohibit oral feeding for all patients, and this should be made clear when discussing the possibility with those patients.

When medications are prescribed to the older dysphagic patient, it is essential that they be administered appropriately. If the patient has difficulty swallowing pills or capsules "whole," a medication that might lose effectiveness or become dangerous if chewed or crushed should be identified before any recommendations are made. For example, a time-release factor (e.g., extended release) may be lost if certain medications are crushed. It is also important to determine if a liquid medication is the right consistency for a dysphagic patient. If it is too thin, it may not be appropriate to use a thickening agent to obtain a better consistency. The patient's pharmacist should be alerted to the patient's needs so appropriate adjustments can be made and instructions given.

Prevention

Prevention measures may be undertaken to help increase and maintain the reserve capacity of the older person. By improving the physical condition of a system, it is hoped that the elderly person's swallow will not be significantly impaired by common illnesses. Before recommending these strategies, however, health factors that might influence the patient's response should be considered.

For promoting healthy oral stage functioning, it is important that that the person maintain good oral hygiene. Poor oral care not only contributes to periodontal disease and eating problems but also threatens overall health. For example, aspiration of bacteria-laden oral secretions increases the risk of aspirate pneumonia. Adequate hydration is important to good oral care. If the older person has reduced saliva, a product to moisturize the mouth may be helpful, such as a saliva substitute, a saliva stimulant, or an antixerostomia dentifrice. Tongue resistance exercises have been found to help maintain tongue strength in the elderly (Robbins et al., 2005). These exercises can be done using the Iowa Oral Performance Instrument (IOPI) or a tongue depressor.

The pharyngeal-stage swallow may be maintained using exercises to promote tongue-base functioning, laryngeal elevation, and UES opening. These exercises include the Shaker exercise, the Mendolsohn maneuver, the tongue-holding maneuver, gargling exercises, and tongue protrusion and retraction. In addition to maintaining swallowing ability, the Shaker exercise may contribute to voice improvement (Easterling, 2008). Conditions such as arthritis, cervical neck fusion, or circulatory problems should be considered before recommending specific exercises.

Risk of esophageal problems may be reduced through small frequent meals, diet control, and maintaining an upright posture after eating. GERD control is a primary factor in preventing significant esophageal disease. A patient handout that provides a discussion of GERD and laryngopharyngeal reflux (LPR) is provided in Appendix 6B.

Dysphagia Intervention

Intervention for a swallowing problem may take the form of rehabilitation strategies or compensatory strategies. Rehabilitation measures promote recovery of certain aspects of the swallow. Some that have met with success include the Shaker exercise and the Mendolsohn maneuver, which improve the pharyngeal response through targeting laryngeal elevation and UES opening. Tongue-base exercises (e.g., gargling, tongue protrusion and retraction) may also be recommended to improve pharyngeal stage efficiency. Preliminary evidence suggests that Lee Silverman Voice Treatment (LSVT) may result in improved swallowing in some patients (Sharkawi et al., 2002).

Deep pharyngeal neuromuscular stimulation (DPNS) and neuromuscular electrical stimulation of the swallowing musculature (NMES) are also examples of rehabilitative strategies. There is a lack of controlled studies to support general use of DPNS. Studies suggest NMES may be effective in treatment of oral and pharyngeal dysphagia following a stroke; however, it has not been found to be more beneficial than traditional swallowing therapy (Bülow, Speyer, Baijens, Woisard, & Ekberg, 2008; Kiger, Brown, & Watkins, 2006). Additionally, clinicians who reported performing NMES did not report use of the same criteria for identifying appropriate patients or use of the same protocol for treatment (Crary, Carnaby-Mann, & Faunce, 2007). Another area of continuing research interest is noninvasive biofeedback methods to facilitate learning of therapeutic strategies. Biofeedback for improvement of swallowing has been provided through surface electromyography to measure muscle effort (Crary, Carnaby, Groher, & Helseth, 2004), accelerometry to measure laryngeal movement (Reddy et al., 2000), and neck force transducers to measure variations in neck circumference (Coulas, Smith, Qadri, & Martin, 2009), with some success reported for each technique.

Rehabilitation measures are typically accompanied by compensatory strategies, and in some cases, only compensatory strategies are recommended. These measures are designed to allow adequate nutritional intake and optimize eating in the presence of swallowing problems. Strategies include positioning, diet change, and feeding modifications. Compensatory strategies should be chosen carefully and their effects monitored. While such strategies can promote a safe swallow, they may have a negative effect on other aspects of the person's health. For example, thickened liquids can reduce risk of aspiration, but if the older person also reduces fluid intake, dehydration may result. Strategies that do not interfere with the person's enjoyment of food should be considered before resorting to recommendations that reduce the acceptability of food or require extreme monitoring by the patient.

It is important that the clinician choose methods that will be most effective for each patient without overwhelming both the patient and family with numerous strategies. For example, an elderly patient with cricopharyngeal dysfunction may be asked to do the Shaker exercise, the falsetto /i/, the Mendolsohn, the Masako/tongue hold, and an effortful swallow, while also receiving thermal and electrical stimulation and being placed on a restricted diet. While some patients may actually try to adhere to the multiple recommendations, the effectiveness of such a treatment approach is questionable and may reduce the patient's motivation and cooperation. Such a regimen would be particularly taxing on a frail, elderly person.

Examples of rehabilitative and compensatory strategies are listed in Table 6.2. Descriptions of some strategies are provided in Appendix 6C.

When no oral feeding is allowed (npo), the physical condition of the elderly patient can deteriorate rapidly and the likelihood of recovery of a functional swallow is reduced. Patients may become dehydrated when recommendations prohibit thin liquids. Recent reports indicate that when used with appropriate npo patients, the Frazier Water Protocol does not increase health complications and may be associated with earlier dismissal from the hospital (Becker, Tewes, & Lemke, 2008; Bronson-Lowe et al., 2008). This protocol permits npo patients to have water or ice chips whenever desired, and patients on diets that restrict thin liquid may have water before and after meals. It is essential that good oral hygiene be maintained in these patients. Patients who demonstrate extreme coughing in response to thin liquids are not appropriate candidates for the Frazier Water Protocol.

TABLE 6.2
Intervention Strategies for Dysphagic Patients

	Strategy	**Disorder**
Exercises	• Shaker • Falsetto • Masako/tongue hold	• UES dysfunction • Poor laryngeal elevation
	• Tongue resistance	• Weak oral stage
	• Tongue base	• Slow pharyngeal stage
	• Effortful sucking	• Weak tongue, cheeks, velum
	• Adduction exercises	• Lack of glottal closure/airway protection
Body positioning	• Lying down/reclining	• Weak oral transit
	• Body slanted to strong side	• Unilateral weakness
	• Remain upright after eating	• Reflux
Positioning head	• Chin tuck	• Poor airway protection • Reduced tongue base action
	• Chin elevated	• Weak oral transit
	• Head turned to weak side	• Unilateral pharyngeal weakness of side of pharynx with reduced airway protection
	• Head tilted to strong side	• Unilateral weakness
	• Push on weak cheek	• Poor bolus control • Pocketing of bolus
Food and diet	• Thickened liquids	• Premature spillage • Slow pharyngeal response
	• Cohesive bolus	• Disorganized manipulation
	• Soft diet	• Reduced strength, poor dentition
	• Enhance taste or smell	• Cognitive impairment • Slow pharyngeal response
Feeding strategies	• Alternate consistencies	• Residue/stasis • Slow pharyngeal response
	• Liquid chaser	• Residue/stasis
	• Placement of bolus	• Scarring • Weakness • Tongue thrusting patterns
	• Control bolus size	• Weakness • Poor oral stage • Cognitive problem

TABLE 6.2 *(continued)*

	Strategy	Disorder
Sensory enhance-ment	• Carbonated/sour bolus	• Slow pharyngeal response
	• Cold liquids	• Slow pharyngeal response
	• Push down with spoon	• Reduced oral response
Safe-swallow strategies	• Supraglottic swallow • Supersupraglottic swallow • Effortful swallow • Mendolsohn	• Poor airway protection
	• Multiple swallows/bolus	• Weakness • Residue/stasis
Feeding imple-ments	• Weighted utensils, cups	• Tremor
	• Straws—one-way flow con-trolled bolus	• Excessive air intake in drinking • Inability to drink from cup

Logically, the best therapy for swallowing is swallowing. Appropriate use of the Frazier Water Protocol provides patients with the opportunity to practice swallowing while promoting hydration and oral health.

Effective long-term implementation of compensatory strategies often relies on the patient or a caregiver. Strategies recommended depend not only on the swallowing disorder demonstrated but also on the care setting and the patient's cognitive state. While it is usually beneficial for a dysphagic person to eat with someone, the setting should be calm and allow for attention to feeding and swallowing strategies. In many long-term care settings, dysphagic patients eat in noisy dining rooms or special feeding rooms. Not only can these settings be highly distracting, but also it may be difficult to provide instructions to residents being fed or to closely monitor compensatory strategies. In those cases, it may be necessary to recommend feeding in the resident's room or dining with one other resident at a less busy time. For all settings, it is important that caregivers be provided with lists of foods that the patient can eat, not just the foods that should be avoided. For any patient, successful intervention relies not only on the actual feeding and swallowing strategies used, but also on preparation of the patient and the environment, careful planning of the meals, and appropriate care after eating. Table 6.3 provides a description of compensatory recommendations that can be provided to caregivers in the home or in a long-term-care setting.

TABLE 6.3
Strategies for Caregivers

Prefeeding

Meal planning and preparation	1. Schedule small, frequent meals or snacks at the same time every day. Allow 45 minutes to an hour for each meal. Do not plan meals to immediately follow physical exercise. 2. Plan to provide maximum calories for "most alert" meal. 3. Encourage self-feeding behaviors by planning foods that do not require utensils. If possible, plan the same foods for everyone with appropriate adjustments in consistency or texture. 4. Enhance sensory characteristics of food, including aroma, visual appearance, temperature, and flavor. 5. If lack of saliva or thick mucous is a problem, plan meals that avoid mucous binders (e.g., dairy products, orange juice, chocolate), dry bread, and foods that require extensive chewing. Increase moisture by adding broth or serving steamed foods.
Patient preparation	1. Be sure person has dentures, glasses, hearing aids, etc. Improve comfort by taking person to the bathroom, washing hands. 2. If allowed, stimulate appetite with a small serving of wine prior to one meal. 3. Reduce "background taste" by oral cleaning prior to meals. Provide artificial saliva if needed. 4. Assure concerned patients that nothing will be hard to eat, hot, poisoned, or big enough to choke them. Allow paranoid patients to watch meal preparation.

Mealtime and eating strategies

Prepare the setting	1. Reduce distractions (no TV or music), remove unnecessary objects on table, and use solid color table and dishes. 2. Have someone eat with the patient, but keep dining groups small or allow patient to eat in separate room. 3. Provide a comfortable room (e.g., appropriate temperature, good lighting). 4. Provide utensils, cups, bowls, and placemats that facilitate eating. Avoid plastic utensils.
Patient preparation	1. Seat the person in the appropriate position, usually upright with head comfortably forward. 2. Allow a "warm up" for feeding: offer small amounts first. 3. Allow pauses during the meal.

TABLE 6.3 *(continued)*

Mealtime and eating strategies, continued

Feeder strategies	1. Offer the food within 5 to 10 minutes of seating the person.
	2. Provide verbal or physical cues for cognitively impaired persons. Meal partner can demonstrate eating.
	3. Facilitate nutritional intake and optimal swallowing by serving high-calorie foods first, reducing the number of food choices, alternating consistencies when feeding, and providing cold or sweet items between bites of the entrée.
	4. Provide encouragement during the meal by using the person's name, offering condiments, assisting with spills, etc.

Post-feeding

Oral care	1. Clean the patient's mouth after eating to remove residue.
	2. Check for pocketed food.
Reflux precautions	1. Ensure patient maintains an upright position for 30 minutes after eating.
	2. Have patient sleep with head elevated.

To promote maintenance of a successful feeding and swallowing program in the patient's home, clinicians should provide structured caregiver education, including recipes and a list of supply sources along with the list of recommended foods. It is also beneficial to offer caregivers information regarding respite services and to schedule follow-up sessions for caregiver support.

In long-term-care facilities, interdisciplinary planning results in better intervention outcomes. Individual plans for each patient should be designed and performance reassessed periodically. To provide better cooperation and prevent unnecessary misunderstandings, both the staff and the resident's family should be knowledgeable of the feeding and swallowing recommendations and procedures. Unfortunately, effectiveness of intervention in many long-term-care facilities is reduced due to the heavy turnover rates in trained staff or a lack of adequate staff to implement the plans.

Reimbursement

A physician must write an order for a specific swallowing evaluation. The requirement for a supervising physician to be present or at least on the premises for different assessment methods varies from state to state. To qualify for reimbursement for instrumental evaluations, clinicians must provide documentation that establishes that the procedure is needed to identify suspected aspiration or that the exact diagnosis of the swallowing disorder cannot be determined through a clinical examination. Clinicians may be concerned that they will not be reimbursed when no disorder is identified during the evaluation; however, the reason for the evaluation should be listed as the primary diagnosis.

Unfortunately, prevention services are not typically reimbursed. To qualify for reimbursement from Medicare and most private insurance companies, intervention services must be considered reasonable and necessary. To meet this criterion, it must be clear that services need to be provided by a qualified therapist or performed under a qualified therapist's supervision. It is also important to demonstrate a reasonable expectation that the procedures will be effective in improving the patient's functioning in a reasonable period of time. This assurance might require documentation that the patient is medically stable and capable of participating in the therapy; for example, evidence of the patient's level of alertness, ability to cooperate, and ability to retain new learning might be provided. The plan of treatment should specify the length and frequency of the recommended intervention (e.g., four 30-minute sessions/week). In the progress report, objective indications of progress should be provided, with an explanation for regressions or plateaus in progress. Reimbursement for establishing a maintenance program may be permitted if the patient's condition can be shown to warrant the clinician's services to manage and periodically reevaluate the effectiveness of the program. If the patient's prognosis for improvement is poor, speech pathology services may not be considered reasonable and necessary, and reimbursement will be denied. Payment may be discontinued if it is determined that the patient's condition is not improving in response to intervention services. Reimbursement denials also result from plans that include repetitive observations or reinforcement of skills that caregivers could be instructed to provide.

Separate Current Procedural Terminology (CPT; American Medical Association [AMA], 2009a) codes are available for physician services and speech–language pathology services. For example, the codes for modified barium swallows are for use by radiologists and are not used for speech–language billing. Separate procedure codes currently exist for swallowing treatment, evaluation of swallowing function, motion fluoroscopy/swallow, FEES, and FEEST. State guidelines may allow the speech–language pathologist to conduct more invasive procedures, such as those requiring endoscopy, only when a supervising physician is on the premises. When these services are provided in an outpatient setting, a modifier should be added that indicates that the service was provided by a speech–language pathologist. Speech–language pathologists should also be aware that some procedure codes are considered mutually exclusive and reimbursement is not typically approved if they are billed on the same day. In some cases, two distinct procedures performed on the same day will be reimbursed if the modifier is added and adequate documentation of the procedures is provided. Healthcare Common Procedure Coding System (HCPCS) codes related to swallowing include a code for dysphagia screening (AMA, 2009b).

When providing treatment, clinicians may provide multiple sessions per day; however, the code for dysphagia treatment is not a time-based code and can be billed only once for each day of service. There is a separate CPT code for treatment using electrical stimulation, but not all insurance carriers cover that procedure. In those cases, clinicians may provide electrical stimulation in addition to traditional swallowing therapy using the general dysphagia treatment code. To be reimbursed, the clinician must document the traditional methods used during each session. When both procedures are covered, the separate codes cannot be billed on the same day.

Key Points

This chapter described the challenges faced by a multidisciplinary team in identifying and remediating the feeding and swallowing problems demonstrated by the elderly population. Major themes included the following:

- Swallowing remains safe and efficient in healthy elderly individuals.
- Changes resulting from normal aging reduce the ability to compensate and put the elderly at higher risk for dysphagia in the event of an illness.
- Exercises to build strength may increase reserve capacity and prevent some swallowing problems.
- Systematic screening programs are effective in early identification of dysphagia and reduction of health complications secondary to swallowing problems.
- Intervention strategies are the same for adults of all ages, but the elderly are more likely to demonstrate physical conditions that prohibit or limit implementation of some strategies.
- Rehabilitation procedures promote recovery of swallowing function.

- Compensation strategies facilitate a safe swallow and are the most common form of intervention for the elderly who develop a feeding swallowing problem.
- Caregivers should be instructed in prefeeding, feeding, and post-feeding strategies.

References

American Medical Association, (2009a). *Current procedural terminology (CPT) 2010.* Chicago: Author.

American Medical Association. (2009b). *Healthcare common procedure coding system 2010: Level II.* Chicago: Author.

Becker, D., Tewes, L., & Lemke, J. (2008, November). *An oral water protocol in rehabilitation patients with dysphagia for liquids.* Paper presented at the American Speech-Language-Hearing National Convention, Chicago, IL.

Bronson-Lowe, C., Leising, K., Bronson-Lowe, D., Lanham, S. Hayes, S., Ronquillo, A., et al. (2008, November). *Effects of a free water protocol for patients with dysphagia.* Paper presented at the American Speech-Language-Hearing National Convention, Chicago, IL.

Bülow, M., Speyer, R., Baijens, L., Woisard, V., & Ekberg, O. (2008). Neuromuscular electrical stimulation (NMES) in stroke patients with oral and pharyngeal dysfunction. *Dysphagia, 23,* 302–309.

Butler, S. G., Stuart, A., Markley, L., & Rees, C. (2009). Penetration and aspiration in healthy older adults as assessed during endoscopic evaluation of swallowing. *Annals of Otology, Rhinology & Laryngology, 118,* 190–198.

Coulas, V., Smith R., Qadri, S., & Martin, R. (2009). Differentiating effortful and noneffortful swallowing with a neck force transducer: Implications for the development of a clinical feedback system. *Dysphagia, 24,* 7–12.

Crary, M., Carnaby, G., Groher, M., & Helseth, E. (2004). Functional benefits of dysphagia therapy using adjunctive sEMG biofeedback. *Dysphagia 19,*160–164.

Crary, M., Carnaby-Mann, G., & Faunce, A. (2007). Electrical stimulation therapy for dysphagia: Descriptive results of two surveys. *Dysphagia, 22,* 165–173.

Easterling, C. (2008). Does an exercise aimed at improving swallow function have an effect on vocal function in the healthy elderly? *Dysphagia, 23,* 317–326.

Grudell, A., Alexander, J., Enders, F., Pacifico, R., Fredericksen, M., Wise, J., et al. (2007). Validation of the Mayo dysphagia questionnaire. *Diseases of the Esophagus, 20,* 202–205.

Hinchey, J., Shephard, T., Furie, K., Smith, D., Wang, D., & Tonn, S. (2005). Formal dysphagia screening protocols prevent pneumonia. *Stroke, 36,* 1972–1976.

Jacobs, J., Logemann, J., Pajak, T., Pauloski, B., Collins, S., Casiano, R., et al. (1999). Failure of cricopharyngeal myotomy to improve dysphagia following head and neck cancer surgery. *Archives of Otolaryngology–Head and Neck Surgery, 125,* 942–946.

Kiger, M., Brown, C., & Watkins L. (2006). Dysphagia management: An analysis of patient outcomes using VitalStim therapy compared to traditional swallow therapy. *Dysphagia, 21,* 243–253.

Lambert, H., Abrahamowicz, M., Groher, M., Wood-Dauphinee, S., & Gisel, E. (2005). The McGill Ingestive Skills Assessment predicts time to death in elderly population with neurogenic dysphagia: Preliminary evidence. *Dysphagia, 20,* 123–132.

Lichtenstein, A. H., Rasmussen, H., Yu, W. W., Epstein, S., & Russell, R. M. (2008). Modified MyPyramid for older adults. *Journal of Nutrition, 138,* 78–82.

Lim. S. H. B., Lieu, P. K., Phua, S. Y., Seshadri, R., Venketasubramanian, N., Lee, S. H., et al. (2001). Accuracy of bedside clinical methods compared with fiberoptic endoscopic examination of swallowing (FEES) in determining the risk of aspiration in acute stroke patients. *Dysphagia, 16,* 1–6.

Manning, L. A., & Gluth, M. B. (n.d.). *Laryngopharyngeal Reflux (LPR).* [Brochure]. Springdale, AR: Author.

Martino, R., Silver, F. Teasell, R., Baylet, M. Nicholson, G., Streiner, D., et al. (2009). The Toronto Bedside Swallowing Screening Test (TOR-BSST): Development and validation of a dysphagia screening tool for patients with stroke. *Stroke, 40,* 555–561.

McHorney, C., Martin-Harris, B., Robbins, J., & Rosenbeck, J. (2006). Clinical validity of the SWAL-QOL and SWAL-CARE outcome tools with respect to bolus flow measures. *Dysphagia, 21,* 140–148.

Nakajoh, K., Nakagawa, T., Sekizawa, K., Matsui, T., Arai, H., & Sasaki, H. (2001). Relation between incidence of pneumonia and protective reflexes in post-stroke patients with oral or tube feeding. *Journal of Internal Medicine, 247,* 39–42.

Nathadwarawala, K. M., McGroary A., & Wiles C. M. (1994). Swallowing in neurological outpatients. *Dysphagia, 9,* 120–129.

Reddy, N. P., Simcox, D. L., Gupta, V., Motta, G. E., Coppenger, J., Das, A., et al. (2000). Biofeedback therapy using accelerometry for treating dysphagic patients with poor laryngeal elevation: Case studies. *Journal of Rehabilitation Research and Development,* 37(3), 361–372.

Robbins, J., Gangnon, R., Theis, S., Kays, S., Hewitt, A., & Hind, J. (2005). The effects of lingual exercise on swallowing in older adults. *Journal of American Geriatrics Society,* 53, 1483–1489.

Roy, N., Stemple, J., Merrill, R., & Thomas, L. (2007). Dysphagia in the elderly: Preliminary evidence of prevalence, risk factors, and socioemotional effects. *Annals of Otology, Rhinology & Laryngology, 116,* 858–865.

Scher, R. L., & Richtsmeier, W. J. (1998). Long-term experience with endoscopic staple-assisted esophagodiverticulostomy for Zenker's diverticulum. *Laryngoscope, 108,* 200–205.

Sharkawi, A., Ramig, L., Logemann, J., Pauloski, B., Rademaker, A., Smith, C., et al. (2002). Swallowing and voice effects of Lee Silverman Voice Treatment (LSVT®): A pilot study. *Journal of Neurology Neurosurgery and Psychiatry, 72,* 31-36.

Steele, C., & Lieshout, P. (2005) Does barium influence tongue behavior during swallowing? *American Journal of Speech-Language Pathology, 14,* 27–39.

Tohara, H., Saitoh, E., Mays, K., Kuhlemeier, K., & Palmer, J. (2003). Three tests for predicting aspiration without videofluorography. *Dysphagia, 18,* 126–134.

Trapl, M., Enderle, M., Teuschl, Y., Matz, K., Dachenhausen, A., & Brainin, M. (2007). Dysphagia bedside screening of acute-stroke patients: The Gugging Swallowing Screen. *Stroke, 38,* 2948–2952.

Turley, R., & Cohen S. (2009) Impact of voice and swallowing problems in the elderly. *Otolaryngology–Head and Neck Surgery, 140,* 33–36.

USC News. (2009). *Keck School surgeons develop new technology to treat gastroesophageal reflux.* Retrieved July 20, 2009, from http://www.usc.edu/uscnews/stories/16383.html

Wakasugi, Y., Tohara, H., Hattori, F., Motohashi, Y., Nakane, A., Goto, S., et al. (2008). Screening test for silent aspiration at the bedside. *Dysphagia, 23,* 364–370.

Wilson, M., &Morley, J. (2004). Nutritional assessment and support in chronic disease management. In C. W. Bales & E. S. Ritchie (Eds.) *Handbook of clinical nutrition and aging* (pp. 77–101). Towata, NJ: Humana Press.

Effects of Medications on Swallowing

Swallowing symptoms	Drug class	Selected common examples
Xerostomia		
Poor bolus movement	Cardiac antiarrhythmics (for abnormal heart rhythm)	• Procainamide (Procan) • Disopyramide (Norpace)
Slow oral and pharyngeal transit	Antidepressants (for mood stabilization)	• Fluoxetine (Prozac) • Paroxetine (Paxil) • Seraline (Zoloft) • Venlafaxine (Effexor)
Increased residue		
Taste change	Antiemetics (for reduction of nausea)	• Meclizine (Antivert) • Metoclopramide (Reglan) • Scopolamine (Transderm Scop)
	Antihistamines (for treatment of allergies)	• Chlorpheniarmine (Chlor-Trimeton) • Diphenhydramine (Benadryl)
	Antihypertensives (for reduction of blood pressure)	• Captopril (Capoten) • Lisinopril (Prinivil, Zestril)
	Antipsychotics/neuroleptics (for psychiatric disorders)	• Chorpormazine (Thorazine) • Closapine (Clozaril) • Haloperidol (Haldol) • Lithium • Risperidone (Risperdal)
	Calcium channel blockers (for heart and vascular disease)	• Amlodipine (Norvasc)
Mucous membrane damage		
Reduced oral intake	Antibacterials	• Erthromycin (E-mycin) • Clindamycin (Cleocin) • Doxycycline (Vibramycin)
Discomfort or pain when eating	Antivirals	• Zidovudine (Retrovir)
Change in preferred food	Bisphosphonates (for osteoporosis)	• Alendronate (Fosamax)

(continues)

137

Effects of Medications on Swallowing (*continued*)

Swallowing symptoms	Drug class	Selected common examples
Mucous membrane damage (continued)		
	Chemotherapeutic agents	• Fluorouracil • Methotrexate
	Nonsteroidal anti-inflammatory drugs (NSAIDS, for pain)	• Aspirin • Ibuprofen (Advil, Motrin) • Naproxen (Aleve, Naprosyn)
	Vitamin supplements	• Iron (Feratab) • Potassium chloride (K-Dur) • Vitamin C
Central nervous system depression and/or reduced muscle coordination and control		
Aspiration Choking Coughing Dehydration or avoidance of liquids	Antidepressants (for mood stabilization)	• Alprazolam (Xanax) • Clonazepam (Klonopin) • Diazepam (Valium) • Lorazepam (Ativan)
	Antiepileptics (for seizures)	• Carbamazepine (Tegretol) • Gabapentin (Neurontin) • Phenobarbital • Phenytoin (Dilantin) • Valproic acid (Depakote)
	Muscle relaxants (for muscle spasms, dystonia)	• Baclofen (Lioresal) • Benzatropine (Cogentin) • Cyclobenzaprine (Flexeril) • Oxybutynin (Ditropan) • Tolterodine (Detrol)
	Narcotics (for pain)	• Codeine sulfate • Fentanyl (Duragesic) • Propoxyphene (Darvon)

Laryngopharyngeal Reflux (LPR)

What Is Laryngopharyngeal Reflux (LPR)?

When you eat something, it reaches the stomach by traveling down a muscular tube called the esophagus. Once food reaches the stomach, acid and pepsin (a digestive enzyme) are added so that digestion can occur. The esophagus has two sphincters (bands of muscle fibers that act as valves to close the tube). These sphincters help keep the contents of the stomach where they belong in the stomach. One sphincter is at the top of the esophagus (at the junction with the upper throat) and one is at the bottom of the esophagus (at the junction with the stomach). When these sphincters are not working properly, a phenomenon termed "reflux" can occur. The term reflux, meaning "backwards flow," usually refers to the regurgitation of stomach contents up through the esophagus and/or into throat (pharynx) and voice box (larynx).

What Is the Difference Between GERD and LPR?

Some people have an abnormal amount of reflux of stomach contents through the lower sphincter, which then pools in the esophagus. This is referred to as GERD, or gastroesophageal reflux disease. If this occurs excessively, irritation and damage to the esophagus can occur—often resulting in prominent heartburn. If the refluxed stomach contents are not held in the esophagus by the upper sphincter, they can leak and cause irritation of the voice box (larynx) and throat (pharynx). This is referred to as LPR, or laryngopharyngeal reflux. The structures in the throat are much more sensitive to stomach acid and digestive enzymes than the esophagus, so even small amounts of reflux into these areas can result in significant

Note. From "Laryngopharyngeal Reflux (LPR)," by Lance A. Manning and Michael B. Gluth. Copyright by the Ear, Nose, and Throat Center of the Ozarks. Reprinted with permission.

damage or irritation. It is important to understand that GERD and LPR are related but distinctly different conditions in regards to cause, symptoms, and treatment. A person can have symptoms of GERD or LPR with or without the other.

Why Don't I have Heartburn or Stomach Problems?

This question is often asked by patients with LPR. Heartburn is generally associated with GERD but may or may not be present with LPR. The fact is that most patients with LPR do not experience significant heartburn. Heartburn occurs when the tissue in the esophagus becomes irritated. More than half the patients with LPR do not experience heartburn because the stomach acid does not stay in the esophagus long enough to irritate the esophagus and cause heartburn symptoms. The threshold for irritating the sensitive tissues of the voice box and throat is much lower than that of the esophagus, so it is possible for these tissues to be irritated while the esophagus is not.

Only irritation of the esophagus causes heartburn; irritation of the throat and voice box causes different symptoms. Most of the reflux events of LPR that can damage the throat happen without the patient ever knowing that they are occurring.

Common Symptoms of LPR
- Hoarseness
- Frequent throat clearing
- Pain or irritation in the throat
- Feeling of lump in throat
- Problems while swallowing
- Bad/bitter taste in mouth (especially in morning)
- Chronic (ongoing) cough
- Asthma-like symptoms
- Excessive post-nasal drip or throat mucous

Some of the symptoms of LPR are related to direct contact of stomach contents with the tissues of the throat and voice box, while other symptoms are indirectly related to LPR such as the adverse consequences of frequent throat clearing and cough. The body's own attempts at protection from LPR can also cause symptoms. Examples of this are increased production of throat mucous or frequent spasm of the muscle of the upper esophageal sphincter (resulting in "lump" in throat or swallowing difficulty).

When Does LPR Occur?

Most prominently, LPR will occur during the daytime within 2 hours after meals—yet it is known to occur throughout the day and night. GERD, if also present, seems to be more pronounced in the evening or at night (particularly while sleeping). LPR will take place independent of body position (very common while sitting or standing upright); however, it might be made worse by lying down flat soon after meals.

Diagnosis of LPR

Your physician can identify various signs of LPR while examining your throat and voice box in the office. The following signs seen by the physician are strong indicators of LPR:

- Redness, irritation, and swelling of the larynx at particular locations
- Small ulcers or growths in larynx (granuloma, polyp, or nodule)
- Swelling of the vocal cords

In some cases, reflux symptoms may prompt the need for further visualization of the esophagus and/or voice box with a scope during a separate procedure performed with sedation or general anesthesia.

If the diagnosis of GERD or LPR is in question, a formal test to evaluate changes in acidity throughout the esophagus may be required. The 24-hour pH monitoring test is the gold standard for monitoring reflux events associated with LPR. This test requires a small tube to be positioned through the nose into the esophagus over 24 hours to monitor the amount and type of reflux during a typical day. If LPR is a concern, it is very important that this test be slightly modified from the usual routine used to test for GERD—specifically a "dual-probe" must be used so that acidity near the throat and voice box can be measured.

Treatment for LPRD

Foods

You should pay close attention to how your system reacts to various foods. Each person may discover which foods cause an increase in reflux symptoms. The following foods have been shown to cause reflux in many people:

- Spicy, acidic, and tomato-based foods like Mexican or Italian food
- Acidic fruit juices such as orange juice, grapefruit juice, cranberry juice, etc.
- Alcoholic beverages (including wine)
- Fast foods and other fatty foods
- Caffeinated beverages (coffee, tea, soft drinks)
- Chocolate
- Mint

Mealtime

- Do not gorge yourself at mealtime.
- Eat meals several hours before bedtime.
- Avoid bedtime snacks.
- Do not exercise immediately after eating.

Stress

Make time in your schedule to do activities that lower your stress level. It has been shown that even moderate stress can dramatically increase the amount of reflux.

Body Weight

Excessive body weight is one of the most important factors associated with reflux. If overweight, consider a realistic, healthy program to reduce body weight over the long term. Your primary care physician can assist with this.

Nighttime Reflux

If are having notable symptoms at night, elevate the head of your bed 4–6 inches with books, bricks, or a block of wood to achieve a 10-degree slant. Do not simply prop the body up with extra pillows.

Tight Clothing

Avoid tight belts and other restrictive clothing.

Smoking

If you smoke, stop! This dramatically worsens reflux and otherwise harms your throat and voice box.

Medications for LPR

Most standard over-the-counter antacid medications (Rolaids®, Tums®, Gaviscon®, Mylanta®, etc.) work by neutralizing acid in the stomach. These medications will not provide any lasting relief of reflux symptoms or reverse chronic irritation in the throat. If needed for immediate symptom relief of heartburn or indigestion, take one dose (as recommended on the label) at meals or at bedtime.

Other types of medications (Prilosec®, Prevacid®, Nexium®, Zantac®, Pepcid®) work by long-term (several hours) reduction of stomach acid production. In most cases, these medications, if properly administered, will successfully reverse many of the symptoms of LPR, yet they do not have an immediate effect. Some of these medications are available over the counter, but generally the most effective medications (called proton-pump inhibitors) and doses require a prescription.

If you are started on a medication for LPR, your physician may prescribe a treatment regimen that is relatively more aggressive or frequent at first, and then taper the treatment back after several weeks. It is essential that you strictly adhere to your prescribed medication regimen for at least 4–6 weeks before any determination can be made about whether or not your medication is beneficial.

Most proton-pump inhibitor medications (Prilosec®, Prevacid®, Nexium®, Protonix®) should be taken in the morning and/or afternoon at least 30 minutes before eating a meal. H2-blocker acid reducing medications (Zantac®, Pepcid®, Tagamet®) are generally taken before bedtime. Be certain to pay close attention to the timing of your medications as prescribed by your physician.

Swallowing Facilitation Strategies

Effortful swallow. Patients are asked to squeeze the bolus forcefully with the tongue and swallow.

Masako/tongue hold. Patients are asked to extend their tongue between their incisors and swallow while holding the tongue in that position. This exercise is not intended to be done while swallowing food or liquid.

Mendolsohn maneuver. When patients swallow, they are asked to hold the larynx in the elevated position for several seconds by tensing the muscles.

Shaker exercise. Patients lie on their back and raise the head until they can see their toes, without raising the shoulders. Head is held in that position for one minute. This is followed by 1 minute of rest. This is done three times. Then, patients raise their head to that level and immediately lower it 30 times. This may be modified for people who are unable to hold their head in the elevated position for 1 minute.

Supraglottic swallow. Patients take a breath and hold it while swallowing, then cough to clear the airway. Super-supraglottic is similar, but patients are asked to hold their breath more forcefully.

Tongue-base exercise. Patients are instructed to protrude the tongue then pull it straight back as far as possible or hold it in the position for gargling or yawning

CHAPTER 7

Cognition and Aging:
Primary and Tertiary Aging Factors

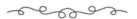

Karee E. Dunn

DUNN ACKNOWLEDGES THAT PRIMARY cognitive aging can be described from multiple perspectives. She begins by discussing cognition as a developmental phenomenon, drawing from work by Piaget and Schaie. She also examines primary aging from the perspective of changes in intelligence, including reference to primary mental abilities and fluid versus crystallized intelligence. Much of the chapter is then built around an information processing model of cognition. Changes in brain structure and activation associated with aging are presented, followed by an explanation of component skills in an information-processing model and changes that are seen in these skill domains. Theories of cognitive aging are described briefly as they relate to observed changes. The chapter closes with discussions of cognitive maintenance and loss prevention, and cognitive growth and potential.

One common myth about aging is that most older people lose their cognitive skills, particularly memory. The realities of cognitive aging contradict this myth. Cognition involves many skills. Older adults actually experience a great deal of stability in some of these skills, along with growth or declines in others. Further, individuals differ with respect to how aging affects their cognitive performance and the rate of changes in cognitive skills. Individual variability is influenced by factors such as education, level of mental activity, emotional state, and physical health. Thus, it is difficult to ascribe exact ages and patterns to changes in cognition as one grows older.

Cognition is critical to any communication activity, so understanding normal cognition is a prerequisite to understanding aging clients and to differentiating between normal (primary) and disordered (secondary) aging. In the past, childhood was seen as a period of growth, adulthood was viewed as a period of stability, and old age was viewed as a time of general loss moving toward death. Contemporary views of cognitive aging describe it as a developmental process, one that reflects an attitude of "not getting older, but getting better."

Cognitive aging can be described from several perspectives. Developmentally, cognition can be viewed in terms of changes either in the way we think across the lifespan or in intelligence. Another perspective examines cognitive aging within the framework of an information processing model and explores what actually happens to component skills such as memory, perception, and attention, and why some cognitive skills decline while others are maintained. Changes in brain structures and pathways and theories of cognitive aging can be considered within the information processing model. These perspectives are discussed in this chapter, which concludes with a review of cognitive growth and potential in later years.

Cognitive Development

One way to look at cognitive aging is to examine how cognitive processing strategies and goals shift as we grow older. This perspective typically takes into consideration the knowledge and experiences gleaned by each individual across the life span. Two such approaches are described briefly.

Cognitive Development Past Adolescence: Postformal Operations

Views of cognitive development tend to focus on the period from childhood into adolescence, with little attention to the adult years. For example, Piaget described a series of stages in the development of intellectual abilities best understood by examining how the quality of a person's thinking changes from early childhood into adulthood (Piaget & Inhelder, 1969). His stages ended with the formal operational stage that begins around 11 years of age. In formal operations, thought is rational, logical, and deductive; it tends to ignore the context for real world problems and the role of emotions in decision making.

Since Piaget's early work, many researchers have suggested that there is a later postformal operational stage that continues through adulthood. This stage is characterized by reasoning that is more relative, flexible, and adaptive, reflecting an understanding that knowledge is temporary and flexible, not absolute (Labouvie-Vief, 1984). Postformal operational thought places relatively less emphasis on acquiring knowledge and greater emphasis on using what is known to answer relevant questions. Because this stage reflects life experience and exposure to higher education, all older adults do not necessarily reach postformal thinking.

For normally aging adults, these developmental shifts in thinking may affect daily cognitive performance, particularly in the problem-solving domain. In facing life changes, adults who have reached the postformal operational stage may actually be more effective in identifying and dealing with these changes than are those who rely primarily on formal operations. They are also more open to new information and more willing to change their worldview based on this information. The fact that education contributes to the acquisition of postformal skills may also explain in part why education is such a critical factor in cognitive aging.

Schaie's Life-Span Model of Postformal Cognitive Development

Another way to view developmental changes in cognition is to look at how shifts in our goals motivate cognitive behavior at different life stages. Schaie and Willis (2000) developed a seven-stage model describing how a person's cognition is the result of social commitments and demands at any particular point in life. As one progresses through these stages, goals shift from the acquisition of knowledge and skills (*I simply need to know*) to practical assimilation of knowledge and skills (*the application of what I know*) to a search for meaning and purpose (*why should I know?*). The later stages are more typical in older adults and reflect postformal thinking. The following are examples of the stages:

1. *Acquisitive stage* (childhood through adolescence). The individual acquires information and skills for their own sake or as preparation for participation in society.
2. *Achieving stage* (late teens to early thirties). Acquired information and skills are used to pursue goals; the individual is no longer learning for the sake of learning.
3. *Responsible stage* (late thirties to early sixties). The individual solves practical problems associated with responsibilities to others, such as employees or family members.
4. *Executive stage* (thirties to middle age). This stage may overlap with the achieving and responsible stages. Individuals at this stage are responsible for societal systems (government

or business) or social movements. They deal with complex relationships on multiple levels.

5. *Reorganizational stage* (late middle age to late adulthood—postformal thought). Retirees reorganize their lives and direct intellectual energy toward meaningful pursuits that replace paid work.

6. *Reintegrative stage* (late adulthood—postformal thought). Biological and cognitive changes lead to greater selectivity with regard to what tasks in which an individual chooses to engage as well as the amount of energy applied to certain tasks. Older adults concentrate their energy on tasks that are most meaningful to them.

7. *Legacy-creating stage* (advanced old age—postformal thought). Older adults may create instructions for the disposition of possessions, make funeral arrangements, share oral histories, or write their life stories as a legacy for their loved ones in preparation for death.

Not everyone passes through all of Schaie's stages, and the time frames are not fixed. Older adults who attain higher levels of education and who remain active mentally, physically, and socially are more likely to progress to the higher stages. Viewing cognitive aging from Schaie's perspective can help clinicians understand better what particular cognitive activities might be a priority for an older client.

Intelligence

Intelligence is often seen as a cornerstone of cognition. It provides another framework for exploring primary cognitive changes in aging and has been studied and debated for the last 50 years. A number of approaches to defining intelligence are summarized here. A central question is whether intelligence decreases with age. In each approach, it is clear that age does not automatically mean a decrease in intelligence.

Primary Mental Abilities

Primary mental abilities is a term used to describe core cognitive skills including spatial analysis, perceptual speed, numerical ability, verbal relations, words, memory, and induction (Thurstone, 1938). Schaie (2005) examined the development of these primary mental abilities over the course of adulthood. In his 21-year study, while individuals experienced mild but important decreases in all of the primary mental abilities by their mid-70s, typical older adults did not fall below the average range of performance for younger adults until their 80s, with less change experienced in verbal abilities. While there was a general trend of decline in old age, age-related peaks were identified for some primary mental abilities. Schaie's data support the premise that cognition is complex and multidimensional, and that there is a dynamic interaction between various cognitive skills and age.

Schaie's data refute the long-standing belief that irreversible, biologically based declines in intelligence are inevitable in early aging (60–70 years of age). However, other factors do influence and potentially predict later cognitive performance in adults, including the sociocultural environment, life experiences, and early (young adulthood) level of language skills. Engaging in exercise has been shown to prevent or ameliorate many cognitive losses, and cohort group (or generation) differences influence cognitive functioning more than age. From the perspective of primary mental abilities, older adults do not systematically decline. Clinical interventions should be designed around an understanding of an individual's current abilities and should avoid stereotypical views of cognitive decline.

Fluid and Crystallized Intelligence

Another way to examine intelligence in older adults is to use the Cattell-Horn model of fluid and crystallized intelligence. *Fluid intelligence* includes abstract reasoning and problem-solving and is independent of acquired knowledge, education, and acculturation. Fluid intellectual skills support an individual's ability to think and act quickly, solve novel problems, and encode short-term memories. *Crystallized intelligence* reflects learning from past experience, acculturation, and acquired knowledge; it supports activities such as test-taking, language use, and acquired skills. While fluid intelligence peaks in adolescence and then declines, crystallized intelligence continues to grow throughout adulthood. This tendency is true in part because crystallized intelligence is greatly influenced by personality and motivation, as well as educational and cultural opportunities, and it is only indirectly affected by the physiological changes that strongly influence fluid intelligence (Horn, 1978; Horn & Cattell, 1967). Adults tend to channel their activities and skills into areas of expertise, which rely more on crystallized and less on fluid intellectual skills. This focus on crystallized intelligence supports higher level reasoning and perhaps underscores the validity of the common saying, "With age comes wisdom."

KnowThis

Information Processing

Previous sections have approached cognitive aging from the perspective of developmental stages in cognitive processing and intellectual abilities. A third common approach is to use information processing theory to discuss specific skills that are or are not affected by aging. Information processing theorists propose that the human mind functions in a fashion similar to a computer. Like a computer, the mind has a limited capacity (i.e., resources) for the type and amount of information it can process at any given time. Also like computers, the brain engages in mechanical processes to manage information. If the human brain changes as we age, changes in various information processing skills might also be expected. It should be possible to examine these skills in order to understand the influence of aging. To do so, it is first necessary to describe what is known about the resources available in aging brain structures and functions.

Age-Related Changes in Neural Structures and Functions

While we now know that brain plasticity continues into adulthood, the brain does undergo a variety of changes as we age. Brain volume decreases, with volume loss beginning as early as age 30 and becoming more pronounced as we reach the 60s, 70s, and older. Volume changes are due in part to neuron-level changes, including neuron shrinkage, loss in myelination, and reductions in dendritic branching. The rate of volume changes varies considerably across different brain regions. The frontal lobe volumes decline most sharply, followed by parietal and temporal lobes, with little decline seen in primary motor or sensory cortex areas. Declines can be quite pronounced; for example, the medial temporal lobe loses close to 2% of brain volume per year past the age of 70 (Christensen, Anstey, Leach, & Mackinnon, 2008; Wingfield, Prentice, Koh, & Little, 2000).

Losses in white matter in the brain far exceed losses in gray matter, with changes most apparent beginning in the 7th decade. White matter has been associated with declines in cognitive performance, particularly in the prefrontal areas of the brain. In addition, there is reduced cerebral blood flow and metabolic activity in general, along with losses in the production of important neurotransmitters like dopamine. All of these changes have been linked to losses in cognitive skills (Christensen et al., 2008; Wingfield et al., 2000).

Several other changes in brain function are of interest in understanding cognitive aging; these relate to where cortical functions are localized.

Generally, cortical function declines more in the back of the brain than in the front (the so-called posterior to anterior shift with aging, or PASA). So occipital activity decreases and prefrontal cortex activity increases as we age. Older adults also show more bilateral activity (more symmetrical) in the prefrontal cortex during language and cognitive tasks. This phenomenon has been termed HAROLD, which stands for hemispheric asymmetry reduction in older adults (Dennis & Cabeza, 2008). This process may be compensatory; older adults with more bilateral activation tend to perform better on cognitive tasks.

The bottom line for cognitive aging is that the brains of older adults may work differently than those of younger adults. If so, it would be reasonable to expect the various cognitive components in our information processing system to respond to aging in highly differentiated ways. To explore what really happens with cognitive skills, it is first necessary to describe the components of this information processing system.

Basic Information Processing Skills

Information processing models of cognition (Atkinson & Shiffrin, 1968) have addressed how the mind receives (input), analyzes, and overtly or covertly responds (output) to information from the environment. The information processing model is illustrated in Figure 7.1. First, external information (a stimulus) enters the sensory store via sight, sound, smell,

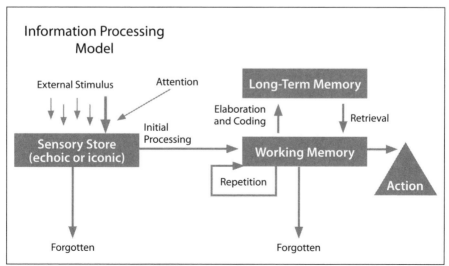

Figure 7.1. The information processing model.

taste, or touch. The sensory store is a very limited, short-term storage unit in which sensory information is held long enough for the brain to perceive it. Information in the sensory store may be either attended to or ignored. If it is ignored, the information drops out of the system and is forgotten. If it is attended, the information is further processed and reaches short-term memory or working memory.

Since the term *short-term memory* is used a number of different ways in the literature, *working memory* will be used here to refer to short-term memory processes sensitive to aging. Working memory is frequently called the mental workbench. It is where individuals consciously or unconsciously manipulate information needed for various cognitive activities. Sensory information is held in working memory for further processing and analysis and may be forgotten or repeated, elaborated, encoded, and then sent to long-term memory (LTM). From LTM, information may be either permanently stored or retrieved and moved back to working memory for additional cognitive operations. While working memory has a limited capacity, the capacity of LTM is unknown and is assumed to be limitless.

LTM is often described as having two primary components, each of which may further be subdivided, as shown in Figure 7.2. It is important to understand these components since they are differentially affected by aging.

Implicit or non-declarative memory is unconscious and is difficult for an individual to verbalize. Two specific types of implicit memory are procedural memory and priming. *Procedural memory* allows us to perform

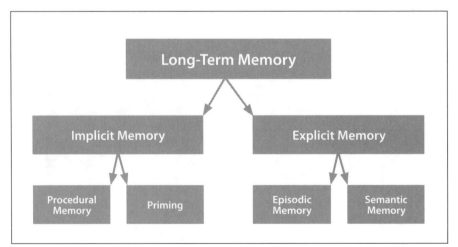

Figure 7.2. Types of long-term memory.

common tasks without the need for conscious recall of how to perform the task. It is "how to" memory. *Priming* refers to memory that is established and triggered by experience. Greater familiarity and experience with information increase the neural pathways linked to that information. This priming increases the likelihood of some responses and decreases the likelihood of others. Priming processes are particularly important in naming. If you are asked to recall the name of a state beginning with the letter *M*, you are more likely to say Missouri (which you have visited frequently) than to say Maine (where you have never traveled).

Explicit or declarative memory requires conscious thought and effort to recall target information; it is what most people mean when they talk about memory. Two specific types of explicit memory are episodic and semantic memory. *Episodic memory* is an autobiographical form of memory that catalogs personal experiences. It helps us remember our first date or what occurred the day our child was born. *Semantic memory* reflects factual or textbook learning about the world. Both types of explicit memories range in strength from recall (strong) to familiarity (weak). The strength of these memories depends on the frequency with which they are retrieved and the context in which they were learned. Memory about the content of a movie will be much greater if that movie was seen on one's first date.

Types of Action Involving Information

In the information processing model, there are many possible cognitive actions. *Action* is what we do with the information we have received or have stored. Of particular interest are higher order cognitive processes such as learning, metacognition, executive functioning, and problem solving. These processes frequently involve the prefrontal cortex, where many changes in brain structure and function are seen in normal aging.

Specific Changes Related to Aging

The following sections describe how components of the information processing model may be affected by aging. Table 7.1 provides an overview of the direction of change (skills improve, maintain, or decline) as well as ways of accommodating any changes in working with older adults.

Sensory Store

The first age-related change that affects information processing in healthy older adults occurs in the auditory and visual sensory store. The internal visual copy is called an *iconic memory,* and the internal auditory copy is

TABLE 7.1

Specific Domains of the Information Processing Models: Age-Related Changes in Those Domains and Means of Ameliorating Those Changes

Domains	Age-related change?	How to accommodate
Sensory store		
Iconic memory	Declines	• Use larger print for instructions on medications and other print material. • Brighten dim lights.
Echoic memory	Declines	• Speak louder or more slowly. • Reduce background noise.
Attention		
Selective attention	Declines	• Decrease distractions by reducing background noises in the environment (e.g., turning down or off the television, closing room door to reduce hallway noise). • Find a room with fewer distractions when working with a client or providing important information or instructions. • Observe behavior closely and ask if the older adult is distracted at the moment by anything. • Increase meaningfulness and personal relevance of tasks. • Explain relevance to treatment activity to older adult's goals.
Divided attention	Declines	• When requiring an older adult to complete a complex task, highlight the personal relevance of the task or draw attention to salient features. • Construct tasks for clients that are interesting, somewhat challenging (but not overly so), clear, and relevant.
Speed and accuracy of perceptual processing	Declines	• Control task complexity. • Provide more time and assistance for complex tasks.
Working memory	Declines	• Identify working memory challenges and priorities unique to each individual. • Help develop strategies to manage consequences (e.g., leaving a reminder note in a regularly visited location such as the bathroom).

∗⫟ **TABLE 7.1** *(continued)*

Domains	Age-related change?	How to accommodate
Long-term memory		
Procedural (implicit)	Stable	
Priming (implicit)	Stable	
Semantic (explicit)	Stable or improves	
Episodic (explicit)	Declines	• Train specific memory strategies, particularly encoding with multisensory information and visualization. • Teach older adults to relate new experiences with past, easily remembered experiences.
Higher order cognitive processes • Learning • Problem solving • Metacognition • Executive functions	Some declines, some changes in strategies	• Help older adults prioritize tasks and component task behaviors. • Alter stimuli for learning to make the information more distinctive and salient. • Reduce the amount of information provided to an older adult for use in problem solving.

called an *echoic memory*. Since both vision and hearing change with primary aging, changes in the sensory store are anticipated. As individuals age, it begins to take longer to register sensory information, there is an increased threshold for stimulus detection, and sensory information fades or is forgotten more quickly after it has registered (Fozard, 1990).

Although sensory losses can be mild in healthy older adults, the effects of any sensory loss may be much greater than the measured loss in sensory acuity. Lindenberger and Baltes (1994) found that visual and auditory acuity in a group of 70- to 100-year-olds explained 50% of the variance in the participants' cognitive scores. This finding suggests that small changes can lead to greater changes in overall cognitive functioning, possibly because of the extra effort required to manage sensory input or to process a flawed stimulus. The idea of effortfulness will be discussed further in the section on theories of cognitive aging.

Attention and Perceptual Processing

Attention plays a major role in determining how information passes through or falls out of the processing mode. It refers to a limited reservoir of cognitive energy that supports information processing (Kok, 2000) and is often affected by aging. While there are many forms of attention, two particularly important ones are selective attention and divided attention. *Selective attention* is the ability to discriminate between relevant and irrelevant information and focus only on the relevant stimuli. Reading a book in the park while blocking out the noise of children playing on the playground illustrates selective attention. Selective attention skills decline with age, and older adults have more trouble than younger adults when tasks are complex. Environments like nursing homes are far from distraction free. Accommodations should be made to reduce irrelevant stimuli.

Engaging in selective attention requires the selective application of one's cognitive energy to one task to the exclusion of others. Older adults have a tendency to conserve effort by being more selective about involvement in tasks that require extended effort and by only exerting energy for tasks that are meaningful, personally relevant, and emotionally salient. These factors must be considered in healthcare interactions.

Divided attention is the ability to process two or more sources of information at one time. Examples of divided attention are talking on the phone and watching a television show, or driving in traffic and reading road signs. When a divided attention task is simple and straightforward, younger and older adults perform similarly (Wickens, Braune, & Stokes, 1987). Both age groups perform more poorly as divided attention tasks become more complex, but once again, the elderly are more affected by task complexity than are younger persons (Madden, 1986; McDowd & Craik, 1988).

Speed and efficiency of perceptual processing decline with aging. *Speed* refers here to signal reception and the time required for initial perceptual processing. Processing speed accounts for 80% or more of age-related variance on memory tasks. Slower performance is not due solely to slowing motor abilities. Younger adults' advantages in reaction time tasks actually increase as the cognitive complexity of a task increases, suggesting that other factors contribute to age differences. Thus, it is important to control the complexity of instructions and tasks for older adults and to provide more time and help as task complexity increases.

Memory

Memory is the storage, retention, and recall of information. Memory problems include inadequate initial storage of information, problems with retention (forgetting), and retrieval deficits. Progressive memory loss does not always accompany advanced age (Jennings & Jacoby, 2003), and there is considerable variability in memory performance between individuals. Of particular interest are normal (primary) changes in working memory and long-term memory, distinguished primarily by how long a memory is expected to last in a particular memory store. Memory challenges in secondary cognitive aging are discussed in the next chapter.

Working Memory. Within the information processing model, working memory is most affected by aging. Some theorists believe that it is the primary source of decline in cognitive operations, including language processing and production, discussed in Chapters 9 and 10.

Losses in working memory affect daily functioning for activities such as processing complicated instructions related to healthcare or retaining and understanding directions to someone's home. The degree of working memory loss is influenced by a number of factors, including cardiovascular fitness, medications, and education. Some working memory tasks are more challenging for the elderly than other tasks. For example, recalling numbers in order (digit span) shows more age-related declines than recalling letters in order (letter span). In general, age differences for spatial working memory are greater than are those for verbal memory span tasks. The way working memory is tested and the relevance of the memory task also influence results and interpretation of age differences. How important is it to older adults to remember the order of a random set of numbers or letters presented to them?

Tests of working memory do not always translate well outside of the confines of a specific experiment. In fact, naturalistic observation may be the best way to identify more practical losses in working memory that affect daily functioning. Family members and friends may also be able to provide information about functional limits due to working memory losses. Some everyday strategies may be useful to minimize the effects of working memory deficits (see Table 7.1).

Long-Term Memory. Age-related differences in LTM are commonplace; however, the presence and magnitude of these differences depend on the type of processing required by a task (e.g., organization vs. semantic elaboration vs. mental imaging). Of the four types of LTM (procedural, priming, semantic, and episodic) described earlier, all but episodic memory processes remain stable or, in the case of semantic memory, may improve. Losses in episodic memory manifest in a variety of ways, such as difficulty remembering newly processed information (Johnson, Reeder, Raye, & Mitchell, 2002) and problems remembering the source of information (Johnson, Hashtroudi, & Lindsay, 1993).

Older adults can use strategies and techniques to reduce, overcome, or even prevent losses in episodic memory. Many of these strategies involve learning to encode new information better or to become more active in encoding activities. In one LTM study, older adults who were *told* to organize new information fared better, when compared to younger adults, than did older adults who were not told to do so and did not do so on their own (Backman, Mantyla, & Herlitz, 1990). Even the negative impact of biological changes to the brain (particularly the hippocampus, used in transferring memories to LTM) can be diminished through mental exercise (Park, Polk, Mikels, Taylor, & Marshuetz, 2001; Schacter, Savage, Apert, Rauch, & Albert, 1996). In healthy older adults, episodic memory is primarily affected for newer experiences, not long-held memories. This finding explains why older adults frequently share detailed stories of their childhood 70 years earlier but have difficulty remembering a phone message received earlier in the day.

Higher Order Cognitive Processes. In an information processing model, all of the previously described components play a role in higher order cognitive processes such as learning, problem solving, metacognition, and executive functioning. Once again, individual differences make it difficult to describe general changes associated with aging. Older adults continue to be able to learn and use new information, although their strategies for doing so are not always as effective or efficient as those of younger adults. Learning and memory are enhanced when the stimuli are distinctive, inconsistent with expectations, or incongruous. Changes in problem-solving behaviors may reflect progression through life stages, as described earlier. In controlled laboratory studies, older adults may not do as well as younger adults, but problem-solving strategies for real-life challenges may remain effective, if somewhat different qualitatively from those of younger persons.

All of these higher order cognitive functions can be considered part of executive functioning, and there are clear differences in the way in which the aging brain activates for various executive functioning tasks. As described earlier, the aging brain is activated more in the front than in the back, and executive processes normally managed in the left prefrontal cortex tend to spill over to the right hemisphere as we age. Some researchers theorize that those who are aging well cognitively are those whose brains can make these transitions as compensations. While more information is needed about executive functions across the lifespan, it is clear that older adults can learn to improve these functions through activities such as prioritizing daily tasks and task components.

Table 7.1 describes the age-related changes in the specific domains of the information processing models. Ways of ameliorating those changes are suggested.

Theories of Cognitive Aging

Individual differences account for some of the heterogeneity of experiences of cognitive aging. Factors affecting a person's cognitive performance include social networks, support systems, relationships, motivation to maintain or maximize performance, personality, health, emotional outlook, life experiences, personal goals, and cultural influences. Cognitive performance is also influenced markedly by how older people view their own cognitive abilities and by negative societal expectations of the elderly and stereotypes about aging. Both personal beliefs and societal perceptions have been shown to disrupt performance on tasks identified as having a memory component (Levy, 2003). Each individual's life experiences can change the brain and thus cognitive functioning. Changes are often adaptive, designed to maintain levels of function despite alterations to the brain itself or to life circumstances.

There are still many unanswered questions about the underlying mechanisms responsible for these observed changes. To answer those questions, a number of theories of cognitive aging have been proposed. While no one theory or combination of theories can explain the uniqueness of each individual's experiences, theories do have the potential to explain some of the seemingly contradictory alterations in mental functioning observed across the lifespan and the uniqueness of each person's cognitive aging. They may also play a role in understanding dementias better and developing more effective interventions.

Theories of cognitive aging and their practical implications are described in more detail in Chapter 9. The current chapter provides only a basic overview of the three most common explanations for age-related cognitive change: (a) resource or reserve limitations, (b) slowing of cognitive processing, and (c) breakdown in normal inhibitory processes.

Resource Capacity Theories

To some degree, virtually all theories of cognitive aging suggest that there is a finite pool of neural or processing resources available for cognitive activity (Burke & Shafto, 2008; Wingfield et al., 2000). As we age, those resources (our reserve capacity) decline. The more complex tasks place greater demands on resources and increase the chances of diminished functioning. There are various definitions of what these resources are. Resources may be actual brain structures. Individuals with more neurons and larger brains (in terms of weight) have more resources to stave off disorders such as Alzheimer's disease. Brain reserve capacity has also been linked to education and intelligence, both of which improve prognosis for recovery from brain damage and provide buffers against cognitive aging. Resources may be described in terms of specific processing components such as working memory capacity, or they may be interpreted broadly to reflect the impact of life changes or stressors on brain reserves and cognitive performance (Burke & Shafto, 2008).

Speed of Processing

Slowing of cognitive and perceptual processing begins in middle age, but it is more noticeable in later years. One of the more obvious age-related changes is an increase in reaction time across the lifespan. Processing of speech signals is perhaps the most time-sensitive of all cognitive behaviors; the longer it takes to complete speech processing, the more likely it is that the signal will decay and subsequent behavior will be inaccurate (Salthouse, 2000).

Inhibition Deficit Hypothesis

A third theory of cognitive aging suggests that, as we age, we experience changes in our brain's ability to inhibit irrelevant information and competing activities, as well as distracting stimuli or thought processes (Hasher & Zacks, 1998). In order to focus attention on one stimulus or activity, we must inhibit attention to other stimuli. In order to engage in problem solving, we must be able to ignore options that are not useful and restrict our thoughts to more appropriate actions. The inhibition deficit theory of cognitive aging is particularly useful in explaining problems with word retrieval.

Cognitive Maintenance and Loss Prevention

The American media typically present a bleak outlook for aging, replete with images of deterioration of cognitive functioning (Carstensen, 2007). It is not surprising that most adults eventually worry about whether they will experience or are experiencing losses in their thinking, remembering, problem-solving, or decision-making abilities. However, there is good news for aging individuals: those with healthy lifestyles can expect few losses in cognition (Carstensen, 2007; Tyas, Snowdon, Desrosiers, Riley, & Markesbery, 2007). It is more likely that reported cognitive losses may actually reflect underlying disease processes that affect both the mind (e.g., depression, Alzheimer's disease) and the body (e.g., metabolic disorders, arteriosclerosis, chronic liver or kidney failure).

Some cognitive losses can be reduced through mental exercises that continue to use and challenge cognitive systems. In other words, the familiar "use it or lose it" refrain applies both to physical functions and to cognitive skills as we age. In the Seattle Longitudinal Study, participants who experienced cognitive decline were given a series of five 1-hour training sessions designed to improve inductive reasoning and spatial orientation. Over half of the participants showed significant improvements, indicating that many cognitive losses are the result of disuse and, more importantly, are reversible (Schaie, 1983).

While this suggests that formal cognitive intervention is required, individuals of all ages can engage in mentally stimulating activities to exercise their brains. The following are some examples of everyday opportunities for mental exercise:

- Test your recall. Make a list of grocery items, things to do, or anything else that comes to mind and memorize it. An hour or so later, try to recall as many items as possible. Make items on the list as challenging as possible for the greatest mental stimulation.
- Draw a map from memory. After returning home from visiting a new place, try to draw a map of the area; repeat this exercise after every trip to a new location.
- Do math in your head. Figure out problems without the aid of a calculator or even pencil and paper. Make this more difficult by walking at the same time.
- Take a cooking class. Learn a new way to cook. Cooking uses a number of senses, all of which exercise different parts of the brain.
- Create word pictures. Mentally visualize the spelling of a word then try to think of any other words that begin or end with the same two letters.
- Refine hand–eye coordination. Learn a new skill that involves fine-motor skills, such as crocheting or painting, or simply work on jigsaw puzzles.
- Learn a new sport. Be sure that any new activity is approved by a doctor or does not result in overexertion.
- Learn a foreign language. Learning a new language stimulates multiple areas of the brain, especially the areas related to listening, hearing, and comprehension.

- Learn how to play a musical instrument, or simply study music. Music stimulates the brain in a number of ways (Melone, 2008).

Later adulthood does not have to be a time in which the mind and body are ravaged by the effects of aging. Instead, the later years can be a time of stability of most cognitive functions, and a time of growth in wisdom and creativity.

Cognitive Growth and Potential

Older adults benefit from a wealth of personal experiences and knowledge that can only be acquired over a lifetime. As a result, they can and often do develop new interests, ways of thinking, and increased wisdom. Maslow (1970) referred to this process as *self-actualization*, the highest level that can be reached in his hierarchy of human needs. Self-actualization occurs when an individual experiences heightened aesthetic, creative, problem-solving, philosophical, and moral understanding. It is a stage more likely to be reached by older rather than younger adults. Similarly, Erikson, Erikson, and Kivnick (1986) noted that older adults are social witnesses to life and possess greater wisdom about the interconnectedness or interdependence of one generation to the next.

Artists

Many older adults develop a greater appreciation for nature and aesthetics as they age. Some may take up a new activity, such as gardening, bird watching, travelling, painting, or playing the piano. A common misconception is that the elderly only engage in these activities because they have nothing better to do. In reality, while they may not have had time for such activities when younger, creative talents do not suddenly arise in late adulthood. Instead, the need to express those talents appears to increase. For those who have used their creative talents throughout their lives, late adulthood is a time of renewed inspiration.

In a study of extraordinarily creative people, Csiksentmihalyi (1996) found that few of the subjects reported feeling that their creative abilities, goals, or quality of work diminished with age. They did report an increased sense of urgency with regard to their work associated with the perception that time, energy, and strength were decreasing. Some examples of older adults who experienced great artistic success in later life include George Burns winning an Academy Award at the age of 80, George Bernard Shaw writing plays at 93, and Grandma Moses still painting at 100 years of age.

Philosophers

As individuals age, many experience a fundamental shift in how they view the world. Some may begin to look back on the time they have spent in lieu of looking forward to time left to spend. In looking back, they may attempt to put their lives in perspective by assessing both failures and successes within the context of their overall life. Butler (1963) named this process *life review* and described it as a final reorganization and integration of one's personality, as well as a final opportunity to come to terms with and resolve conflicts that occurred earlier in life to prepare for death.

Erikson (1959) described a similar process in the last of his eight stages of personality development; each stage is marked by a specific psychosocial crises. The final crisis is *integrity versus despair*, and the process involves reflecting back on one's life. Those older adults who find that their lives were well spent emerge with a sense of integrity and are prepared to accept death. If they find that their lives were not well spent, they may emerge with a sense of despair and are unprepared to accept death. Life review does not always cross the threshold of awareness. Not all older adults are actively and consciously attempting to engage in a life review or resolve this psychosocial crisis.

In some instances, life review takes on the simple form of reminiscence, nostalgia, or storytelling, which can be natural healing processes that promote mental health in the elderly (Butler, Lewis, & Sunderland, 1998). The importance of reminiscence provides a rationale for setting up programs called *reminiscence groups*; they are most often found in long-term-care (nursing home) settings. Such programs are designed to provide more formal structure for helping elders engage in life review.

The increased introspection and reflectivity experienced as people age may also lead to or intensify attempts to expand one's life perspective historically, socially, and culturally. Productivity for historians, philosophers, and other scholars frequently does not peak until these individuals reach their 60s or 70s. For example, Cervantes published *Don Quixote* at the age of 68, and Will and Ariel Durant published *The Lessons of History* and *Interpretations of Life* in their 80s. These works demonstrate how continuing cognitive development, and particularly life review, can lead to great cognitive accomplishments, not simply losses, as we age.

Sages

Increased wisdom is reportedly one of the positive consequences of grow-ing older. There are many definitions of wisdom; most refer to insight into the human condition or to knowledge about the best ways to live one's life (Baltes & Staudinger, 2000). Wisdom can be broken down into two types —philosophical wisdom and practical wisdom (Dittmann-Kohli & Baltes, 1990). *Philosophical wisdom* reflects an understanding of the abstract rela-tionship that exists between one's self and the rest of humankind. *Practi-cal wisdom* reflects expert knowledge, superior judgment, and exceptional insight with regard to the fundamental pragmatics of real life (Baltes & Staudinger, 1993). Collectively, wisdom requires the interplay of knowl-edge, understanding, and experience as well as the capacity to apply these qualities to problem solving.

Earlier sections of this chapter used different approaches to concep-tualizing cognition in aging individuals. The final example provided here is Baltes and Smith's (1990) work on age-related changes in wisdom. They proposed that the mind possesses two fundamental dimensions: the me-chanics of mind and the pragmatics of mind. The *mechanics of mind* in-volves the basic operations of information processing (mental hardware) already discussed; age-associated losses are most commonly seen in this dimension. The *pragmatics of mind* represents mental software that in-cludes factual and strategic knowledge acquired across the lifespan, as well as the ability to retrieve this information and apply it to solving real-life problems. Pragmatics of mind also reflects motivations and emotions. Wisdom is associated with the pragmatics dimension, and it is defined as the development of strategies to navigate the major and minor obstacles of everyday life.

Because culture and experience, rather than biology, affect the prag-matics of mind, aging may be associated with cognitive growth in wisdom, not a decline or stagnation (Harppe, Winner, & Brownell, 1998; Rybash, Roodin, & Hoyer, 1995). However, chronological age alone does not bring wisdom, and describing all older persons as wise would actually be a form of stereotyping, although admittedly a positive one. Other conditions con-tribute to the development of wisdom, including personality-related dis-positions (e.g., openness to new experiences or generativity) and life ex-periences (e.g., training, good guidance, or mentoring in dealing with life's challenges; Baltes & Staudinger, 1993, p. 77).

Overall, it appears that the mechanics of cognition in late adulthood may not be as efficient as cognition in younger adulthood, but mental processes in late adulthood can be more creative, adaptive, and appropriate to the final chapter of life. As older adults move forward, they may have the requisite experiences to take on new roles as artists, philosophers, and sages. Consequently, they also have a great deal to offer their respective communities. Engagement in new cognitive roles reflects the fact that cognitive development is multidirectional and that while some abilities may decrease, others emerge and grow well into old age.

Key Points

This chapter highlights two primary factors: (a) Cognitive aging is extremely complex, and (b) there is more to cognitive aging than loss of cognitive functioning. Key points about cognitive aging are as follows:

- Primary cognitive aging consists of both loss and growth in different cognitive skills.
- Older adults' intelligence does not begin to decline until the mid-70s, with more noticeable declines in the 80s.
- Semantic knowledge is relatively spared.
- The greatest changes are seen in how information is processed as adults grow older, particularly affecting working memory, episodic memory, sensory processing, and aspects of attention.
- Changes in brain structure and function contribute to cognitive aging.
- Possible underlying factors also contribute, such as limited resources or slowing or loss of inhibition.
- Cognitive performance in older adults is influenced by reduced resource capacity, slowing of processing, and loss of inhibition.
- Engagement in cognitively stimulating activities and strategy training can help maintain skills and reduce decline.
- Areas of cognitive growth across the lifespan can include application of acquired knowledge, creativity, and wisdom. Culture, not biology, determines wisdom.
- Old age, as with any other stage of life, is a time of great potential and vulnerability. Elderly individuals may end life either with a positive outlook, viewing their life as well spent, or with a negative outlook, feeling their life was wasted.

References

Atkinson, R. C., & Shiffrin, R. M. (1968). Human memory: A proposed system and its control processes. In K. W. Spence & J. T. Spence (Eds.). *The psychology of learning and motivation* (Vol. 2, pp. 89–195). New York: Academic Press.

Backman, L., Mantyla, T., & Herlitz, A. (1990). Psychological perspectives on successful aging: The optimization of episodic remembering in old age. In P. B. Baltes & M. M. Baltes (Eds.), *Successful aging* (pp. 118–163). New York: Cambridge University Press.

Baltes, P. B., & Smith, J. (1990). Towards a psychology of wisdom and its ontogenesis. In R. J. Sternberg (Ed.), *Wisdom: Its nature, origins, and development.* Cambridge, UK: Cambridge University Press.

Baltes, P. B., & Staudinger, U. M. (1993). The search for a psychology of wisdom. *Current Directions in Psychological Science, 2,* 75–80.

Baltes, P. B., & Staudinger, U. M. (2000). Wisdom: A metaheuristic (pragmatic) to orchestrate mind and virtue toward excellence. *American Psychologist, 55,* 122-136.

Burke, D. M., & Shafto, M. A. (2008). Language and aging. In F. I. M. Craik & T. A. Salthouse (Eds.), *The handbook of aging and cognition* (3rd ed., pp. 373–443). New York: Psychology Press.

Butler, R. N. (1963). The life review: An interpretation of reminiscence in the aged. *Psychiatry, 26,* 65–75.

Butler, R. N., Lewis, M., & Sunderland, T. (1998). *Aging and mental health: Positive psychological and biomedical approaches* (5th ed.). Austin, TX: PRO-ED.

Carstensen, L. L. (2007). Growing old or living long: Take your pick: Research to understand the psychological and emotional process of aging is essential to creating a society in which the elderly can thrive. *Science and Technology, 23,* 41–54.

Christensen, H., Anstey, K. J., Leach, L. S., & Mackinnon, A. J. (2008). Intelligence, education and occupation as indices of brain reserve. In F. I. M. Craik & T. A. Salthouse, (Eds.), *The handbook of aging and cognition* (3rd ed., pp. 133–189). New York: Psychology Press.

Csiksentmihalyi, M. (1996). *Creativity.* New York: Harper Collins.

Dennis, N. A., & Cabeza, R. (2008). Neuroimaging of healthy cognitive aging. In F. I. M. Craik & T. A. Salthouse (Eds.), *The handbook of aging and cognition* (3rd ed., pp. 1–54). New York: Psychology Press.

Dittmann-Kohli, F., & Baltes, P. B. (1990). Toward a neo-functionalist conception of adult intellectual development: Wisdom as a prototypical case of intellectual growth. In C. N. Alexander & E. J. Langer (Eds.), *Higher stages of human development* (pp. 54–78). New York: Oxford University Press.

Erikson, E. H. (1959). Identity and the life cycle: Selected papers. *Psychological Issues, 1,* 50–100.

Erikson, E. H., Erikson, J. M., & Kivnick, H. Q. (1986). *Vital involvement in old age.* New York: Norton.

Fozard, J. L. (1990). The significance of work friends in late life. [Special issue: Process, change and social support]. *Journal of Aging Studies, 4,* 123–129.

Hasher, L., & Zacks, R. T. (1998). Working memory, comprehension and aging: A review and a new view. *The Psychology of Learning and Motivation, 22,* 193–225.

Harppe, F. G. E., Winner, E., & Brownell, H. (1998). The getting of wisdom: Theory of mind in old age. *Developmental Psychology, 34,* 358–362.

Horn, J. L. (1978). Human abilities: A review of research and theory in the early 1970s. *Annual Review of Psychology, 27,* 437–486.

Horn, J. L, & Cattell, R. B. (1967). Age differences in fluid and crystallized intelligence. *Acta Psychologica, 26,* 107–129.

Jennings, J. M., & Jacoby, L. L. (2003). Improving memory in older adults: Training recollection. *Neuropsychological Rehabilitation, 13,* 417–440.

Johnson, M. K., Hashtroudi, S., & Lindsay, D. S. (1993). Source monitoring. *Psychological Bulletin, 114,* 3–28.

Johnson, M. K., Reeder, J. A., Raye, C. L., & Mitchell, K. J. (2002). Second thoughts versus second looks: An age-related deficit in selectively refreshing just-active information. *Psychological Science, 13,* 64–67.

Kok, A. (2000). Age-related changes in involuntary and voluntary attention as reflected in components of the event-related potential (ERP). *Biological Psychology, 54,* 107–143.

Labouvie-Vief, G. (1984). Logic and self-regulation from youth to maturity: A model. In M. L. Commons, F. A. Richards, & C. Armon (Eds.), *Beyond formal operations* (pp. 52–83). Cambridge, UK: Cambridge University Press.

Levy, B. R. (2003). Mind matters: Cognitive and physical effects of aging self-stereotypes. *The Journals of Gerontology, 58B,* P203–P211.

Lindenberger, U., & Baltes, P. B. (1994). Sensory functioning and intelligence in old age: A strong connection. *Psychology and Aging, 9,* 339–355.

Madden, D. J. (1986). Adult age differences in the attentional capacity demands of visual search. *Cognitive Development, 1,* 335–363.

Maslow, A. H. (1970). *Motivation and personality* (2nd ed.). Princeton, NJ: Van Nostrand.

McDowd, J. M., & Craik, F. I. M. (1988). Effects of aging and task difficulty on divided attention performance. *Journal of Experimental Psychology: Human Perception and Performance, 14,* 267–280.

Melone, L. (2008). Brain exercises that boost memory and may fight Alzheimer's. *Everyday Health.* Retrieved May 4, 2008, from http://www.everydayhealth.com/longevity/mental-fitness/brain-exercises-for-memory.aspx

Park, D. C., Polk, T. A., Mikels, J. A., Taylor, S. F., & Marshuetz, C. (2001). Cerebral aging: Brain and behavioral models of cognitive function. *Dialogues in Clinical Neuroscience, 3,* 151–165.

Piaget, J., & Inhelder, B. (1969). *The psychology of the child.* New York: Basic Books.

Rybash, J. M., Roodin, P. A., & Hoyer, W. J. (1995). *Adult development and aging* (3rd ed.). Dubuque, IA: Brown and Benchmark.

Salthouse, T. A. (2000). Steps towards the explanation of adult age differences in cognition. In T. Perfect & E. Maylor (Eds.), *Models of cognitive aging* (pp. 19–49). Oxford, UK: Oxford University Press.

Schacter, D. L., Savage, C. R., Apert, N. M., Rauch, S. L., & Albert, M. S. (1996). The role of the hippocampus and frontal cortex in age-related memory changes: A PET study. *Neuroreport, 7,* 1165–1169.

Schaie, K. W. (2005). *Developmental influences on adult intelligence: The Seattle Longitudinal Study* (2nd ed.). Oxford, UK: Oxford University Press.

Schaie, K. W. (1983). The Seattle Longitudinal Study. A twenty-one year investigation of psychometric intelligence. In K. W. Schaie (Ed.), *Longitudinal studies of adult psychological development.* New York: Guilford.

Schaie, K. W., & Willis, S. L. (2000). A stage theory model of adult cognitive development revisited. In B. Rubinstein, M. Moss, & M. Kleban (Eds.), *The many dimensions of aging: Essays in honor of M. Powell Lawton* (pp. 175–193). New York: Springer.

Thurstone, L. L. (1938). *Primary mental abilities.* Chicago: University of Chicago Press.

Tyas, S. L., Snowdon, D. A., Desrosiers, M. F., Riley, K. P., & Markesbery, W. R. (2007). Healthy ageing in the Nun Study: Definition and neuropathologic correlates. *Age and Ageing, 36*, 650–655.

Wickens, C. D., Braune, R., & Stokes, A. (1987). Age differences in the speed and capacity of information processing: A dual-task approach. *Psychology of Aging, 2*, 70–78.

Wingfield, A., Prentice, K., Koh, C. K., & Little, D. (2000). Neural change, cognitive reserve and behavioral compensation in rapid encoding and memory for spoken language in adult aging. In L. T. Connor & L. K. Obler (Eds.), *Neurobehavior of language and cognition: Studies of normal aging and brain damage honoring Martin L. Albert* (pp. 3–21). Boston, MA: Kluwer Academic.

CHAPTER 8

Cognitive Aging: Secondary Aging Factors—Cognitive Disorders of Communication in Older Adults

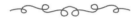

Gina L. Youmans and Scott R. Youmans

YOUMANS AND YOUMANS BUILD on Chapter 7's overview of primary cognitive aging, presenting common secondary cognitive disorders, which are typically described within speech–language pathology as *cognitive communication disorders*. The disorders discussed in this chapter include the dementias, right-hemisphere damage, and traumatic brain injury. In considering evaluation, the authors emphasize the need for person-centered functional assessments. Treatment sections of this chapter underscore differences and similarities in approaches to managing the cognitive communication problems associated with secondary aging. Finally, reimbursement challenges are described.

As discussed in the previous chapter, there are many positive age-related changes in cognition, including broader life experience, enhanced wisdom, greater cultural understanding, and creativity. However, most normally aging individuals also experience some decline in cognitive functions such as sensory processing, memory, and efficiency of information processing. These primary aging factors are usually subtle and do not generally affect the person's ability to engage in daily activities. Unfortunately, as individuals age they are also more likely to experience secondary disorders of cognition. Some develop a progressive brain disease known as *dementia*, which gradually degrades cognitive functioning. Others may suffer acute, sudden brain damage caused by a stroke or traumatic brain injury. Individuals with these types of secondary aging disorders often present with what are called *cognitive communication disorders*: communication problems that are secondary to disrupted memory, attention, executive functioning, and mental processing speed.

This chapter focuses on the dementias, given their prevalence in older populations. It also provides an overview of right-hemisphere brain damage and traumatic brain injury, for which older individuals are at an increased risk. Diagnostic principles and techniques are discussed, with emphasis on elderly-friendly and functional assessment. The chapter closes with a summary of treatment goals and approaches. Aphasia, which results from damage exclusively to language centers of the brain, is discussed in Chapter 10.

Dementia

Mild Cognitive Impairment

Normal, age-associated cognitive decline is often very difficult to distinguish from the initial stages of dementia; however, it is important to identify this subtle form of secondary cognitive aging as early as possible. Mild cognitive impairment (MCI) is a diagnostic category for those individuals whose cognitive difficulties appear more serious than expected in the course of normal aging but not serious enough for a diagnosis of dementia. It is a boundary category that does not differentiate between primary and secondary aging. Many individuals who are categorized as having MCI are experiencing normal, age-associated decline, or are normally aging individuals who have performed at lower levels on cognitive tests throughout their lifespan. However, some persons with MCI are in the early stage of dementia (Smith & Rush, 2006). Any medical professional involved in the care of elderly individuals should monitor those classified with MCI for cognitive or behavioral decline.

To be categorized as having MCI, individuals must present with normal general cognitive function, normal activities of daily living, and no diagnosis of dementia, while demonstrating abnormal difficulty in at least one cognitive domain: memory, attention, language, executive function, or visuospatial ability (Petersen et al., 2001). MCI may also be diagnosed if a person has impairment in two cognitive domains but continues to function well in daily life.

Definition of Dementia

Dementia is a general term for a group of chronic, degenerative brain dis-eases that progress gradually over time from mild to severe impairment. All dementias involve significant cognitive and memory impairments. How-ever, the type and degree of cognitive, behavioral, and motor impairment seen in aging individuals varies widely across dementia etiologies. Specific types of dementia are often difficult to diagnose definitively. Many types, such as Alzheimer's-type dementia and frontotemporal dementia, can only be formally diagnosed upon autopsy. The American Psychiatric Association (APA; 2000) has established strict diagnostic criteria for dementia in the *Diagnostic and Statistical Manual of Mental Disorders* (*DSM-IV-TR*). These criteria include an impairment of memory concurrent with impairment of at least one other cognitive area, such as language or executive functioning. These cognitive impairments must decline over time and must not be tran-sient. The criteria for dementia are more comprehensive and strict than are those for MCI. One notable difference is that dementia criteria require that an individual's social or professional functioning be significantly af-fected. In addition, medical professionals must systematically rule out all other possible causes of cognitive impairment, such as substance abuse, psychiatric illness, or brain injury, in order to differentially diagnose de-mentia in general and to establish physiological and cognitive evidence of a particular neurodegenerative disease that is the cause of the dementia.

Medical and Neurocognitive Assessment of Dementia

This process of differential diagnosis of dementia is complex and involves a team of medical experts. It is complicated by the fact that individuals ex-periencing mild memory or cognitive impairment often attempt to deny or compensate for their difficulties. Eventually, if the impairment persists or worsens, they or their family members seek help from a family physician, neurologist, mental health professional, and/or speech–language patholo-gist. Sometimes participation in a community memory screening may be the first step.

   If an initial assessment indicates the possibility of dementia, indi-viduals should be referred for a comprehensive medical and cognitive evaluation (see Bourgeois & Hickey, 2009, for additional information). The diagnostic team has two goals: first, to determine whether dementia is present; and second, to identify if possible which specific neurodegenera-tive disease process is causing the dementia.

During the medical examination, a physician confirms the gradual and progressive nature of the cognitive impairment, completes a neurological assessment, and collects individual and family medical history. The physician rules out other possible medical causes of cognitive impairment (e.g., liver and renal disease, diabetes, urinary tract infection) and affective disorders (e.g., depression, anxiety) that can masquerade as dementia. Risk factors for certain heritable types of dementia are also assessed. It is fairly routine for neuroimaging tests such as magnetic resonance imaging (MRI) or computed tomography (CT) to be performed, as well as blood tests and a review of current medications and their possible side effects or interactions.

The neurocognitive examination, which is usually performed by a cognitive or neuropsychologist, provides a comprehensive assessment of an individual's cognitive, behavioral, and social–emotional functioning. Performance across different cognitive domains, such as attention, memory, spatial planning, language, and executive functioning, is compared to age-appropriate norms. A thorough examiner considers cultural, educational, and age-related factors to distinguish between normal age-related cognitive decline and suspected MCI or dementia. The examiner also looks for specific patterns of impairment that can discriminate between dementia types.

This description of the components of assessment for persons with suspected dementia reflects what is considered to be appropriate and necessary. Unfortunately, many individuals with dementia-like behaviors do not receive a thorough evaluation. Typically, for considerably older individuals with limited family and financial support, it is likely that assessment will be limited to a basic evaluation by a family physician. Labels such as "memory loss" or "confusion" may be applied, and the individual may not be referred for additional testing.

Types of Dementia

Many different neurological diseases cause chronic, progressive dementia. The following sections provide a review of cognitive–behavioral profiles, clinical progression, incidence statistics, and diagnostic information for the most prevalent dementia types, particularly those that may include cognitive-communication impairments that require speech–language intervention.

Alzheimer's-Type Dementia

Incidence and Risk Factors. Alzheimer's dementia (AD) accounts for 50% to 60% of all dementia cases, and it affects approximately 40% to 60%

of adults over age 85 (National Institute of Aging, 2003). AD appears late in life, usually in individuals 65 years and over. The risks associated with developing AD are advanced age, low education, low socioeconomic status, living alone or being single, a family history of AD, and history of a head injury. Toxins such as aluminum, pesticides and lead, and alcohol have been implicated as AD risk factors, but current research is inconclusive (Munoz, Ganapathy, Eliasziw, & Hachinski, 2000; Richter, 2004).

Diagnosis and Brain Pathology. Based on a thorough medical and neurocognitive assessment, individuals may receive a diagnosis of possible or probable AD. Upon autopsy, if a pathologist identifies characteristic neuritic plaques of Beta A4 amyloid protein and neurofibrillary tangles in anterior and medial temporal lobes, a definitive diagnosis of AD is made.

Cognitive Impairment Profile. Memory impairment is the hallmark feature and the earliest symptom of AD. In early stages of AD, individuals may experience mild episodes of forgetfulness and word-finding difficulties due to memory impairment. Sensory memory (particularly visual memory) appears to be disrupted early on and becomes progressively worse. Visual perceptual difficulties may be the underlying cause of the visuospatial impairments typical of AD, and they may contribute to difficulty recognizing familiar items or people (visual agnosia) later in the illness. Short-term memory, or working memory, is particularly impaired in AD; as the disease progresses, individuals experience significant difficulty encoding daily events and new information.

In contrast, long-term memory is relatively spared until the later stages of the illness. For example, individuals with AD frequently retell familiar, personal stories from their childhood accurately but forget what they just had for breakfast and may not even recall having eaten. They also are likely to recognize old friends and family members but not attendants or clinicians they see daily but have only interacted with since suffering short term memory loss. This difficulty recalling recent events and encoding new information frequently causes disruptive behaviors such as repetitive questioning, agitation, and wandering. If a person does not recall asking a personally important question, such as when her son will arrive, she is likely to repeat the question over and over. When a person does not recognize his surroundings, he is likely to become nervous, anxious, and disoriented. He may wander off seeking familiar surroundings, or even become frightened and combative.

Language abilities are a relative strength for individuals with AD until the later stages of the illness. Expressive speech is generally fluent and syntactically correct, with no articulation difficulties. The ability to hold a fairly normal sounding conversation often masks memory difficulties, especially early in the illness. In addition, reading comprehension, writing, and pragmatic skills such as turn taking and topic appropriateness are relatively spared until AD approaches later stages (Bourgeois & Hickey, 2009).

However, word-finding impairment occurs early in AD and becomes progressively worse; this difficulty does increasingly affect speech output, subtly at first. Closer examination of conversation usually reveals relatively empty speech characterized by lack of specific content and information, frequent use of indefinite pronouns, and repetition of the conversational partner's remarks. In addition, individuals with AD have difficulty with comprehension of abstract language and complex conversation. It is likely that these apparent language difficulties are memory-related, rather than true language problems, and are attributed to deterioration of semantic information stored in long-term memory (Hodges & Patterson, 1995). In late-stage AD, language problems do finally become pervasive, and individuals may be echolalic, noncontingent, or even mute (Bourgeois & Hickey, 2009).

High-level executive function abilities are also relatively spared in AD compared to the significant memory impairment; however, minor difficulties often exist early in the illness. Problems with inhibiting inappropriate responses or behaviors, flexible problem solving, and organization may be present early in AD, and they may have a subtle effect on pragmatic appropriateness. Along with language and memory impairments, executive functions become significantly impaired in middle and late stages of the illness. Attention difficulties may also contribute to information processing, executive functioning, and memory problems, as well as apparent pragmatic difficulties in conversation.

In addition to these cognitive impairments, individuals who present with AD often exhibit problem behaviors that may contribute to their communication difficulties. Early in the illness, these individuals may become depressed, anxious, and easily agitated. As AD progresses, behaviors such as aimless wandering, hoarding, repetitive questioning and repetitive vocalizations often appear, as well as psychiatric disturbances such as delusions of persecution and hallucinations. These behaviors often increase late in the day, a condition known as *sundowners' syndrome*.

Frontotemporal Dementia

Incidence and Risk Factors. Frontotemporal dementia (FTD) is less common than AD, accounting for 8% to 20% of progressive dementias (Gustafson, Brun, & Passant, 1992). FTD occurs earlier in life than does AD, most typically in individuals in their 40s and 50s. However, symptoms occasionally begin as early as age 35 (Franczak, Kerwin, & Antuono, 2004). Researchers suggest that 25% to 40% of FTD cases are inherited, and that men are more at risk for developing FTD than are women (Bird et al., 2003).

Diagnosis and Brain Pathology. FTD is also diagnosed provisionally until autopsy, when the cognitive and behavioral profile can be confirmed. Atrophy is present in anterior frontal and temporal lobes, and pathological markers for other dementias, such as the neurofibrillary tangles and plaques of AD, must be absent. Pick's disease, a specific subtype of FTD, is diagnosed if a pathologist observes Pick bodies in the affected lobes (Dickson, 2001; Morris, 2003).

Cognitive Profile. FTD initially causes deterioration of the anterior frontal lobe, an area of the brain that supports executive functions such as appropriate inhibition of behaviors, mental flexibility, judgment, perspective-taking, reasoning, planning, and self-monitoring. The first complaints of individuals affected by FTD, and more commonly of their family members, relate to personality changes and inappropriate behavior. These may include compulsive lying, inappropriate humor, sexually explicit comments, lack of concern for others, apathy, and depression. The communication of individuals with FTD is pragmatically impaired early in the illness as individuals lose their ability to inhibit and monitor what they say; to appreciate nuances of conversation, such as sarcasm and humor; and to understand that the knowledge, beliefs, and emotions of their communication partner differ from their own. As FTD progresses, significant memory, attention, and language impairments also appear, and these further exacerbate communication difficulties. Memory impairments vary widely across individuals; sustained and selective attention deteriorates significantly. Language comprehension and naming tend to be preserved until late in the illness relative to spoken language, which often becomes repetitive or echolalic, and may progress to mutism (Franczak et al., 2004).

Dementia With Lewy Bodies

Incidence and Risk Factors. Dementia with Lewy bodies (DLB) is the second most frequent cause of chronic, progressive dementia; it is implicated in 20% to 30% of all dementia cases. Males who are 70 years and older are those most commonly diagnosed with DLB (Barber, Newby, & McKeith, 2004).

Diagnosis and Brain Pathology. DLB is provisionally diagnosed based on a characteristic pattern of cognitive, behavioral, and motor deterioration.

A pathologist definitively diagnoses DLB if characteristic Lewy bodies are present in the brain upon autopsy.

Cognitive Profile. Individuals with DLB initially have difficulty with attention, executive function such as reasoning and problem solving, and visuospatial abilities. Cognitive communication impairment in early DLB is caused primarily by these executive function deficits and is similar to individuals with FTD. Language and memory are relatively spared; however, difficulties do develop primarily in long-term episodic memory and word finding in conversation and verbal fluency tasks. Cognitive impairment and mental processing speed fluctuates markedly across time. In addition to this pattern of cognitive difficulties, individuals with DLB typically exhibit psychiatric disturbances such as mood changes, depression, and delusions, along with motor impairments such as tremor and gait disturbances (Galasko, Salmon, Lineweaver, Hansen, & Thal, 1998).

Dementia in Parkinson's Disease

Incidence and Risk Factors. Parkinson's disease (PD) is a degenerative motor disorder caused by decreased production of the neurotransmitter dopamine by the substantia nigra. Individuals with PD exhibit tremor, rigidity, poor initiation of movement, and a general paucity of movement. Speech–language clinicians frequently become involved to address speech intelligibility issues caused by the hypokinetic dysarthria found in this population. PD develops primarily in older, white males between the ages of 50 and 79 years. It is diagnosed in approximately 1.5% to 2.5% of the population, and only a subset of individuals with PD (18% to 30%) develops dementia (Cummings, 2003). A small number of PD cases are thought to be hereditary, and exposure to pesticides and herbicides may increase the risk of developing PD (Warner & Schapira, 2003).

Diagnosis and Brain Pathology. PD is clinically diagnosed based on motor, cognitive, and behavioral patterns of impairment. PD pathological markers include Lewy bodies, neurofibrillary tangles, and decreased substantia nigra pigmentation, all of which are also present in other neurodegenerative diseases. Thus, a definitive diagnosis may only be made when histological evidence from an autopsy is combined with a characteristic PD clinical profile (Cummings, 2003).

Cognitive Profile. When it occurs, PD-related dementia appears to be associated with cortical and subcortical degeneration of the frontal lobe areas, which connect to the substantia nigra. Cognitive difficulties reflect this frontal lobe involvement and include general slowing of cognitive processes, executive function deficits, and problems processing emotional information such as vocal inflection and facial expressions. Language and memory are relative strengths; however, short-term memory and pragmatic language difficulties may develop (Litvan et al., 1991). Individuals with PD may also exhibit behavioral changes, including hallucinations, agitation, and depression (Cummings, 2003).

Vascular Dementia

Incidence and Risk Factors. Vascular dementia (VaD), also known as multi-infarct dementia, is relatively common and causes approximately 20% of all cases of chronic dementia (O'Brien et al., 2003). VaD is caused by multiple small cerebrovascular accidents (CVAs), or strokes, that occur across time. The risk factors for VaD are the same as those for stroke and heart disease: hypertension, smoking, high cholesterol, diabetes, and a family history of heart disease or stroke.

Diagnosis and Brain Pathology. Although VaD causes chronic and gradually increasing cognitive impairment, it may begin with a marked, sudden onset, which differs from the gradual, insidious onset of other dementias. VaD usually progresses in a stepwise pattern with intermittent periods of slight recovery, rather than the gradual deterioration seen in most other chronic dementias. This pattern is caused by the individual suffering small areas of stroke-induced brain damage over time. VaD is differentially diagnosed when this pattern of onset and progression is noted. Further, many individuals with VaD show obvious signs of CVA, such as unilateral hemiparesis and unilateral facial weakness. In addition, CT and MRI images may reveal small brain lesions caused by repeated CVAs. Lesions that are very small may not be detected. Medications that regulate blood pressure and prevent blood clots can significantly reduce or even prevent progression of this dementia; therefore, it is important that VaD be correctly diagnosed.

Cognitive Profile. The cognitive profile of VaD varies widely across individuals because the locations of focal brain lesions are different in each case. However, individuals with several small cortical lesions often have the memory impairments, word finding difficulties, and disorientation that mimic AD symptoms. They may also have signs of depression, agitation, and anxiety that can appear similar to the characteristics of some individuals with AD. In fact, VaD is easily confused with AD until illness progression has been determined (Nagaratnam, Phan, Barnett, & Ibrahim, 2002).

Right-Hemisphere Disorder

Right-hemisphere disorder (RHD) is an acquired cognitive-communication disorder associated with damage to the nondominant hemisphere of the brain (typically the right). It can result from any insult to the cerebral cortex, such as head injury, inflammation, or brain tumor. Due to the high incidence of stroke in the older population, elderly individuals are particularly at risk for secondary aging impairments due to RHD. One in 100 individuals over the age of 70 will suffer a stroke or CVA, and 75% of individuals who have a stroke are 65 or older (National Stroke Association, 2002). RHD is frequently the result of these CVAs. Elderly individuals who are affected have slower recovery of cognitive functions and suffer a higher degree of permanent cognitive impairment than do younger individuals. In addition, elderly individuals are more likely than their younger counterparts to be experiencing pre-existing age-linked cognitive declines that may exacerbate the cognitive-communication impairments associated with RHD (Brookshire, 2007).

RHD can cause a broad range of changes in a person's cognition, behavior, perception, and communication, and it may be accompanied by speech impairments (dysarthria) and swallowing disorders (dysphagia). RHD characteristics present in each individual with different degrees of severity. The resulting behavior also reflects the individual's unique personality; background and experiences; degree of familial or community support; degree of normal cognitive aging; as well as divergent cognitive, behavioral, perceptual, and communication abilities.

Cognitive Impairment in RHD

Attention is typically impaired in RHD and is also an underlying factor contributing to other problems experienced by these individuals. One such problem is *anosognosia, a denial of (or inattention to) illness, which can cause considerable challenges in treatment*. Another common difficulty likely caused by impaired attention is a neglect of the left side of space. A client with left neglect may only eat from the right side of a plate or only read the right half of a book, ignoring the left, and may insist that the left half of the world does not exist. The issue underlying neglect is inattention, not visual blindness. Cognitive deficits are also common, including problems with memory and executive functions such as reasoning, problem solving, and judgment. In addition, cognitive inflexibility and difficulty integrating information are often seen (Brookshire, 2007; Davis,

2000; Haynes & Pindzola, 1998). These cognitive impairments frequently underlie the communication difficulties associated with RHD.

Behavioral Impairment in RHD

Behavioral symptoms can include a lack of initiation or a reduced level of motivation. As a result, people with RHD may appear less ambitious and energetic, with less personal drive than seen prior to RHD. They may also be impulsive and have a decreased ability to self-monitor. Some persons with RHD seem to react to others with apparent indifference and show reduced sensitivity to overt emotions, facial expressions, gestures, and other nonverbal cues. These deficits also appear to be byproducts of impairments to attention (Brookshire, 2007; Davis, 2000; Haynes & Pindzola, 1998).

Perceptual Impairment in RHD

Persons with RHD can have problems with auditory and especially visual perception. Auditory perceptual impairments may include difficulty with musical and sound recognition and pitch and loudness discrimination. Visual perceptual deficits may cause difficulties with recognition of objects, recognition of faces, recognition of geographic location, construction and visuospatial tasks, color perception, and depth perception (Davis, 2000; Murray & Clarke, 2006). Again, these perceptual problems are the result of underlying attentional deficits; however, a stroke can also damage visual pathways and cause visual field cuts, or blindness, in one or more visual quadrants. Since older persons may already be experiencing changes in visual and auditory perception due to primary aging, RHD impairments may be overlooked. The distinction between normal aging and RHD perceptual deficits must be considered in assessment.

Cognitive-Communication Impairment in RHD

Unlike aphasia, which results from damage to language centers in the brain, RHD causes individuals to experience problems with complex language comprehension and production because of cognitive impairments. Communication problems are also related to the behavioral and perceptual impairments previously described.

Persons with RHD have difficulty with the production and comprehension of prosody. Their speech is sometimes characterized as monotonous and robotic, lacking normal pitch and loudness variability. Thus the information normally conveyed via prosodic features is not available to listeners. These prosodic deficits can impair language comprehension (Brookshire, 2007), as can other cognitive impairments.

In terms of language production, persons with RHD typically have significant difficulty maintaining a conversation. They exhibit problems with organizing and integrating their speech, resulting in rambling, repetitive, and excessive discourse. They may answer questions impulsively, with inadequate thought, and may speak in unnecessary detail without providing much relevant information. They may focus on irrelevant or tangential details with no central theme or cohesion. In addition, speakers with RHD may show little perspective-taking ability or regard for their conversation partners. Poor eye contact, failure to take turns, and a paucity of nonverbal cues also exacerbate communication difficulties for these individuals (Brookshire, 2007; Davis, 2000).

Language comprehension difficulties mirror conversation impairments. Persons with RHD appear to be more literal and less able to understand subtleties of spoken and written language, such as figurative language, humor, and sarcasm (in part due to prosodic deficits). Some individuals with RHD also misjudge the appropriateness of facts and statements. Their judgments may be impulsive, and they have difficulty shifting their thinking once they have made a judgment. Finally, people with RHD may have difficulty inferring information, such as the themes or morals of stories (Brookshire, 2007; Davis, 2000).

The attentional, pragmatic, and integration-based difficulties that generally characterize RHD are often subtle and may seem minimal compared to the more obvious language impairments of the aphasias and the significant memory and behavioral difficulties of the dementias. However, RHD may significantly affect the quality of life of affected individuals. RHD often disrupts professional and social relationships. This can be extremely detrimental to elderly individuals, as an issue of quality of life and as a risk factor for developing additional illnesses such as dementia (Bourgeois & Hickey, 2009). In addition, mild RHD, like early stages of dementia, may be difficult to diagnose accurately and may be misattributed to normal cognitive aging.

Traumatic Brain Injury

Traumatic brain injury (TBI) simply means damage to the brain caused by a sudden, external event. TBI can be either an open injury, such as a bullet wound, or a closed-head injury, such as occurs in a car accident when a sudden impact damages the brain. In closed-head injury, the brain moving forcefully back and forth in a person's skull damages neuronal axons with a shearing, twisting force. This force causes diffuse injury throughout the brain and is responsible for many of the resulting cognitive and behavioral problems. In addition, the brain impacts the front and back of the skull, causing more focal damage. The anterior frontal lobe and temporal lobe poles are particularly vulnerable to focal damage, as is the occipital lobe at the back of the brain. Additional consequences of TBI include intracranial hemorrhaging, swelling, and hydrocephalus, all of which can create more brain damage. When these changes occur within the fixed space of the skull, pressure is placed on brain tissue. *Ischemia* (brain cell death due to oxygen loss) is common. All of these concomitant conditions contribute to the diffuse and complex nature of TBI outcomes (Brookshire, 2007). Thus, persons with TBI may have aphasia, RHD, dysarthria, dysphagia, cognitive impairments, or any combination of these disorders.

Individuals over age 60 have the second highest risk of suffering a closed-head TBI (following young adult males). In comparison to their younger counterparts, the elderly are at greater risk due to their high incidence of falls, increased chance of brain hemorrhage, and slower neurological recovery following falls (Brookshire, 2007; Murray & Clark, 2006). Elderly individuals who have suffered only mild closed-head TBI may still have significant long-term difficulty with word fluency, verbal memory, visual memory, and higher level language skills such as inferencing (Goldstein et al., 1994). They are more likely to have pre-existing problems, such as stroke, diabetes, or dementia, which may exacerbate the effects of brain injury. Further, for many older persons, long-term cognitive-communication impairment may be mild and difficult to differentiate from the effects of normal aging.

Since there is considerable overlap between cognitive-communicative disorders, only those characteristics unique to TBI are discussed. Recovery from a head injury depends on the nature and extent of the injury, as well as other personal and environmental factors, such as premorbid intelligence and cognitive abilities, familial support, and age. Some stages of recovery are common to TBI, although the starting point may differ from one client to the next. Not all clients progress through these stages in a linear fashion or at a similar rate. Overall survival rate following TBI is lower for the elderly, and rate of recovery across the common stages is slower and results in greater long-term difficulties. Many individuals do not recover to an independent level of functioning.

The earliest and most life-threatening stage in recovery from TBI is a coma or period of unconsciousness. If a client is comatose following a

TBI, the length of the coma is roughly correlated with the severity of the injury and the amount of recovery to be expected. Clients then recover into a semicomatose state in which they are awake but unresponsive, or move into a more responsive state of recovery. Clients with TBI often go through stages in which they are initially agitated, distractible, restless, and impulsive, and then they progress into stages in which their behavior is more appropriate. They become better oriented and more independent but may still exhibit residual problems (Murray & Clark, 2006). Again, clients do not necessarily follow a predictable sequence of stages in a predictable time frame, but many have similar persistent problems of cognition and communication.

Cognitive Impairment in TBI

Memory and attention are commonly impaired. Clients can experience significant amnesia in which they forget memories that occurred before or after their injury. Complete amnesia often resolves; however, memory problems are a typical and long-lasting by-product of a TBI. The inability to remember new information (anterograde amnesia) is a particular hindrance to therapy. Like RHD, attention impairments in TBI can cause additional deficits, such as anosognosia. Also similar to RHD, clients may exhibit poor reasoning, problem solving, and judgment (Davis, 2000). Recovery in the elderly is slower, and long-term deficits are more severe. Many of the cognitive problems associated with TBI are similar to those seen in dementia, creating challenges for assessment and diagnosis.

Behavioral Impairment in TBI

Behaviors are quite variable, depending on stage and severity of the TBI. Similar to persons with RHD, individuals with TBI may have poor or reduced initiation and motivation. Common symptoms also include impulsivity and disinhibition (may be sexually or socially inappropriate). Individuals may be aggressive, restless, agitated, or distractible, and they may exhibit reduced sensitivity to others. During the intermediate stages of recovery, persons recovering from a TBI may appear confused and disoriented. Indeed, behavioral impairments associated with TBI are sometimes significant obstacles to therapy.

Perceptual Impairment in TBI

The perceptual problems common to persons with RHD are also typical problems seen in persons with TBI. In addition to reduced visual sensitivity due to normal aging, focal damage to the occipital lobe may cause blindness, field cuts, or an inability to recognize or interpret visual stimuli in the brain regardless of visual acuity.

Cognitive-Communication Impairment in TBI

Unless the person with a TBI also has dysarthria, aphasia, or another related disorder, he or she is most likely to exhibit communication problems that are directly related to the cognitive impairments. Some of these common cognitive-communication impairments are similar to those observed in individuals with RHD, although persons with TBI often have more severe memory impairments. Similarities with RHD are seen in impairments of understanding and using prosody as well as in pragmatic skills such as eye contact, turn taking, and topic maintenance. Excessive, disorganized, tangential, irrelevant language output is frequently observed. In some stages of TBI, it is common to see *confabulation, which is the fabrication* and embellishment of information often associated with gaps in memory. Impulsivity may inhibit thoughtful responses in conversation.

In the absence of aphasia or other pre or postmorbid impairments, the language comprehension of persons with TBI can resemble that seen with RHD, although the memory challenges in TBI create more severe language comprehension deficits. Clients are more concrete and less subtle than their former selves, with difficulty comprehending complex and abstract oral and written language. Their judgments regarding the correctness of information, their tendency to jump to conclusions, and their inability to infer information contribute to impairments in comprehension of complex information.

Evaluation of
Cognitive-Communication Disorders

Individuals in early to middle-stage dementia and those with mild to moderate TBI or RHD impairments often sound relatively normal. Their clearly articulated, fluent output may mask subtle underlying memory, attention, and executive functioning difficulties that affect daily communication. Many healthy adults of all ages have short attentions spans, are relatively concrete, and are somewhat vague in conversations. When these types of behaviors occur in older adults, they are usually just assumed to be the result of normal aging. Thus, diagnosing mild cognitive-communication impairments can be difficult.

Cognitive-Communication Assessment in the Elderly Population

Assessment of elderly individuals with cognitive-communication impairment is similar to that of younger populations in many ways. As with any communication assessment, a clinician should obtain a cognitive-linguistic impairment profile, a functional communication profile, baseline data, and a determination of a client's stimulability for treatment. For clients with dementia, clinicians should identify specific problem behaviors that are affecting communication and daily functioning, troubleshoot repair strategies, and probe stimulability for specific treatment approaches. Bourgeois and Hickey (2009) provided excellent, specific advice about tailoring an assessment so that the stage is set for reimbursable cognitive intervention planning for individuals with dementia.

Person-Centered Evaluation

Older individuals who experience a loss of function after a full, active life may be particularly distressed by assessments designed to uncover their weaknesses. They may also be less likely to advocate for themselves than are younger individuals, and they may already feel devalued by our youth-oriented society. Older individuals may have more test anxiety than their younger counterparts, who often have more school-based experience with standardized testing.

One way to alleviate some of these fears and frustrations is to use a person-centered style of assessment. Clinicians should clearly communicate that they are interested in the person in front of them, not just his or her impairments. This reassurance can be accomplished simply by admiring the client's profession, hobbies, or accomplishments. When a client has discussed his career as a musician and has shared his love and knowledge of gardening, he may have more confidence in the clinician's ability to treat him as a unique, experienced individual rather than just a communication impairment. The elderly client may be less distressed when cognitive difficulties are uncovered, and may also trust the clinician enough to see past defenses he may have constructed to compensate for his cognitive difficulties. Such a person-centered focus on wisdom and life experience may also capitalize on the strength of crystallized intelligence, which is thought to increase with advanced age (see Chapter 7).

A person-centered approach also involves talking directly to the client about the reasons for each activity and test. An ongoing conversation about difficulties and strengths during testing, and asking the clients' opinion of their own performance, allow individuals to participate in their assessment rather than experiencing it as something being done to them. In addition, information is gained about the client's insight, or lack thereof, into his or her difficulties.

A person-centered assessment focuses on the client's well-being throughout testing. When tasks are difficult or frustrating, the clinician should try to support the client so that she becomes successful. Also, it is important to keep in mind that very rarely must a certain test be completed or a certain test score obtained. Finishing a test or activity should never be more important to clinicians than the person sitting in front of them.

Accommodations

As mentioned in the chapter on cognitive aging, even normally aging elderly individuals can experience decreased attention, memory, and sensory and information processing abilities. Clinicians must compensate for these normal changes to identify actual impairments accurately. Elderly individuals tend to focus their more limited attention on topics and activities that they find personally engaging or important. Including clients in the diagnostic process, relating diagnostic activities to important daily activities or skills, and encouraging conversation on topics of interest should help maintain the clients' focus and interest in the assessment. Normal cognitive aging may also degrade selective attention, so the room in which testing takes place should be well lit, quiet, and as free of distractions as possible. Test instructions should be clear and brief but not condescending, and clinicians should confirm understanding of instructions.

Visual changes also occur with normal aging. In addition, clinicians must keep in mind that yellowing of the lens of the eye in normal aging may cause difficulties with color identification that have nothing to do with a cognitive impairment. Clinicians should be aware of the client's visual and auditory status, as well as the presence or absence of visual neglect. If clients have glasses or use hearing aids, they should wear these during testing. Enlarging print and pictures can promote testing accuracy. Sometimes outside referrals to audiologists, ophthalmologists, or neuropsychologists are necessary to obtain this information about visual functioning if it is not available. To ensure a valid diagnosis, clinicians should make certain the specialist to whom they refer their client has experience with persons with acquired neurogenic disorders.

Clinicians must also consider testing fatigue in cognitive evaluation of older individuals. Cognitive impairment can be significantly exacerbated when clients are tired, and older individuals often fatigue more quickly during cognitively demanding activities. Simply asking a client how he or she is feeling is always a good idea and may reveal testing variables such as fatigue and illness. The time of day when an evaluation occurs may also affect test performance, particularly for individuals with dementia, who may experience an exacerbation of cognitive-behavioral impairment late in the day.

Assessment Materials

Evaluation materials should be age appropriate. Even if a test or activity suits the client's abilities, if it is geared toward children, it is not appropriate for older adults. Treating this population with proper respect is vital to accurately assessing their abilities and forming a productive therapeutic relationship. Materials that are personally relevant or of interest to the client should be used when possible. Many aging clients with cognitive-communication impairment have difficulty encoding new information, so it is very important for clinicians to wear nametags that are clearly visible and in large print. Nametags clearly printed with the clinician's first name may be most appropriate for individuals with dementia.

Standardized Evaluation of Cognitive-Communication Disorders

A thorough assessment of cognitive-communication impairment should evaluate memory, attention, executive function, orientation, language, and conversational-pragmatic abilities, in addition to probes of problem behaviors and treatment options. Formal standardized evaluations of cognition and communication can aid in the diagnosis and treatment planning of cognitive-communication impairments. Screening measures can quickly assess general cognitive and linguistic abilities, indicate the need for further testing, and guide assessment planning. Comprehensive assessment batteries test across many cognitive and linguistic domains affected by TBI, RHD, and dementia. Standardized activity-based assessments are also available to determine cognitive-communication strengths in functional contexts. Finally, standardized domain-specific measures can probe more deeply impairment in a single cognitive or linguistic behavior, such as word-finding or memory.

While standardized evaluations have their place in the diagnostic process, they are not always normed appropriately for the client being evaluated. Many instruments do not include norms for individuals ages 80 and above, and some do not even have norms for individuals in their 70s. Because aspects of cognition often decline with advanced age, elderly individuals may be incorrectly diagnosed with a pathology when their test performance is compared to norms from a younger age group. In addition, most standardized tests are not broadly normed across cultures and socioeconomic classes and do not properly assess bilingual speakers and non-native English speakers. Standardized comprehensive batteries are quite long, and clients with neurological disorders may have difficulty tolerating extensive testing. Appendix 8A provides examples of potentially age-appropriate standardized screening tests, comprehensive assessment batteries, functional activity instruments, and domain-specific tests.

Nonstandardized, Dynamic Assessment of Cognitive-Communication Disorders

Standardized assessment is useful because it compares one client's performance to a larger population, and because standardized re-testing allows formal tracking of a client's abilities across time. In contrast, nonstandardized, dynamic assessments can be more flexible, client-tailored, and functional; they provide additional valuable information to guide functional treatment planning. However, dynamic assessment lacks normative comparison, allows more room for clinician bias, and does not readily allow replication to track changes in performance across time.

Dynamic assessment may involve nonstandardized diagnostic activities or the flexible use of standardized instruments. A dynamic assessment approach allows clinicians to probe underlying reasons for cognitive-communication difficulties, and actively identify strategies that improve a client's performance. Because dynamic assessment is tailored to each individual, the clinician can collaborate with a client and relevant others to identify problem behaviors such as repetitive questioning or angry outbursts, and probe strategies to help repair these difficulties.

Nonstandardized assessment usually includes conversation during which a clinician can identify communication strategies and behaviors that are helpful or detrimental, and evaluate the effect of different types and levels of partner support. Asking for advice in a client's area of expertise has been found particularly useful in engaging individuals with mild to moderate dementia and increasing the informativeness of their conversation (Dijkstra, Bourgeois, Youmans, & Hancock, 2004). Videotaping a conversation is recommended when possible to provide baseline data for use in treatment and to make observations of behaviors, such as turn-taking, eye contact, and communicative gestures, easier and less subjective.

Treatment of Cognitive-Communication Disorders

Many of the problems that persons with dementia experience are a result of their underlying memory impairment. Attention and executive functions also cause communication difficulties in this population. These same cognitive domains contribute to cognitive-communication impairments associated with TBI and RHD. Thus, there is some overlap in treatments used with all three of these disorders, despite differences in primary neurological diagnoses (Tompkins, 1995). Unlike RHD and TBI, dementia is characterized by decline in functioning. Thus, dementia treatment should focus on maintaining social engagement, interpersonal communication, and independent functioning in a preferred environment for as long as possible in a manner that is functionally tailored to each individual (Bourgeois & Hickey, 2009).

Memory Interventions

Environmental Modification

Memory impairment can be compensated for by organizing the client's life into predictable routines that take place in well-organized and familiar surroundings, and, in particular, by modifying the environment with salient memory cues. For example, labels can be used to identify the content of drawers and cupboards. It is important to remember that even individuals with significantly advanced dementia are still able to benefit from written text, and single-word labels can be particularly beneficial. Keys and other necessary items should be kept in the same place consistently. Lists, calendars, clocks, pill boxes, and schedules that are neatly organized and in obvious and visible places can also compensate for memory difficulty. Salient cues, such as brightly colored flowers or favorite photographs, can be purposefully associated with specific locations, such as a client's new room in assisted living or the bathroom at home. If the memory impairment is caused by a progressive dementia, environmental memory cues should be put in place as early as possible, so that these cues are familiar as memory deteriorates.

Memory Books

Memory books and wallets can provide excellent memory support for clients, and, in doing so, can enhance the communication and socialization of individuals with significant memory loss. Memory books are tailored to individuals, so the size and complexity of pictures and text, the size of the book itself, and the involvement of the client in the creation of the book is different for each individual. Memory books and wallets have been particularly effective for individuals with dementia. For this population, memory books usually focus on relevant life-history events, such as weddings, vacations, photos of past homes, pets current and past, and family members. This content capitalizes on preserved long-term memories for this population, and simple text accompanying these pictures capitalizes on relatively preserved reading ability.

Documented benefits of memory book use for individuals with dementia include increases in specific conversational information and initiation of conversational interactions, decreases in empty speech and repetitions, and expanded amount and quality of social interactions (Bourgeois, Dijkstra, Burgio, & Allen-Burge, 2001). Individuals with dementia who previously appeared uninterested in conversation may use their memory books to actively engage staff and other residents in conversation. Frequently they point to pictures, read aloud the simple caption, and then augment this interaction with further comments on the photo. As pointed out throughout this text, social isolation is detrimental to cognitive functioning. Social engagement is extremely important for elderly individuals, particularly those with cognitive impairment. Simply creating a memory book for a client is often insufficient. Books tend to be lost or remain unused unless the staff, family members, and the client (possibly through spaced retrieval) are made aware of the book and practice using it to support conversation.

Individuals with RHD and TBI can also benefit from having well-organized, personally relevant information at their fingertips and often become actively involved in the creation of memory books and wallets. For these persons, a memory book may serve more as an organizational strategy. It is important to note that, particularly in these populations, some individuals are averse to the idea of using physical memory aids. For that reason, the development of such external memory aids should be discussed with each client.

Spaced Retrieval

In the last decade, compelling research on the memory technique of spaced retrieval has established that individuals with dementia are able to learn new information (Bourgeois et al., 2003). Spaced retrieval has been used to teach individuals to recall and use new functional strategies (Bourgeois & Hickey, 2009). It has also been successfully used with individuals who have significant memory impairment secondary to TBI (Bourgeois & Melton, 2005). *Spaced retrieval* is a formal memory-training procedure in which the clinician elicits a specific target response from the client by systematically manipulating the time interval preceding recall. Intervals are increased or decreased as a consequence of the correctness of a client's response, and training occurs in an errorless learning fashion. Once successfully trained, the strategy is deployed automatically in response to the trained stimulus cue, so strategy use does not require conscious application.

This technique can be very powerful when used to put a functional strategy in place to decrease a problem behavior or increase the independence and quality of life of someone with significant memory loss. Strategies can include learning to stop and take a deep breath when angry, re-learning a grandchild's name, or recognizing a room number. For example, an individual with dementia who is disrupting staff with repetitive questioning can be trained to refer to a cue card on which the answer to the question has been written. In this case, the clinician would repeatedly ask the same question, such as, "What do you do when you need to know when your wife is coming to pick you up?" and would require the client to answer, "I look at my card," and then actually follow through and read the card aloud. Many clients with dementia have learned to independently pick up a card and read it every few minutes, each time becoming settled after reading the answer to an important question. As a result, staff members become much less frustrated and residents appear less anxious.

Internal Memory Strategies

Clients who can self-monitor their memory difficulties and consciously apply repair strategies or information encoding strategies may benefit from one or several well-known memory techniques. Encoding strategies such as repeating information over and over (rehearsal) or mentally linking an item of information to a salient cue (association) may be helpful and can be overtly trained in therapy. Some clients benefit from closing their eyes and mentally visualizing the action they need to recall in a future situation. Clients may also close their eyes and visualize a past event to help recall information, and some clients benefit greatly from visualizing the first letter or the overall shape of a word. Mnemonics such as rhymes and acronyms are also commonly used memory techniques that can be overtly taught in therapy. Because these techniques are familiar to most of us, it is easy to overlook them as too simple or obvious. However many clients benefit from overt training and practice in using these techniques functionally. It should be noted that individuals with even mild dementia may not have the ability to apply such internal strategies, and external environmental cues may be more appropriate (Bourgeois & Hickey, 2009).

Attention and Engagement

Environmental Modification

Individuals with dementia are often easily distracted and overwhelmed by their environment. This difficulty attending to the environment often leads to limited social engagement. Environments should be simplified and de-cluttered, and this need for simplicity must be kept in mind when adding environmental cues and supports. A speech–language pathologist can work with home caregivers or residential staff to optimize environmental light-ing, particularly in nursing homes. Lighting is often found to be inadequate (Bourgeois & Hickey, 2009); however, an overly illuminated environment can also overwhelm limited attentional and perceptional resources. Like individuals with RHD and TBI, those with dementia are better able to con-centrate when auditory distractions are removed. Simply moving a client to a quiet, calm location can increase social and communicative involvement. In addition to removing distracting elements, speech–language patholo-gists can work with staff and caregivers to create opportunities for active engagement. Individuals with dementia can be oriented around a table or sitting area, facing each other, rather than side by side, as often occurs in residential settings. Personally relevant objects and pictures can be added to a central table to aid attentional focus and engagement. In addition, individuals with dementia who are agitated or easily distracted can benefit from simple, functional activities that focus their attention, such as sorting coins or folding towels. Ideally, activities are purposeful and mirror past interests or occupations (Bourgeois & Hickey, 2009).

Direct Attention Treatment

For individuals with RHD and TBI, direct intervention to improve attention is often appropriate. It can be particularly important to address attention issues in elderly individuals who suffer stroke or brain injury because their attention, perception, and sensory memory may already be compromised through normal aging. Preexisting changes in these cognitive domains may exacerbate problems attending to the environment. Many different exer-cises can be used for each of the types of attention: focused, selective, alter-nating, and divided. Sohlberg and Mateer (2001) suggested activities that address multiple types of attention. Focused attention can be improved by asking the client to attend to a narrative and indicate when a specific word is mentioned. Paragraph comprehension can also address focused atten-tion and is often easy to tailor to the interests of the individual. Selective attention can be treated by asking a client to participate in an activity while distractions (competing stimuli) are presented. To treat alternating atten-tion, the clinician can ask a client to switch back and forth between two activities. As with individuals with dementia, visual aids such as written task reminders or instructions can help reorient the client, maintain focus on key topics during conversations, and keep conversational strategies in mind. Modifying the environment to reduce the number of distractions can help reduce distractibility. As previously discussed, it is particularly important to focus on topics and activities of personal relevance for elderly individuals and to clearly explain the reasons for more abstract, less obviously functional exercises.

Executive Functions

Inferencing and Abstract Thinking

Difficulties with inferencing, including the ability to understand figurative language, incongruencies, humor, and implied meanings, can be caused by an underlying executive functioning impairment, particularly in perspective taking. Such difficulties are typical of individuals with frontotemporal dementia, Pick's disease, RHD, TBI, and mild to moderate AD. Brookshire (2007) lists several treatment possibilities for treating inferencing problems. For humor, a joke can be told and the client can attempt to describe why it is funny or can be asked to provide the punch line from a closed set of choices. Metaphors and idioms can also be explained by the client, or their meanings selected from a closed set. For individuals with mild to moderate dementia, as well as RHD and TBI, difficulties in perspective taking may impair conversational abilities. Specifically informing clients about a communication partner's beliefs, emotions, intentions, and prior knowledge may support conversation for these individuals.

Reasoning, Judgment, and Problem Solving

To address problem-solving and reasoning abilities, the clinician can create hypothetical situations and ask the client what to do. Additionally, the client may be asked to list and sequence steps involved in complex tasks of personal interest. It is sometimes beneficial to teach structured problem-solving approaches to avoid impulsive answers. For example, the client can engage in role-playing activities with others to simulate real-life situations for which impulse control is required. Planning activities and engaging in time-management tasks can be used to target reasoning and judgment difficulties (Brookshire, 2007; Sohlberg & Mateer, 2001). Some of the problem-solving activities involve generating acceptable responses to actual situations in which the clients will be involved.

Individuals who have problems with impulsivity might find themselves frequently acting out inappropriately without thought to the consequences of their behavior. Solutions can be generated for ongoing or frequent situations, and strategies can be formed to deal with unique situations in which the client does not know how to handle himself or herself.

Clients can learn to "self-talk" through difficult situations by rehearsing a memorized checklist of problem-solving strategies that can be used when a problem arises (Sohlberg & Mateer, 2001). For example, if a client with TBI frequently becomes agitated and aggressive when under strain, a solution might be to help that client identify the onset of anxiety and to remove himself or herself from the situation, take a deep breath, or use other stress-reducing strategies.

Additional Treatment Concerns for Individuals With Cognitive-Communication Impairment

Anosognosia

A common problem—and a particular barrier to the treatment of clients with cognitive-communication disorders—is *anosognosia*, a denial or minimizing of disorders. For clients who deny they have problems or who lack insight into their limitations, it is sometimes necessary to "prove" to them that they have something they need to work on. This should be done in a gentle, nonconfrontational manner, but it is necessary that the client accept that there is a disorder prior to any real commitment to therapy. Videotaping sessions and analyzing them with the client tends to meet this goal effectively.

For clients who do not have a realistic view of their impairments or who have difficulty with abstract thinking, direct memory and attention exercises may be too abstract initially. To help clients "buy into" therapy, clinicians may first have them identify something that they feel is a problem for them. For example, a client might deny most of her impairments but acknowledge difficulty following conversations with her spouse. The clinician could then focus on language comprehension, particularly in a conversational context, and thus demonstrate the benefits of therapy. Once a trusting relationship has been established, the client may be more motivated to try therapy activities that are less obviously relevant to her.

Pragmatic Impairment

Pragmatic difficulties and ineffective conversational strategies are best remediated by videotaping and analyzing conversation. This approach allows for a natural conversation to take place at the time without continually halting and dissecting it. The clinician can provide concrete examples of the client's successes and areas that need improvement that might otherwise be missed. The ability to rewind and view an exchange several times allows for a more comprehensive analysis of the conversation. At times, it is best to begin by analyzing videotapes of others who are having similar problems. Some of the more spirited talk shows tend to provide ample examples of problematic pragmatics.

Visual Perceptual Impairment

The client's visual perceptual difficulties can be addressed by copying simple or complex figures either outright or from memory. The client can also be engaged in visual scanning activities to address visual processing and neglect. In addition to treating the underlying impaired attention, the client needs to be made aware of his neglect and taught strategies to compensate for it. For example, clients can be encouraged to attend to both sides of their visual space systematically, or to run their finger or an index card along a line of text until they locate the left margin of a passage. For a more salient cue, the left side of a text can be marked with a red line and the client can be trained to begin reading only after locating the red mark.

Caregiver Involvement

Caregivers often want to help their loved one, and they may be able to encourage the client to follow through with homework and strategies outside of therapy. Caregivers may also help identify goals that uniquely appeal to the client, and they may learn strategies to aid them as a communication partner for their loved one. The involvement of significant others in the therapy process can be a powerful force for client well-being and recovery. However, there are times when the involvement of caregivers is not beneficial. Some clients may strongly prefer to leave their friends and family out of therapy, and their privacy should be respected. In addition, involving a spouse or child in therapy can undermine a client's traditional role in a family. This addition may exacerbate a preexisting sense of loss of independence and identity already in place because of other age-related changes.

A clinician must also be aware that caring for persons with cognitive-communication disorders is stressful for family members and significant others. It is particularly so for those who care for individuals with dementia, due to the progressively worsening nature of the disease and the personality and behavioral changes that accompany it. Rather than becoming involved in therapy, caregivers may need respite from caregiving and support for themselves. A knowledgeable clinician recognizes these needs and refers caregivers to available community resources such as senior center dementia programs, adult daycare, and caregiver support groups.

Group Therapy

Group therapy can be extremely beneficial to individuals with cognitive-communication disorders, particularly for older clients with limited social interactions. Groups enhance communication by providing opportunities to practice strategies in a judgment-free environment. There are social and emotional benefits as well. Whether an elderly person is coping with the abrupt loss of ability and independence due to stroke or dealing with progressive decline, depression and social withdrawal are common. Group therapy involving others who are in similar situations can add comfort, socialization, informational resources, and several sympathetic ears. Groups may combine individuals with various diagnoses such as RHD and dementia or may be specific to a single diagnosis.

The benefits of communication and problem-solving groups for individuals with TBI and RHD are widely recognized; however, clinicians may be less aware of group therapy options for individuals with dementia. One such group activity, question-asking reading (QAR), promotes social participation, reading comprehension, and communication through text and cue-card-supported discussion of current events (Stevens, King, & Camp, 1993). Poetry groups, in which a group leader records theme-based comments and feelings from individuals with dementia and then reads the group output aloud as poetry, have enhanced clients' sense of self-esteem and their communication with staff and family members (Hagens, Beaman, & Ryan, 2003). Another group approach is the Breakfast Club (Boczko, 1994), which uses sensory stimulation and a structured routine to return positive social interactions and increased interpersonal communication to institutional mealtimes. Individuals with dementia may also benefit from many of the problem-solving and communication activities common to TBI and RHD groups, including musical bingo, scrabble, timeline discussions, categorical naming, and sharing of personal photos; however, they often need more individualized support to participate.

Reimbursement

Medicare only reimburses speech–language pathologists for *skilled* services. Clinicians must ensure that their specific skilled training is necessary for all evaluation and treatment activities—that their services could not have been provided by someone without speech–language training. Reimbursement for cognitive-communication therapy requires documentation that a client's *communication* (not just memory or attention) is problematic and in need of intervention. This means that clinicians must document exactly how underlying cognitive impairments are directly affecting their client's functional communication.

In the past, cognitive-communication therapy was often not reimbursed for individuals with dementia. However, the Federal Nursing Home Reform Act of 1987 now mandates that communication therapy be provided for those individuals with dementia who require it, and Medicare does reimburse. Clinicians must carefully document the need for skilled communication intervention and take baseline data on specific, measurable behaviors and strategies that will be targeted in therapy. Treatment should directly enhance functional communication and participation or train strategies that facilitate communication. The client's progress in treatment should be clearly documented. Clinicians should not target improvement or restoration of cognitive functioning for individuals with progressive diseases, but maintenance of skills and facilitation of optimal strategies are appropriate goals.

Medicare Part A covers in-patient medical care in acute and rehabilitation hospital settings, home health settings, and skilled nursing facilities. Reimbursement is based on a prospective payment system in which the amount of funding depends on the rehabilitation team's initial prognosis, treatment goals, and estimated time needed for a client to meet his or her treatment goals. Medicare Part B covers out-patient care in hospitals, clinics, and long-term care facilities. Reimbursement funds are currently limited to $1,780 per client for physical therapy and speech–language services combined. However, clinicians may exceed this limit if they can demonstrate that a client's needs are complex or medically necessary and justifiable. Bourgeois and Hickey (2009) discuss these reimbursement issues further and give practical advice for navigating the Medicare system.

International Classification of Diseases–Clinical Modification, 9th revision (ICD-9-CM), codes describe a client's diseases, injuries, symptoms, and conditions (National Center for Health Statistics [NCHS], 2009). The ICD-9-CM codes for hereditary and degenerative diseases of the central nervous system or cerebrovascular disease usually describe the general medical diagnosis of clients with cognitive communication impairment. The appropriate ICD-9-CM codes must be included on all paperwork: evaluations, treatment plans, daily notes, and so on. Medical care providers should note that the expanded and updated 10th revision of these codes (NCHS, 2010) will come into mandated use in the United States, with a currently planned implementation date of October 13, 2013.

Key Points

Cognitive disorders common in the elderly were described. Assessment and intervention strategies appropriate for individuals with these disorders were discussed. Key elements included the following points.

- Older individuals have an increased risk of experiencing cognitive-communication disorders associated with dementia, RHD, and TBI.
- Mild forms of these disorders may be difficult to differentiate from normal aging changes in cognition.
- Cognitive-communication assessments of older individuals must accommodate primary age-related changes in cognition, sensory systems, and health.
- A person-centered approach, which clearly values the strengths associated with life experience, is highly recommended for assessment and treatment of older individuals.
- Environmental modifications and memory books are excellent functional treatment options for older individuals experiencing memory difficulties.
- Use of appropriate strategies can help older individuals with reasoning, judgment, and pragmatic and behavioral difficulties, and spaced retrieval can help train useful strategies for individuals who have significant memory difficulty.
- Direct treatment of cognitive impairments in memory, attention, and executive functioning should be made as functionally relevant as possible for older individuals.
- Caregiver involvement in therapy can be very beneficial; however, family members or significant others may be overburdened or unable to take on a teacher role.
- Reimbursable services are skilled, communication-oriented, and clearly documented. Treatment for progressive illnesses must focus on functional communication and strategy training rather than restoration of cognitive functioning.

References

American Psychiatric Association. (2000). *Diagnostic and statistical manual of mental disorders* (4th ed., text rev.). Washington, DC: Author.

Baines, K. A., Martin, A. W., & Heeringa, H. M. (1999). *Assessment of language-related functional activities.* Austin, TX: PRO-ED.

Barber, R., Newby, J., & McKeith, I. (2004). Lewy body disease. In R. Richter & B. Richter (Eds.), *Alzheimer's disease: A physician's guide to practical management* (pp. 127–135). Totowa, NJ: Humana Press.

Bayles, K. A., & Tomoeda, C. K. (1994). *Functional linguistic communication inventory.* Tucson, AZ: Canyonlands Publishing.

Bernstein, J. H., & Waber, D. (1994). *Rey-Osterrieth complex figure.* Lutz, FL: Psychological Assessment Resources.

Bird, T., Knopman, D., VanSwieten, J., Rosso, S., Feldman, H., & Tanabe, H. (2003). Epidemiology and genetics of frontotemporal dementia/Pick's disease. *Annals of Neurology, 54,* S29–S31.

Boczko, F. (1994). The breakfast club: A multi-modal language stimulation program for nursing home residents with Alzheimer's disease. *The American Journal of Alzheimer's Care and Related Disorders and Research, 9,* 35–38.

Bourgeois, M., Camp, C., Rose, M., White, B., Malone, M., Carr, J., et al. (2003). A comparison of training strategies to enhance use of external aids by persons with dementia. *Journal of Communication Disorders, 36,* 361–378.

Bourgeois, M., Dijkstra, K., Burgio, L., & Allen-Burge, R. (2001). Memory aids as an AAC strategy for nursing home residents with dementia. *Augmentative and Alternative Communication, 17,* 196–210.

Bourgeois, M., & Hickey E. (2009). *Dementia: From diagnosis to management—A functional approach.* New York: Taylor & Francis.

Bourgeois, M., & Melton, A. (2005). Training compensatory memory strategies via the telephone for persons with TBI. *Aphasiology, 19,* 353–364.

Brookshire, R.H. (2007). *Introduction to neurogenic communication disorders* (7th ed.). St Louis, MO: Mosby-Year Book.

Bucks, R. S., Willison, J. R., & Byrne, L. M. T. (2000). *Location learning test.* Bury St. Edmunds, Suffolk, England: Thames Valley Test Company.

Cummings, J. L. (2003). *The neuropsychiatry of Alzheimer's disease and related dementias.* London: Martin Dunitz.

Davis, G.A. (2000). *Aphasiology: Disorders and clinical practice.* Needham Heights, MA: Allyn & Bacon.

Delis, D. C., Kaplan, E., & Kramer, J. H. (2001). *Delis–Kaplan executive function system.* San Antonio, TX: Psychological Corp.

Dickson, D. W. (2001). Neuropathology of Pick's disease. *Neurology, 56*(Suppl. 4), S16–S20.

Dijkstra, K., Bourgeois, M., Youmans, G., & Hancock, A. (2006). Implications of an advice-giving and teacher role on language production in adults with dementia. *The Gerontologist, 46,* 357–366.

Folstein, M. F., Folstein, S. E., & McHugh, P. R. (1975). "Mini-mental state": A practical method for grading the cognitive state of clients for the clinician. *Journal of Psychiatry Research, 12,* 189–198.

Franczak, M., Kerwin, D., & Antuono, P. (2004). Frontotemporal lobe dementia. In R. Richter & B. Richter (Eds.), *Alzheimer's disease: A physician's guide to practical management* (pp. 137–143). Totowa, NJ: Humana Press.

Galasko, D., Salmon, D. P., Lineweaver, T., Hansen, L., & Thal, L. J. (1998). Neuropsychological measures distinguish patients with Lewy body variant from those with Alzheimer's disease. *Neurology, 50,* A181.

Goldstein, F. C., Levin, H. S., Presley, R. M., Searcy, J., Colohan, A. R. T., Eisenberg, et al. (1994). Neurobehavioural consequences of closed head injury in older adults. *Journal of Neurology, Neurosurgery and Psychiatry, 57,* 961–966.

Gustafson, L., Brun, A., & Passant, U. (1992). Frontal lobe degeneration of non-Alzheimer type. In M. Rossor (Ed.), *Unusual dementias* (pp. 559–582). London: Balliere Tindall.

Hagens, C., Beaman, A., & Ryan, E. (2003). Reminiscing, poetry writing, and remembering boxes: Personhood-centered communication with cognitively impaired older adults. *Activities, Adaptation, and Aging, 27,* 97-112.

Haynes, W.O., & Pindzola, R. H. (1998). *Diagnosis and evaluation in speech pathology* (5th ed.). Needham Heights, MA: Allyn & Bacon.

Helm-Estabrooks, N. (2001). *Cognitive linguistic quick test.* San Antonio, TX: Psychological Corp.

Hodges, J. R., & Patterson, K. (1995). Is semantic memory consistently impaired early in the course of Alzheimer's disease? Neuroanatomical and diagnostic implications. *Neuropsychologia, 33,* 441–459.

Holland, A., Frattali, C., & Fromm, D. (1999). *Communicative activities of daily living* (2nd ed.). Austin, TX: PRO-ED.

Litvan, I., Mohr, E., Williams, J., Williams, J., Gomez, C., & Chase, T. (1991). Differential memory and executive functions in demented patients with Parkinson's and Alzheimer's disease. *Journal of Neurology, Neurosurgery, & Psychiatry, 54,* 25–29.

Mattis, S. (2001). *Dementia rating scale* (2nd ed.). Lutz, FL: Psychological Assessment Resources.

Morris, J. C. (2003). Dementia update 2003. *Alzheimer Disease and Associated Disorders, 17,* 245–258.

Munoz, D. G., Ganapathy, G. R., Eliasziw, M., & Hachinski, V. (2000). Educational attainment and SES in patients with autopsy-confirmed AD. *Archives of Neurology, 57,* 85–89.

Murray, L. L., & Clark, H. M. (2006). *Neurogenic disorders of language: Theory driven clinical practice.* Clifton Park, NY: Thompson Delmar.Learning.

Nagaratnam, N., Phan, T. A., Barnett, C., & Ibrahim, N. (2002). Angular gyrus syndrome mimicking depressive pseudodementia. *Journal of Psychiatry and Neuroscience, 27,* 364–368.

National Center for Health Statistics. (2009). *International classification of diseases* (9th Rev., clinical modification) Retrieved June 20, 2010, from http://www.cdc.gov/nchs/icd/icd9cm.htm

National Center for Health Statistics. (2010). *International classification of diseases* (10th Rev., clinical modification). Retrieved June 20, 2010, from http://www.cdc.gov/nchs/icd/icd10cm.htm

National Institute of Aging. (2003). *Alzheimer's disease progress report 2001–2002* (NIH Publication No. 03-5333). Washington, DC: U.S. Department of Health and Human Services.

National Stroke Association. (2002). *All about stroke.* Retrieved June 20, 2010, from: http//www.stroke.org

O'Brien, J. T., Erkinjuntti, T., Reisberg, B., Roman, G., Sawada, T., & Pantoni, L. (2003). Vascular cognitive impairment. *The Lancet: Neurology, 2,* 89–98.

Petersen, R., Stevens, J., Ganguli, M., Tangalos, Cummings, J., & DeKosky, S. (2001). Practice parameter: Early detection of dementia: Mild cognitive impairment (an evidence-based review). Report of the Quality Standards Subcommittee of the American Academy of Neurology. *Neurology, 56,* 1133–142.

Randolph, C. (1998). *Repeatable battery for the assessment of neuropsychological status.* San Antonio, TX: Psychological Corp.

Richter, B. Z. (2004). Potential and established risk factors for Alzheimer's disease. In R. Richter & B. Richter (Eds.), *Alzheimer's disease: A physician's guide to practical management* (pp. 65–71). Totowa, NJ: Humana Press.

Robertson, I. H., Ward, T., Ridgeway, V., & Nimmo-Smith, I. (1994). *The test of everyday attention.* Gaylord, MI: Northern Speech Services.

Ross-Swain, D., & Fogle, P. (1996). *Ross information processing assessment–geriatric.* Austin, TX: PRO-ED.

Schretlen, D. (1997). *Brief test of attention.* Lutz, FL: Psychological Assessment Resources.

Smith, G., & Rush, B. (2006). Normal aging and mild cognitive impairment. In D. Attix and K. Welsh-Bohmer (Eds.), *Geriatric neuropsychology: Assessment and intervention* (pp. 27–55). New York: Guilford Press.

Sohlberg, M. M., & Mateer, C. A. (2001). *Cognitive rehabilitation: An integrative neuropsychological approach.* New York: Guilford Press.

Stern, R. A., & White, T. (2003). *Neuropsychological assessment battery: Administration, scoring and interpretation manual.* Lutz, FL: Psychological Assessment Resources.

Stevens, A., King, C., & Camp, C. (1993). Improving prose memory and social interaction using question asking reading with adult day care clients. *Educational Gerontology, 19,* 651–662.

Tompkins, C. A. (1995). *Right hemisphere communication disorders: Theory and management.* San Diego, CA: Singular.

Warner, T. T., & Schapira, A. H. V. (2003). Genetic and environmental factors in the cause of Parkinson's disease. *Annals of Neurology, 53,* S16–S25.

Wechsler, D. (1997). *Wechsler adult intelligence scales* (3rd ed.). San Antonio, TX: Psychological Corp.

Wiig, E. H., Nielsen, N. P., Minthon, L., & Warkentin, S. (2002). *Alzheimer's quick test: Assessment of parietal function.* San Antonio, TX: Psych Corp.

Wilson, B. A., Alderman, N., Burgress, P., Emslei, H., & Evans, J. J. (1996). *Behavioural assessment of the dysexecutive syndrome* (BADS). Bury St. Edmunds, Suffolk, England: Thames Valley Test Company.

Wilson, B. A., Cockburn, J., & Baddeley, A. (2003). *The Rivermead behavioural memory test* (2nd ed.). Bury St. Edmunds, Suffolk, England: Thames Valley Test Company.

Assessment Instruments for Cognitive-Communicative Disorders

Instrument	Normative age range (in years)	Contents/subtests	Administration time/specific group
Screening instruments for general cognitive abilities			
Mini-mental State Examination (MMSE; Folstein, Folstein & McHugh, 1975)	18–85	Orientation, attention, calculation, immediate memory, delayed memory, visuospatial construction	10m General
Modified Mini-mental State Examination (3MS; Jones et al., 2002)	60–84	Orientation, attention, calculation, immediate memory, delayed memory, visuospatial construction, object relations	10m General
The Alzheimer's Quick Test (AQT; Wiig, Nielsen, Minthon, & Warkentin, 2002)	15–72	Timed naming tasks, scored for response accuracy and response time	10m Alzheimer's dementia
Cognitive Linguistic Quick Test (CLQT; Helm-Estabrooks, 2001)	18–89	Orientation, attention, verbal memory, visual memory, naming, auditory comprehension, executive functions	30m General
Assessment batteries			
Dementia Rating Scale–2 (DRS-2; Mattis, 2001)	56–105	Attention, initiation-perseveration, construction, conceptualization, memory recall, memory recognition	45–60m dementia
Repeatable Battery for the Assessment of Neuropsychological Status (RBANS; Randolph, 1998)	20–89	Immediate memory, visuospatial-constructional, language, attention, delayed memory	30–45m General use, but developed for dementia
Ross Information Processing Assessment–Geriatric (RIPA-G; Ross-Swain & Fogle, 1996)	65–98	Orientation, short-term memory, long-term memory, auditory comprehension, reasoning	40–60m General, elderly

(continues)

Assessment Instruments for Cognitive Communication Disorders (*continued*)

Instrument	Normative age range (in years)	Contents/subtests	Administration time/specific group
Neuropsychological Assessment Battery (NAB; Stern & White, 2003)	18–97	Attention, language, memory, spatial, executive functions; Includes functional activities	4 hours, can use subtests individually General use
Wechsler Adult Intelligence Scales–III (WAIS-III; Wechsler, 1997)	16–89	Language comprehension, vocabulary, auditory verbal memory, visuoconstruction, executive functions	90m General
Functional communication activity-based assessments			
Communicative Activities of Daily Living–2 (CADL-2; Holland, Frattali, & Fromm, 1999)	26–90	Reading, writing, using numbers, social interaction, divergent communication, contextual communication, sequential relationships, humor/metaphor/absurdity	30–40m RHD, TBI
Functional Linguistic Communication Inventory (FLCI; Bayles & Tomoeda, 1994)	Not specified	Greeting and naming, writing, following commands, gestures, sign and picture comprehension, word reading, answering questions, reminiscing, conversation	30–40m Dementia
Assessment of Language-Related Functional Activities (ALFA; Baines, Martin, & Heeringa, 1999)	16–95	Telling time, checkbook and money skills, addressing an envelope, math, medicine labels, calendar use, telephone use, taking messages	30–90m
Specific domain measures			
Memory			
Rey-Osterrieth Complex Figure Test (Bernstein & Waber, 1994)	6–93	Non-verbal memory, visuospatial construction, strategy use, organization	10m, excluding recall delays General

Assessment Instruments for Cognitive Communication Disorders (*continued*)

Instrument	Normative age range (in years)	Contents/subtests	Administration time/specific group
Memory (*continued*)			
Rivermead Behavioural Memory Test–II (RBMT–II; Wilson, Cockburn, & Baddeley, 2003)	11–94	Long term memory, recognition, immediate recall, delayed recall, orientation	25–60m General
Location Learning Test (Bucks, Willison, & Byrne, 2000)	50–96	Functional non-verbal memory, visuospatial recall, visual-perceptual abilities	25m dementia
Executive Functions			
Behavioural Assessment of the Dysexecutive Syndrome (BADS; Wilson, Alderman, Burgess, Emslei, & Evans, 1996)	16–87	Mental flexibility, inhibition, working memory, organization and planning, strategy use, abstract thinking, apathy, unconcern for social rules	30–45m General
Delis–Kaplan Executive Function System (D-KEFS; Delis, Kaplan, & Kramer, 2001)	8–89	Verbal and nonverbal fluency, inhibition, mental flexibility, problem-solving, categorical processing, deductive reasoning, planning, rule use, metaphors	90m General
Attention			
Test of Everyday Attention (Robertson, Ward, Ridgeway, & Nimmo-Smith, 1994)	18–84	Selective attention, attentional switching, sustained attention, divided attention, working memory	45–60m General
Brief Test of Attention (Schretlen, 1997)	17–84	Brief attention screen using alphanumeric lists (controls for confounds of memory, visual scanning, and motor impairments)	5–10m General

CHAPTER 9

Language and Aging: Primary and Tertiary Aging Factors

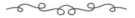

Barbara B. Shadden

SHADDEN PRESENTS AN OVERVIEW of primary and tertiary aging factors affecting language systems. The chapter begins with a discussion of perceptions of the language of older adults, then moves into age-related changes in language systems such as semantics and syntax. Much of the remaining chapter describes discourse comprehension and production in normally aging adults. General factors influencing discourse behaviors (e.g., discourse goals and emotional content) are identified, followed by review of key measures of discourse performance and summary of changes that may be seen in the elderly. An overview of changes in reading and writing is also provided. Primary changes in language systems are related to models of cognitive aging. The chapter closes with discussions of tertiary factors affecting language performance in normally aging adults and possible prevention approaches designed to maintain language and communicative skills.

Language is at the heart of daily communication. Cognitive skills such as memory and problem solving rely so heavily on language that they cannot function adequately in its absence. While cognition and language are discussed as though they are distinct processes, the reality is that language is one component of cognition, and what we know about cognitive aging often comes from studies of language. Like cognition, language is incredibly complex and undergoes many changes across the lifespan. Some of these changes are predictably related to aging processes; others are the result of the unique characteristics of the individual, including intelligence and its component cognitive skills, education, physical health, personality, and life experience and current circumstances.

Variability in language skills is present throughout the lifespan. Some people possess exceptional language skills, while others fall at the low end of what is considered normal. Although most elderly individuals continue to use their language effectively, those with limited language skills have fewer resources to cope with changes in brain structure and function. As a result, they are likely to experience more difficulties as they age.

Language in normally aging adults has been studied extensively. Some of what has been learned relates to specific language systems like semantics or syntax. Primary aging changes in these systems are described briefly in this chapter. True communication, however, takes place through discourse. Discourse behavior is sensitive to many variables, including primary changes in other cognitive systems, and is discussed in greater detail. Before reviewing normal changes in language, however, clinicians should consider the perceptions of older adults and their conversational partners. These perceptions are critical to the success of any communicative interaction.

Primary Aging in Language Systems

Primary Aging: Perceptions of Language

Older adults value communication as much as or more than younger adults. Keeping in touch with family and friends is an important aspect of daily living, as are staying current with news and engaging in social activities. Reading and writing are reported to be valued more by the elderly than by younger adults. The Internet and its information and e-mail communications are used by many older individuals. For most elderly, the only communication problems they describe are by-products of other aspects of aging, such as vision and hearing loss, altered voice quality, and possibly some hearing impairment.

A voice may sound old, and a hearing loss can be easy to identify. However, primary aging changes in language skills are much less obvious, both to the elderly and to their communication partners. Changes are less obvious in part because of the wide range of what is considered acceptable or normal. Further, we do not typically listen to someone talk and judge the complexity of that person's syntax or the adequacy of his or her vocabulary.

In everyday situations, the effects of primary aging on language are neither noticeable nor particularly impairing. Frequently, only the language of the *old-old* (i.e., individuals 85 and older) is identified as somehow different.

When a normal change is noticed, it is often related to word retrieval or a breakdown in discourse comprehension and production. How these changes are interpreted depends on a variety of factors. For communication partners, perceptions are influenced by the relationship with the older person (e.g., family member, friend, healthcare provider). Within families, adult children of aging parents are most likely to identify even minor alterations in language and communication. They may be distressed by perceived changes because they fear these are signs of emerging cognitive deficits (such as those associated with dementia). They may also find it difficult to acknowledge and accept the role reversals that can occur when adult children become caregivers to their parents.

Other factors affecting partner perceptions include prior experiences with older adults, the apparent age of a specific older partner, and the content of the conversation. Partners are more likely to focus on communicative content, style, and perceived overall effectiveness. For example, an older person may be perceived as somewhat verbose and dominating in conversations, with content that is perhaps more egocentric or restricted. Most judgments of the effectiveness of older adults' communications are strongly influenced by attitudes and stereotypes related to the elderly and to aging in general. If the expectation is that the elderly are somewhat incompetent, any changes in language and communication appear to confirm that incompetence. Perceptions of incompetence lead to use of potentially demeaning language, such as elderspeak, which will be discussed in Chapter 12.

When older adults recognize language difficulties, they too may fear the implications of changes. For example, as people age, they become more sensitive to everyday instances of trouble finding the specific word or name they want to say. The closer people get to age 65, the greater these concerns become. In fact, what might have been an amusing lapse at age 30 becomes a potential symptom of mental failing at 55. The elderly person may fear that any memory loss might signal the beginning of cognitive decline, similar to the concerns of adult children.

In addition, some elderly individuals are aware that they are experiencing more trouble understanding complex information presented verbally or in writing. Before an important doctor's appointment, for example, a patient may be concerned about being able to understand and remember what the doctor is going to say. After the appointment, the patient may leave feeling somewhat confused or overwhelmed by the information provided. Similar concerns may arise when complex instructions are given very rapidly. In these instances, difficulties processing detailed information can be perceived once again as a sign of failing cognition.

Finally, normally aging older adults may find their perceptions of their own communicative competence influenced by the behaviors and attitudes of their communication partners, as noted earlier. When communication partners "talk down" to healthy elderly people, the message is that the older person is less competent. While older persons may not always be conscious of these messages of incompetence, they can often sense that their communication is not valued.

Given concerns about language behaviors as possible indicators of cognitive decline, it is important to examine what actually occurs with primary aging. Many of the changes described in the following sections have little functional impact under optimum communication conditions. However, they assume greater importance when circumstances are more challenging and there is greater pressure on the older person to communicate. Clinically, what we really need to know are how aging alters language behavior, why alterations occur, and how language behaviors associated with primary aging can be distinguished from secondary language disorders such as aphasia. Normal changes in syntax and semantics are described first, followed by a discussion of discourse comprehension and production. Table 9.1 provides an overview of changes in specific language systems, along with factors that influence language behavior.

Primary Aging: Semantics

The term *semantics* refers to the meaning aspects of language. Semantics involves vocabulary recognition and knowledge, strategies for remembering new semantic information, and speed and accuracy in retrieving words. Lexical and semantic changes associated with primary aging are of considerable interest to clinicians because word finding deficits are observed in most of the communication disorders experienced by the elderly.

Vocabulary and Lexical Recognition and Comprehension

Basic vocabulary knowledge and recognition are relatively spared as we age. These skills are sometimes referred to as *passive vocabulary*. At the word level, passive vocabulary actually improves across the lifespan, with declines seen only after the age of 70 or 75 (Verhaeghen, 2003). For example, when given a choice, an older adult can pick the correct word to name a picture, select correct definitions for words, and identify synonyms and antonyms. Lifespan improvement is observed for sentence-level semantic comprehension as well (Burke & Shafto, 2008; Thornton & Light, 2006).

TABLE 9.1

Changes in Semantic and Syntactic Performance Associated With Primary Aging

Language domain	Age-related (primary) aging changes	Influences on language performance
Lexical and semantic skills		
Recognition and comprehension	• Passive vocabulary and sentence-level comprehension improve until 70+	• Cohort life experiences • Educational levels ↑
Encoding and retention of new information	• Encode fewer words; use less imagery, elaboration, and organization • Rely more on semantic encoding strategies	• Time pressure ↓ • Distractors ↓
Active word retrieval		
Naming tasks	• Decline in word finding • Respond differently from younger adults when given a priming cue	• Type of word (e.g., proper vs. common noun) • Complexity of visual stimulus ↓ • Word frequency ↓ • Imageability ↓ • Abstraction ↓ • Distractors ↓ • Increased density of word target ↓
Verbal fluency	• Slower to generate word lists • Access and use fewer categories • Categories with real-life value show little decline • Fluency tasks using letters are less susceptible to aging	• Type of category • Type of word
Tip-of-the-tongue (TOT)	• Increased frequency of TOT experience • More problems with names and other proper nouns	• Type of word • Fewer neural connections to other words ↑
Slip-of-the-tongue	• More slip-of-the-tongue errors • More omissions than younger persons have	• Increasing speech rate ↑

(continues)

TABLE 9.1 (continued)

Language domain	Age-related (primary) aging changes	Influences on language performance
Syntactic processing	• Generally spared (basic syntax) • More difficulty with complex sentences	• Syntactic ambiguity ↓ • Availability of lexical context information ↑ • Presence of distractors ↓ • Rapid rate of presentation ↓
Syntactic production	• Some reduction in utterance length • Reduced use of grammatically complex syntax • More errors in producing complex syntax	• Diminished vocabulary (for utterance length) ↓ • Working memory demands ↓ • Education ↑ • Cognitive status ↑ • Physical functioning ↑

Note. Both personal and task variables are listed. Direction of influence is shown by ↑ (improves performance) and ↓ (detracts from performance). When change is variable, there is no arrow.

Although there is normal age-related slowing in recognition and comprehension of words and sentences, the problem is not at the level of word meanings. In studies of brain activation during language tasks, delays are associated with initial perceptual processing of speech stimuli and with higher level understanding of sentences, not with semantic processing of actual words (Federmeier, Van Petten, Schwartz, & Kuras, 2003). Apparently, sensory and perceptual processing places greater demands on the aging brain than on the brains of younger adults, but the basic semantic organization of the brain is relatively untouched by aging.

Retention of New Semantic Information

Although passive vocabulary is spared, the aging brain is less effective at storing, retaining, and retrieving new lexical or semantic information (Burke & Shafto, 2008; O'Hanlon, Kemper, & Wilcox, 2005). A typical retention task might involve asking a person to listen to a long list of words, remember them, and then tell all the remembered words. Most adults use a variety of strategies to accomplish this task, including organizing the list into categories or visualizing some of the words. Older adults retain and retrieve fewer words and use less imagery, elaboration, and organization than do younger adults. They rely more on semantic encoding strategies (e.g., unconsciously linking all words with related meanings). Factors influencing performance are listed in Table 9.1.

Active Word Retrieval

Aging does affect *word retrieval*, which is the ability to find the words we want when talking. Measurable declines in word finding begin relatively early in adulthood and extend across the lifespan (LaGrone & Spieler, 2006; Spieler & Balota, 2000). As people move into their 70s, they become slower in naming objects or pictures, name fewer items, and make more errors (typically semantic errors such as circumlocutions, visual errors, and "don't know" responses). A variety of factors affect an older individual's ability to retrieve words (see Table 9.1). These factors affect people of all ages but are more disruptive to the elderly. In addition, older adults demonstrate increased frontal lobe activation during naming (Wierenga et al., 2009), consistent with the hemispheric asymmetry reduction in older adults (HAROLD) model described in Chapter 7.

When we learn new vocabulary, words are stored in our brains with numerous connections to other words based on meaning, sound, and word structure. These connections are considered the word's neighborhood (Thornton & Light, 2006). Some connections should be strengthened as people age, and word finding should be helped by providing priming cues from the target word's neighborhood. A *priming cue* is a stimulus presented immediately before a person is asked to name items. For example, for the word *forest*, a phonological cue might be *form* since it begins with the same sound. A semantic cue for the same word would be *tree,* and a syllable cue could be *farthest.* When compared with young adults, older adults benefit similarly when primed with first syllables and more when primed with semantic information. However, if the priming cue has numerous potentially related words and neural connections, older adults do more poorly.

Active word retrieval is required in verbal fluency and generative naming tasks that require a person to list as many words in a category (e.g., animals, transportation) as possible during a fixed time frame. Performance is usually measured by looking at the number of accurate different words produced, the categories (if any) used to create the list, and other observed strategies for recall. In general, verbal fluency tasks show moderate and reliable age-related declines, although letter naming declines more slowly. Other changes in word fluency are shown in Table 9.1. When elderly individuals are asked to generate information relevant to daily activities, age differences are reduced (Hough, 2007).

Tip-of-the-tongue (TOT) experiences also shed light on aging and word retrieval (Thornton & Light, 2006). When a speaker cannot think of a desired word, the sense that the word is "almost there" is what is called the *TOT phenomenon.* Everyone has TOT experiences, and people can often provide information about the target word, like its meaning or grammatical function. Older adults report more daily TOT experiences than younger adults. Proper nouns are more affected than common nouns; the elderly have greater difficulty retrieving target words that have fewer associations in the brain. TOT experiences are associated with activation of brain regions responsible for phonological production, so the breakdown is partly at the sound level (Shafto, Burke, Stamatakis, Tam, & Tyler, 2007).

All of us also occasionally mix elements of two words together when we speak (e.g., saying "dood gog" for "good dog"), insert the wrong sound in a word, or experience a breakdown in speech fluency. These slips of the tongue can provide clues about what is going on in the brain and how speakers plan phonologically and motorically for expressing semantic content (MacKay & James, 2004). The speech of older adults has more of these errors and different types of errors when compared with the speech of younger adults (see Table 9.1).

Primary Aging: Syntax

Syntactic Processing (Comprehension)

Under optimal conditions, basic syntactic processing is relatively spared in aging. However, when presented with complex sentences with multiple embedded clauses, older adults do not process syntax as well as younger individuals do. Syntactic processing difficulties increase when speech rate increases or when distractors are present. The elderly appear to rely more on lexical meaning to interpret sentences with syntactic ambiguity (Burke & Shafto, 2008).

Age-related syntactic processing delays and errors are associated directly with declines in working memory (Kemper & Sumner, 2001). Problems occur when the task requires holding an early part of a sentence in working memory while processing the remainder of a sentence. Consider the following sentence: "After he went to the ball park to watch his friends who were playing softball, the boy stopped by his favorite ice cream store where they always had mint chocolate chip cones." To understand this sentence, the listener must hold both of the initial subordinate clauses in mind until it is clear that "he" is "the boy" and must then interpret the rest of the sentence in this context.

Syntactic Production

Utterance length is highly variable across the lifespan. Most studies show some reduction in length in older adults, possibly because of an increase in sentence fragments. Sentence length is not related to underlying working memory problems but is instead more directly related to a person's vocabulary (Kemper & Sumner, 2001).

Older adults have the necessary skills to use a range of syntactic forms. Despite this, use of complex forms decreases consistently with advancing age across a wide range of tasks (Thornton & Light, 2006). Changes are seen at both the sentence and paragraph level. When asked to use highly complex forms, older persons make more errors. However, all but the oldest are able to recognize errors. Once again, syntactic complexity is linked to working memory. Working memory is needed to hold complex sentence structures in active storage while ideas and words are selected and arranged. Other factors affecting expressive syntax are seen in Table 9.1.

Primary Aging: Discourse Behaviors

In daily activities, we pay little attention to the words and sentences people use to communicate. Instead, our language is produced and understood as discourse. *Discourse comprehension* and *discourse production* are terms that describe language in units longer than words, phrases, or sentences. Understanding the discourse behaviors of the elderly helps us understand how language and cognition come together to frame a message.

Emotional Regulation and Goals

Discourse comprehension and production are influenced by lifespan changes in emotional regulation and in goals and priorities, as summarized in Table 9.2. When compared with younger adults, the elderly assign greater weight to emotional and interpersonal factors in problem solving and in discourse. They often insert more personalized and autobiographical comments into discourse and elaborate more on emotional themes. They are also more likely to be influenced by emotional content and nonverbal cues in recall and interpretation of stories. Across the lifespan, there is a shift toward more positive emotions and words.

Personal goals also change across the lifespan and may influence an individual's specific choices about what to include in discourse, as well as his or her general goals for discourse. Differences in choice of discourse content are seen primarily in more autobiographical (personal) discourse samples. More broadly, the use of narratives (in the sense of life stories) may become more important to some adults as they age. Personal narratives help older adults express values, participate in decision making, maintain a sense of self, and set goals in end-of-life care.

TABLE 9.2
General Factors Influencing
Discourse Comprehension and Production

Factor	Influence on discourse performance
Emotional regulation	• Emotional and interpersonal factors influence problem solving • Emotional factors more important in interpreting and framing discourse • Emotional themes elaborated more • Personalized comments and topics may intrude more • Increased use of positive words
Personal goals for discourse	• More autobiographical • Broader goals regarding purpose of discourse • More use of life stories for personal meaning-making, expression of values, end-of-life decision making
Task	• Narrative discourse better understood and used than expository discourse • Narratives judged more interesting and clear than those of younger adults • Basic conversational skills maintained but highly variable

Note. Data in the table were adapted from the following sources: Beaman, Pushkar, Etezadi, Bye, and Conway, 2007; Brady and Sky, 2003; Hunt and McHale, 2008; Lewis and Rogers, 2007; Löckenhoff, Costa, and Lane, 2008; Randall, 2008; Riediger, Li, and Linderberger, 2006; Stine-Morrow, Miller, and Hertzog, 2006; Thompson, Aidinejad, and Ponte, 2001; Thompson, Garcia, and Mallow, 2007; Trunk, 2008; Tun, 1989; Young and Rodriguez, 2006.

Types of Discourse

There are different discourse types based on the goals or functions served by the language. Discourse types include narrative (stories), procedural (instructions), expository (informing), and conversation (social interaction). Older adults typically understand and use narratives (stories) better than expository (e.g., instructions, medical information) discourse. They also retain basic pragmatic conversational skills well into old age.

The distinction between discourse comprehension and production of narrative versus expository speech is an important one. From a comprehension perspective, the narrative structure of episodes and story grammar is familiar and well learned. If you recognize that a story is being told, you can anticipate that something will happen to the characters, they will respond, and there will be consequences. Familiarity with this structure allows older persons to use cognitive resources more efficiently to process discourse information. Not surprisingly, they do well when asked about the basic themes or moral of a story, which is referred to as *macrostructure*. They are more likely than younger adults to be creative in interpreting narrative, although they are also more likely to interpret stories in the context of their own life experiences (Adams, Smith, Nyquist, & Perlmutter, 1997).

In contrast, expository speech has less organizational structure, is less predictable, and often requires processing of large chunks of relatively new information. The resulting greater cognitive load can lead to problems with understanding important forms of expository discourse, such as written information for healthcare or taking medicines (Kim, Bayles, & Beeson, 2008).

Similar patterns are seen in discourse production. Familiarity with narrative structure of episodes and story grammar helps older adults produce coherent, well-formed stories throughout the lifespan. In fact, clear, simple language in storytelling may be a strength for some elderly people. While some older-old individuals display qualitative changes in their choice of information or organizational style, they can still be distinguished from persons with Alzheimer's disease based on narrative organization (Cannito Hayashi, & Ulatowska, 1988). In general, the elderly can explain the main points or gist of a story (Olness, 2000).

For any type of discourse task, performance deteriorates with advanced age, complexity, and time constraints. It is also positively influenced by higher education, vocabulary skills, and overall cognition.

Discourse Comprehension

There are slight but consistent declines in language and discourse comprehension across the lifespan, beginning as early as the 30s and escalating in the 70s and later. There is also tremendous variability (Burke & Shafto, 2008; Thornton & Light, 2006; Ulatowska & Chapman, 1991). The factors known to affect discourse comprehension are those related to (a) subject (i.e., older adult) characteristics, (b) task demands, (c) spoken or written content and organization, and (d) instructions (Von Eye, Dixon, & Krampen, 1989). Table 9.3 summarizes what is known about the effects of these variables on comprehension. One consistent pattern in aging is that comprehension declines as complexity increases or as normal cues are altered or removed in some fashion. Another pattern is that changes are most evident in people who are old-old. Education frequently influences performance.

TABLE 9.3

Factors Affecting Discourse Comprehension in Older Adults

Major variables	Specific factors	Examples of impact on older adults
Individual characteristics	• Chronological age • Education • General level of verbal ability • Sensory impairments • Personal interests or goals • Life experiences • Beliefs • Cultural values • Cognitive skills and level of mental activity	*Education* • Those with higher education perform better. • Higher education helps older adults access more strategies to maximize performance. *Advanced age, typically 75 or older* • Associated with poorer discourse performance *Age and education combined* • Response profile of old-old with limited education looks like that of neurologically impaired person.
Task (and response) demands	• Recognition • Comprehension • Recall • Generation of new information • Generation of macrostructural overviews • Attentional challenges • Simultaneous processing demands • Presence of distractors • Time limitations	• Performance more accurate for multiple-choice questions (recognition) than for retelling tasks (generation) • Macrostructural interpretation accurate until asked to generate alternate explanations • Comprehension declines when time pressure is introduced, distracting stimuli are present, or task is more complex
Content and organization of written or spoken discourse	• Type of discourse • Length • Personal relevance and emotional valence • Syntactic complexity and ambiguity • Speech rate • Semantic familiarity, abstraction, or frequency of occurrence • Idea (propositional or informational) density • Familiarity of content • Discourse modality (visual, auditory)	• Narrative discourse comprehension better than expository discourse • Text factors that improve younger adults' comprehension help older adults even more (e.g., emotional valence and personal relevance). • Text factors that disrupt the performance of younger people have a greater negative effect on older people (e.g., any form of complexity including syntactic, semantic, and idea density). • Greater benefit from cues like prosody and multiple modalities

TABLE 9.3 *(continued)*

Major variables	Specific factors	Examples of impact on older adults
Content and organization of written or spoken discourse *(continued)*	• Information load (how much is conveyed in how many words or over what time period) • Compression of speech signal • Manipulation of prosody (without and with normal and exaggerated cues, as in elderspeak)	• More disrupted by speech compression, increased rate, etc.
Instructions	• What to attend to • What to disregard • What will be asked	• Greater benefits from information about what will be important in text • Greater impairment when instructions are misleading or irrelevant

Discourse Production

Discourse production is as variable as discourse comprehension and is influenced by many of the same factors (Burke & Shafto, 2008; Thornton & Light, 2006). Table 9.4 provides an overview of these factors. For example, the syntactic complexity used in spoken and written discourse declines in later years and is tied closely to working memory and education. Syntactic complexity in written discourse actually differentiates low- and high-ability adults, as well as normal elderly from those with mild cognitive impairment (Fleming & Harris, 2008; Mitzner & Kemper, 2003). Reduced syntactic complexity may be a strategy used to preserve quality of communication. When older adults use less complexity, their narratives are often judged to be clearer and more interesting than those of younger adults (Kemper, 1990, 2006). Older adults also experience declines in semantic performance for discourse tasks (e.g., type-token ratio). Decline can be explained by underlying word retrieval difficulties coupled with increased cognitive demands, particularly on executive functions (Fleming, 2009).

The language of normally aging adults is less fluent than that of younger adults. The most common disfluencies are interjections, followed by revisions and repetitions. These breaks in fluency (*verbal fragmentation*) are interpreted as uncertainty behaviors, probably related to word retrieval problems or to cognitive organizational demands (Bortfeld, Leon, Bloom, Schober, & Brennan, 2001; Schiller, Ferreira, & Alario, 2007).

TABLE 9.4

Age-related Changes in Discourse Production
and Factors Influencing Performance

Discourse production	Age-related (primary) changes	Influences on discourse production
Core language skills	• Syntax: Grammatic complexity reduced • Semantics: Word finding decline	• Same variables seen in sentence-level syntax and semantics also seen in discourse
Fluency of language	• More verbal fragmentations in form of different disfluencies (interjections, then revisions and repetitions) • Fluency breakdown is cue to speaker age	• Cognitive demands of task ↓ • Time pressure ↓
Cohesion/coherence	• Increase in use of pronouns without adequate cohesive reference • Global thematic maintenance sometimes declines	• Advanced age ↓ • Working memory demands ↓ • Executive function demands ↓
Information	• Declines in amount, type, and efficiency of information produced • Quantity: Less information • Quality: Reduced relevance, reduced accuracy • Efficiency: Less information produced per number of words or for time period sometimes affects perceptions of effectiveness. • OTS or verbosity: Increased OTS in subgroup of older adults	• Advanced age ↓ • Task complexity ↓ • Type of discourse task—variable effects; OTS more commonly seen in discourse with personal theme • Cognitive skills ↑ • Poorer ADLs and IADLs* ↓ • Psychosocial factors: Reduced social networks, increased self-focus ↓
Organizational structure	• Discourse structural organization relatively well-preserved, particularly narrative skills • Generating macrostructures (gist, moral, summary, theme) also well-preserved under optimum conditions	• Age ↓ • Education ↑ • Vocabulary↑ • Cognitive skills↑ • Text complexity ↓ • Time constraints ↓ • Increase in new information ↓

TABLE 9.4 *(continued)*

Discourse production	Age-related (primary) changes	Influences on discourse production
Pragmatics	• Topic skills: Topic regulation and turn-taking well preserved • Speech style accommodations: Used by older persons but less often than younger • Social perspective taking: Slight decline • Content: Broad range of topics and partners, typically focus on positive, use stories to communicate messages • Prosody and other nonverbal skills: Maintained, although some declines in right-hemisphere mediated skills (for metaphor, inference, humor) • Rely more on prosody in conversation than do younger adults	• Topic skills: Breakdown in underlying cognitive processes like memory ↓ • Accommodations: Partner, task—variable effects • Content: Setting, partner—variable effects • Content: Personal and positive content ↑ overall quality ↑ • Nonverbal: Vision and hearing losses ↓ • Partner elderspeak: All aspects of pragmatics ↓

Note. ADL = abilities of daily living; IADL = instrumental activities of daily living; OTS = off-topic speech. Direction of influence is shown by ↑ (improves performance) and ↓ (detracts from performance). When change is variable, there is no arrow.

There is also a decrease in referential cohesion across the lifespan (Glosser & Deser, 1992; Pratt, Boyes, Robins, & Manchester, 1989). *Cohesion* is the use of words to refer back to information in previous sentences. In the following example, the pronoun "she" in the second sentence clearly refers back to Jill and helps link the two sentences:

1. Bob went to the store, where he saw Jill.
2. She was there buying some orange juice.

If the first sentence had been, "Susie went to the store, where she saw Jill," the reference would be unclear and the sentence would confuse a listener. For the elderly, there is a pattern of inaccurate or vague pronoun referencing, increased use of indefinite terms (*this, that, it, something*), and other ambiguous language (*the one people usually use* to refer to what is needed to hang a picture on the wall). As a discourse task becomes more complex, cohesion problems escalate. Cohesion is most commonly disrupted in the old-old group (85 and above), and young-old (typically, 65–75 years of age) and old-old can be differentiated on the basis of cohesive adequacy. Discourse coherence also declines across the lifespan (Korolija, 2000). *Coherence* refers to a speaker's ability to maintain the thematic unity of the discourse passage.

Information exchange is at the core of discourse production. Information can be measured in many ways, including important elements in a picture description, steps in explaining how to do something, or core elements of a story. In general, slight declines in the amount, type, and rate of communicating information are seen as people age (Juncos-Rabadán, Pereiro, & Rodríguez, 2005; Ulatowska & Chapman, 1991). The oldest individuals produce the least information, with less efficiency and accuracy and reduced relevance. There is also age-related decline in propositional (idea) density and in communicative efficiency. Typically, these changes in information content of the old-old are apparent to conversational partners and may interfere with the everyday effectiveness of communication.

Inefficient communication of information is associated with the concept of *verbosity* or *off-topic speech* (OTS). OTS usually begins as appropriate topic-relevant comments in a conversation but relatively quickly becomes sidetracked into language that is unnecessarily extended, lacking in structure, and irrelevant (Arbuckle, Nohara-LeClair, & Pushkar, 2000). OTS can affect the global coherence of a conversational turn because partners often have difficulty following the twists and turns of the topic. About 20% of adults over the age of 60 produce extreme off-target verbosity (Thornton & Light, 2006). While chronological age does not predict OTS (Pushkar et al., 2000), it has been linked to other cognitive, situational, and personality attributes (see Table 9.4). OTS usually appears in discourse with a clear personal theme (e.g., a personal story, autobiographical material).

Conversation partners may view a verbose older adult as less desirable (and less competent), effectively reducing opportunities for social interaction. However, not all OTS is judged negatively. In some situations, people using OTS are seen as more interesting and informative, as well as more talkative and less focused (James, Burke, Austin, & Hulme, 1998). There are many possible explanations for OTS. It may simply reflect changes in communicative goals and priorities (Trunk, 2008). Some older persons may place greater value on social interactions; others may lack social contacts and thus crave additional conversation when the opportunity arises. OTS may also occur when conversation is used to seek validation or to teach and share life experiences.

Pragmatics

Pragmatics refers to use of language in social contexts and is typically described in reference to conversations. Successful pragmatic understanding and use require a complex interaction of cognitive and linguistic skills. In general, basic pragmatic skills remain functional for older adults (in the absence of other aging variables or pathology), although many elderly have trouble following conversations in a group (Murphy, Daneman, & Schneider, 2006). Several aspects of pragmatics are described here.

Conversational topic regulation and orderly *turn taking* are maintained well by older communicators, who are often more effective than young adults at latching one turn to the next. *Latching* involves use of reference to the past or to common events in order to smoothly integrate topics; it often takes advantage of content from the partner's turn to shift topics. Appropriate topic maintenance and switching skills and turn-taking behaviors are even seen in cognitively intact older nursing home residents. On occasion, attempts to hide memory breakdowns in conversation may create what appear to be topic maintenance issues on the surface (Ryan, Bieman-Copland, Kwong See, Ellis, & Anas, 2002).

Some common stereotypes exist about who older people talk with and what they talk about. Older adults are believed to talk primarily about their family, their health, the past, and the weather, and they are believed to talk mostly to family members. These perceptions are not supported in topic analyses of real conversations. The elderly are sometimes described as master storytellers. Their discourse in general shows highly effective use of historical events and social experiences as a topic-organizing framework. These strategies may function to express life experience and wisdom in an effective and functional manner.

Other aspects of *content* and *style* also differentiate older and younger communicators in discourse interactions. It was suggested earlier that older communicators tend to select more positive topics and use more positively framed language. This does not mean that all conversational content with all conversational partners is positive. Particularly within families, it is common to find that an aging parent may share negative feelings and interpretations of events more with one family member than another. Elderly individuals may also be relatively positive in conversations with acquaintances or healthcare providers while being much more negative in discussing similar topics with family members.

Successful use of pragmatics in conversation depends in part on the understanding and use of nonverbal information. Prosody provides powerful cues for understanding complex syntactic language as well as ambiguity, humor, metaphor, and similar language aspects. In general, older adults are able to use these cues to help in conversational processing (assuming no interference from hearing or vision impairment). In fact, they may rely even more on nonverbal cues than younger individuals do. They attend more closely to features such as facial expression and prosody in order to interpret discourse (Thompson, Aidinejad, & Ponte 2001). When understanding and use of nonverbal skills are affected by aging, changes relate to aspects of cognition mediated in the right hemisphere (e.g., humor perception, understanding written metaphor and inference). These right-hemisphere decrements are not seen until the 70s (Zanini, Bryan, De Luca, & Bava, 2005).

Finally, pragmatic success in conversation depends heavily on communication partners' abilities to understand each other's characteristics and perspectives. This partner sensitivity or perspective taking can be seen in the ways that a person's speech is accommodated to different partners. We use short, simple sentences in talking with young children or perhaps slow our rate of speech for someone who is not a native speaker of English. Older people typically accommodate appropriately when communicating with younger partners, at least in controlled research tasks. However, social perspective-taking skills show some decline with age, and the elderly may not make as many adjustments in their communications as do younger adults (Horton & Spieler, 2007). When conversational partners make inappropriate accommodations (e.g., use elderspeak), the pragmatic behavior of the older person may change. Some people become frustrated or irritated by elderspeak and will avoid similar interactions in the future. Others may become more hesitant and reluctant to engage in shared turn taking or topic initiation. Chapter 12 describes what triggers elderspeak, when it may and may not be helpful, and implications for clinical practice (Kemper & Harden, 1999).

Reading and Writing

Reading and writing serve many functions for all adults (Meyer & Pollard, 2006). For the elderly in particular, reading is a source of pleasure and entertainment. It is also an important tool in health communication and health literacy. *Health communication* refers to activities such as reading and understanding health information as an informed consumer, or complying with written health instructions or information on prescription bottles. Literacy skills are also important because they can predict cognitive behavior in aging and may be a more powerful indicator of brain reserve in older adults than years of education. Low levels of literacy skills early in one's life are associated with a much steeper decline in memory tasks over the lifespan (Soederberg, 1997). In fact, it appears that literacy skills may protect against memory decline in elderly individuals who do not have dementia (Mitzner & Kemper, 2003).

Primary aging affects reading and writing in ways similar to what is seen in other language systems. In addition, literacy requires knowledge of the symbol code of letters and the spelling conventions used in printed text. Reading and writing tap into the pool of life experiences and the knowledge of the reader or writer; they can play a role in quality of life and adaptation to age-related life change. Alterations in reading and writing and factors affecting performance are described in Table 9.5.

Reading. On the National Adult Reading Test (Ferraro & Sturgill, 1998), timed written word processing remains relatively intact across most of the lifespan. Reading comprehension competency extends through age 74, and then begins a gradual decline. Written narrative understanding

TABLE 9.5
Reading and Writing Across the Lifespan

Written language	Age-related (primary) changes	Factors influencing behavior
Reading	• Timed written word processing relatively intact across lifespan • Reading comprehension for discourse intact into 60s and then gradual decline • Comprehension of narrative better than expository	• Increased syntactic complexity • Increased propositional (idea) density • Visual acuity and perception • Education • Type of text • Familiarity of content • Functionality of content and form • Ethnic group • Working memory • Executive function
Writing	• Reduced syntactic complexity • Slowing associated with retrieving orthographic knowledge • Decline in idea density • Shift toward more positive content	• Education • Cognitive status • Physical functioning • Working memory demands

Note. Data in the table were adapted from the following sources: DeBeni, Borella, and Carretti, 2007; MacKay and Abrams, 1998; Ryan, Anas, Beamer, and Bajorek, 2003; Scialfa, 2002; Stine-Morrow, Milinder, Pullara, and Herman, 2001; Tun, 1989; Wingfield, Prentice, Kohl, and Little, 2000.

is maintained better than written expository text, for reasons discussed earlier. Factors affecting reading performance are listed in Table 9.5. Working memory is critical to reading, and visual sensory and perceptual changes can create particular challenges for the older reader. Vision can be affected by low illumination and contrast, visible distractors, and retinal blurring. These factors can make the initial processing of written stimuli more difficult and demanding, even though the individual can actually read the material.

Writing. Across the lifespan, individuals experience reductions in syntactic complexity in writing. Spelling errors increase with age, while awareness of such errors lessens. However, spelling changes do not seem to be connected to other cognitive skills or to factors such as education. Idea density in writing declines, and emotional content tends to shift, with positive emotions becoming increasingly prominent in later years. As with spoken discourse, overall written language performance is associated with other age-related cognitive changes.

Primary Aging Changes in Language: Theoretical Explanations

While the effects of primary aging on language behaviors are complex, they are not random. Instead, recurring patterns explain why performance is affected by some variables but not others. If we can explain those patterns, we can better understand the challenges faced by normally aging adults in everyday communication, as well as adults with acquired language disorders, such as aphasia. We can also develop more appropriate assessments and interventions, ones that maximize communicative functioning by taking into consideration premorbid linguistic and cognitive strengths as well as limitations.

Chapter 7 outlined how aging affects brain structures and functions and the common theories of cognitive aging (e.g., loss of processing resources, slowing of cognitive processes, breakdown in inhibition). The following sections describe the ways in which these theories can explain primary aging in language systems (Burke & Shafto, 2008; Thornton & Light, 2006).

Resource Capacity Theories

The resource capacity theories of cognitive aging all propose that the brain loses some capacity as it ages, and this loss is reflected in performance whenever there are increased demands on cognitive and linguistic skills

(Burke & Shafto, 2008). Adults of all ages perform more poorly when fatigued, sick, experiencing major stress, or coping with life changes and social losses. To the extent that older adults are at greater risk for some of these life challenges and have fewer brain resources, cognition may fluctuate and show decrements that are related to diminished reserves.

Virtually every age-related decline in language functions identified in this chapter can be explained by reduced resource or reserve capacity. For example, the most common factor affecting language comprehension and production is complexity. More complex language tasks show more age-related declines because of the resources required to carry them out. Expository speech was also described as being more difficult than narrative for older persons to process because it requires managing a large amount of new information without a familiar organizational structure. Education is another factor that routinely influences language performance. Those individuals with higher education presumably have more cognitive and linguistic resources and thus are less vulnerable to age changes.

There are variations of the resource capacity theories. Each further defines the resource or capacity that is reduced, specifically working memory, stimulus degradation, and transmission deficits.

Working memory (WM) capacity declines and becomes less efficient as we age, particularly into and beyond the 70s. Some researchers suggest that this is the primary cognitive resource lost as we age. Certainly, losses in WM are the main reason that aging adults have increased difficulty understanding and using grammatically complex sentences. Older adults with syntactic processing difficulties display more symmetrical frontal lobe activation as compensation and rely more on semantic skills for syntactic processing than do younger people. However, older individuals whose syntactic processing is similar to that of younger individuals show asymmetrical brain activation and WM capacities comparable to those of younger adults. WM losses also account for some of the challenges faced by the elderly in understanding all kinds of discourse, including written material (Carpenter, Miyake, & Just, 1994). Changes in working memory capacity should be considered when designing health communication materials (e.g., instructions for taking medications).

Signal degradation theories target breakdown in the initial processing of visual or auditory language material to explain loss of resource capacity (McCoy et al., 2005; Wingfield, Tun, & McCoy, 2005). It has been known for years that age-related hearing impairment (presbycusis) can affect speech–language comprehension. Even when older adults with a hearing loss can accurately recognize a spoken word or sentence, they do not perform well on some recall tasks. Adults without hearing loss also experience delays in auditory perception of speech. In effect, the stimulus is degraded in some fashion, and processing takes more effort, which then limits cognitive resources for subsequent comprehension and retention of language. This theory can also explain why auditory distractors disrupt language processing more in the elderly than they do in younger adults; they further degrade the incoming language signal (Schneider, Daneman, & Murphy, 2005). Changes in visual perception are similarly linked to reading comprehension. Visual challenges make initial processing more difficult and deplete cognitive reserves (Burke & Shafto, 2008).

The transmission deficit theory of cognitive aging suggests that it is changes in *how* information is transmitted neurologically that cause cognitive breakdown (MacKay & Abrams, 1998; MacKay & James, 2004). Throughout our lives, brain development and learning occur in part because connections between neurons and neuron networks are strengthened with increased activation and usage. Aging weakens these connections. More complex tasks require access to multiple points of information. Any weakening of the connections among these points would require committing more cognitive resources, leading to predictable declines in cognitive and linguistic functioning. The idea of weakened connections (and thus resources) can be used to predict which language systems are more likely to be affected. In the semantic system, for example, the meaning of words is stored in many locations with many connections (e.g., apples are red, can be eaten, grow on trees). Weakening of one set of connections can be compensated for by others. In contrast, the syntactic system has fewer stored representations and alternate neural connections, resulting in predictable declines.

Speed of Processing

A core characteristic of cognitive aging is slowing of mental processes and of neural transmission. This slowing begins in middle age but is more noticeable in later years. The degree to which speed is a factor in daily performance varies from one cognitive system to the next (Burke & Shafto, 2008; Hartley, 2006; Salthouse, 2000). Processing of speech signals is perhaps the most time-sensitive of all cognitive behaviors, and slowing in initial speech processing may cause further decrements in subsequent language operations (Caplan, Waters, & Alpert, 2003). While we would not expect impaired functions for basic word recognition or understanding simple sentences, more complex language activities are associated with multiple small delays. The longer it takes to complete the needed linguistic processing, the more likely it is that the signal will decay and language behavior will be affected. All of these effects are seen in older adults. Further reductions in speed of processing are seen in persons with aphasia and other secondary disorders of communication.

Inhibition Theories

One of the more intriguing theories of cognitive aging suggests that, as we age, we experience changes in our brain's ability to inhibit irrelevant information and competing activities, as well as distracting stimuli or thought processes. This is the *inhibition deficit hypothesis* (Hasher & Zacks, 1998). The effects of reduced inhibition can be seen in a variety of language behaviors. For example, word retrieval can actually be disrupted in the elderly if a prompt or priming word triggers too many connections in the brain. In the search for the word *azalea*, success in word retrieval may be disrupted by the triggering of other flower names (*daisy, aster*), other garden-related thoughts and words (*dirt, planting*), words that sound similar (*azure, aspen*), and even visual images. The differential impact of certain distracting stimuli can also be blamed on triggering neural connections that the aging brain cannot inhibit. If irrelevant speech is used as a distractor and the aging brain cannot inhibit the associations triggered by that speech, decrements in language performance will be observed. Even OTS in conversation can be explained in part by an inability to inhibit other thoughts and irrelevant information triggered during the conversation (Bell, Buchner, & Mund, 2008).

Tertiary Aging Effects on Language

Many of the variables that affect primary aging are part of what can be considered tertiary effects of aging on language and communication. Older adults who do not have a language or cognitive-communicative disorder still experience life changes that can affect understanding and use of language in daily contexts, primarily pragmatics. Given the fact that pragmatics is relatively well preserved in primary aging, any factors that undermine pragmatic performance impair an older adult's ability to use communication as an adaptive tool.

Older adults may be experiencing losses in their social networks due to death of family and friends or geographical dispersal. They may be coping with chronic health conditions such as arthritis, diabetes, and heart disease that limit their engagement in activities or may make them more dependent on others for assistance. Sensory losses in hearing and vision limit social interactions and enjoyment of activities such as reading and watching movies or television. Hearing impairment also directly affects communication strategies (Heine & Browning, 2004).

Many elderly persons move from family homes to other residential settings. These moves are considered major life stressors, particularly when precipitated by a health problem or loss of a spouse (even when the decision was made by the older person). For some individuals, this relocation may be a move to a retirement community of other older adults who maintain an active and engaged lifestyle. Language skills are typically unaffected in these circumstances, and language continues to be a tool for successful adaptation to these changes. For others, the move may be to an assisted living or long-term-care facility. In such environments, older persons are viewed and treated as less competent and more needy. Other residents may have dementia or severe health problems that limit opportunities for satisfactory interactions. Auditory and visual sensory deficits are common, and the physical environment of a nursing home makes it difficult to overcome these sensory impairments in conversation (Brink & Stones, 2007). Some older adults with normal language skills may still be able to use their skills to reduce communication barriers, while others may reduce their efforts to communicate or instead may become very demanding and pragmatically inappropriate in social interactions.

Although most elderly cope well with life changes and stresses and maintain communicative functioning, some do not. All of these changes affect quality of life and may lead to depression or a diminished sense of well-being. The effects of tertiary aging on pragmatics in interpersonal interactions are variable. Some elderly individuals withdraw from interactions; others may struggle to maximize social contacts by talking too much or demanding time and attention from communicative partners. Younger adults and caregivers may seem less interested in interacting and appear demeaning when they do interact.

Prevention

Given the vulnerability of older adults to factors disrupting communication, preventive interventions should be considered. Prevention takes many forms. It can refer to efforts to eliminate or reduce risks for specific health problems. In the context of stroke-related language disorders such as aphasia, prevention targets diet, exercise, smoking, and other factors that increase risk of cardiovascular disease. However, there is also a need for preventive interventions that can help vulnerable older adults maintain communication skills, prevent decline in language functions, and improve interactions. Only a few examples are provided here.

Cognition Enhancement

In Chapter 7, Dunn described ways that older adults can continue to stimulate and use their cognitive skills. Cognitive training programs such as Advanced Cognitive Training for Independent and Vital Elderly (ACTIVE) improve memory and retrieval, speed of response, and executive function, all of which are vital to language performance (Ball et al., 2002). Physical exercise also helps maintain physical health and cognitive skills (e.g., executive functions), which benefit language and communication (Kramer, Fabiani, & Colcombe, 2006). Programs that increase socialization also increase opportunities for communicative interactions. While we need to know more about the connections between preventive cognitive programs and language skills, there is reason to believe they can help seniors maintain language tools as they are. Older adults with relative strengths in cognition prior to a stroke have more tools for recovery after the stroke occurs.

Education and Training for Healthcare Providers

A number of programs have been designed to teach people to interact appropriately with the elderly. Training has been designed for residential care staff, certified nursing assistants, volunteers in meal delivery programs, counseling professionals, family of elderly nursing home residents, and faculty and students in professions serving the elderly. Other programs target communication between family and nursing home staff. Although outcomes vary, most programs result in improved communicative interactions, particularly reductions of patronizing speech or elderspeak (Williams, Kemper, & Hummert, 2003).

Communication Programs for Older Adults Without Communication Disorders

Some preventive programs have been developed to help healthy older adults maintain or improve their communication skills and interactions. One example is the "Keep on Talking" program. The 5-hour program has helped participants retain skills and reduce social isolation (Worrall, Hickson, Barnett, & Yiu, 1998). Other programs target development of skills for interpersonal effectiveness, improved communication in group interactions, and social engagement and support through Internet-based communication. All of these programs were developed specifically for the elderly.

Key Points

This chapter described the normal changes in language skills experienced as individuals age, as well as tertiary factors influencing language behaviors. Major themes included the following:

- Some language and communication skills remain intact or even improve across the lifespan.
- When declines in language performance exist, they are most commonly associated with complex activities that require rapid processing and extensive use of cognitive resources. Some declines produce no noticeable effect on communication.
- The old-old are most affected by primary aging changes in language.
- Tertiary aging factors can affect how, when, and with whom the elderly use their language and how they are judged by others.
- Some older adults are at risk for impaired daily communication even though a communication disorder is not present.
- Subtle normal changes in language may be difficult to differentiate from disorders like mild cognitive impairment or mild aphasia, which is why clinicians must understand normal aging.

References

Adams, C., Smith, M. C., Nyquist, L., & Perlmutter, M. (1997). Adult age-group differences in recall for the literal and interpretive meanings of narrative text. *Journal of Gerontology: Psychological Sciences, 52B,* 187–195.

Arbuckle, T. A., Nohara-LeClair, M., Pushkar, D. (2000). Effect of off-target verbosity on communication efficiency in a referential communication task. *Psychology and Aging, 15,* 65–77.

Ball, K., Berch, D. B., Helmers, K. F., Jobe, J. B., Leveck, M. D., Marsiske, M., et al. (2002). Effects of cognitive training interventions with older adults: A randomized controlled trial. *Journal of the American Medical Association, 288,* 2271–2281. Retrieved August 1, 2009, from http://jama.ama-assn.org/cgi/content/full/288/18/2271

Beaman, A., Pushkar, D., Etezadi, S., Bye, D., & Conway, M. (2007). Autobiographical memory specificity predicts social problem solving ability in old and young adults. *The Quarterly Journal of Experimental Psychology, 57,* 1275–1288.

Bell, R., Buchner, A., & Mund, I. (2008). Age-related differences in irrelevant-speech effects. *Psychology and Aging, 23,* 377–391.

Bortfeld, H., Leon, S. D., Bloom, J. E., Schober, M. F., & Brennan, S. E. (2001). Disfluency rates in conversation: Effects of age, relationship, topic, role, and gender. *Language and Speech, 44,* 123–149.

Brady, E., & Sky, H. (2003). Journal writing among older adults. *Educational Gerontology, 29,* 151–163.

Brink, P., & Stones, M. (2007). Examination of the relationships among hearing impairment, linguistic communication, mood, and social engagement of residents in complex continuing-care facilities. *The Gerontologist, 47,* 663–641.

Burke, D. M., & Shafto, M. A. (2008). Language and aging. In F. I. M. Craik & T. A. Salthouse (Eds.), *The handbook of aging and cognition* (pp. 373–443). New York: Psychology Press.

Cannito, M. P., Hayashi, M. M., & Ulatowska, H. K. (1988). Discourse in normal and pathological aging: Background and assessment issues. *Seminars in Speech and Language, 9,* 117–134.

Caplan, D., Waters, G., & Alpert, N. (2003). Effects of age and speed of processing on rCBF correlates of syntactic processing in sentence comprehension. *Human Brain Mapping, 19,* 112–131.

Carpenter, P. A., Miyake, A., & Just, M. A. (1994). Working memory constraints in comprehension: Evidence from individual differences, aphasia, and aging. In M. A. Gernsbacher (Ed.), *The handbook of psycholinguistics* (pp. 1075–1122). San Diego, CA: Academic Press.

DeBeni, R., Borella, E., & Carretti, B. (2007). Reading comprehension in aging: The role of working memory and metacomprehension. *Aging, Neuropsychology, and Cognition, 14,* 189–212.

Federmeier, K. D., Van Petten, C., Schwartz, T. J., & Kuras, M. (2003). Sounds, words, sentences: Age-related changes across levels of language processing. *Psychology and Aging, 18,* 858–872.

Ferraro, F., & Sturgill, D. (1998). Lexical effects and lexical properties associated with National Adult Reading Test (NART) stimuli in healthy young adults and healthy elderly adults. *Journal of Clinical Psychology, 54,* 577–584.

Fleming, V., & Harris, J. (2008). Complex discourse production in mild cognitive impairment: Detecting subtle changes. *Aphasiology, 22,* 729–740.

Fleming, V. B. (2009, May). *Comprehension and aging: The mediating effects of executive function.* Paper presented at the annual Clinical Aphasiology Conference, Keystone, CO.

Glosser, G., & Deser, T. (1992). A comparison of changes in macrolinguistic and microlinguistic aspects of discourse production in normal aging. *Journal of Gerontology, 47,* 266–272.

Hartley, A. (2006). Changing role of the speed of processing construct in the cognitive psychology of human aging. In J. E. Birren & K. W. Schaie (Eds.), *Handbook of the psychology of aging* (6th ed., pp. 183–207). Burlington, MA: Elsevier Academic Press.

Hasher, L., & Zacks, R.T. (1998). Working memory, comprehension and aging: A review and a new view. *The Psychology of Learning and Motivation, 22,* 193–225.

Heine, C., & Browning, C. (2004). Communication and psychosocial profiles of older adults with sensory loss—A focus group study. *Aging and Society, 24,* 113–130.

Horton, W., & Spieler, D. (2007). Age-related differences in communication and audience design. *Psychology and Aging, 22,* 281–290.

Hough, M. (2007). Adult age differences in word fluency for common and goal-directed categories. *Advances in Speech Language Pathology, 9,* 154–161.

Hunt, N., & McHale, S. (2008). Memory and meaning: Individual and social aspects of memory narratives. *Journal of Loss & Trauma, 13,* 42–58.

James, L., Burke, D., Austin, A., & Hulme. E. (1998). Production and perception of 'verbosity' in younger and older adults. *Psychology and Aging, 13,* 355–367.

Juncos-Rabadán, O., Pereiro, A., & Rodríguez, M. (2005). Narrative speech in aging: Quantity information content, and cohesion. *Brain and Language, 95,* 423–434.

Kemper, S. (1990). Adults' diaries: Changes in written narratives across the lifespan. *Discourse Processes, 13,* 207–223.

Kemper, S. (2006). Language in adulthood. In E. Byalystok & F. I. M. Craik (Eds.), *Lifespan cognition: Mechanisms of change* (pp. 223–238). Oxford, UK: Oxford University Press.

Kemper, S., & Harden, T. (1999). Experimentally disentangling what's beneficial about elderspeak from what's not. *Psychology and Aging, 14,* 656–670.

Kemper, S., & Sumner, A. (2001). The structure of verbal abilities in young and older adults. *Psychology and Aging, 16,* 312–322.

Kim, E., Bayles, K., & Beeson, P. (2008). Instruction processing in young and older adults: Contributions of memory span. *Aphasiology, 22,* 753–762.

Korolija, N. (2000). Coherence-inducing strategies in conversations amongst the aged. *Journal of Pragmatics, 32,* 425–462.

Kramer, A. F., Fabiani, M., & Colcombe, S. J. (2006). Contributions of cognitive neuroscience to the understanding of behavior and aging. In J. E. Birren & K. W. Schaie (Eds.), *Handbook of the psychology of aging* (6th ed., pp. 57–83). Burlington, MA: Elsevier Academic Press.

LaGrone, S., & Spieler, D. (2006). Lexical competition and phonological encoding in young and older speakers. *Psychology and Aging, 21,* 804–809.

Lewis, T., & Rogers, R. (2007). Family stories and the life course: Across time and generations. *Discourse and Society, 18,* 225–230.

Löckenhoff, C., Costa, P., & Lane, R. (2008). Age differences in descriptions of emotional experiences in oneself and others. *Journals of Gerontology: Series B: Psychological Sciences and Social Sciences, 63B,* 92–99.

MacKay, D., & Abrams, L. (1998). Age-linked declines in retrieving orthographic knowledge: Empirical, practical, and theoretical implications. *Psychology and Aging, 13,* 647–662.

MacKay, D., & James, L. (2004). Sequencing, speech production, and selective effects of aging on phonological and morphological speech errors. *Psychology and Aging, 19,* 93–107.

McCoy, S. L., Tun, P. A., Cox, L. C., Colangelo, M., Stewart, R. A., & Wingfield, A. (2005). Hearing loss and perceptual effort: Downstream effects on older adults' memory for speech. *Quarterly Journal of Experimental Psychology, 58A,* 22–33.

Meyer, B. J. F., & Pollard, C. K. (2006). Applied learning and aging: A closer look at reading. In J. E. Birren & K. W. Schaie (Eds.), *Handbook of the psychology of aging* (6th ed., pp. 233–260). Burlington, MA: Elsevier Academic Press.

Mitzner, T., & Kemper, S. (2003). Oral and written language in late adulthood: Findings from the Nun Study. *Experimental Aging Research, 29,* 457–474.

Murphy, D., Daneman, M., & Schneider, B. (2006). Why do older adults have difficulty following conversations? *Psychology and Aging, 21,* 49–61.

O'Hanlon, L., Kemper, S., & Wilcox, K. (2005). Aging, encoding, and word retrieval: Distinguishing phonological and memory processes. *Experimental Aging Research, 31,* 149–171.

Olness, G. (2000). Expression of narrative main-point inferences in adults: A developmental perspective. *Dissertation Abstracts International: Section B: The Sciences and Engineering, 61,* 3302.

Pratt, M. W., Boyes, C., Robins S., & Manchester, J. (1989). Telling tales: Aging, working memory, and the narrative cohesion of story retellings. *Developmental Psychology, 25,* 628–635.

Pushkar, D., Basevitz, P., Arbuckle, T., Nohara-LeClair, M., Lapidus, S., & Peled, M. (2000). Social behavior and off-target verbosity in elderly people. *Psychology and Aging, 15,* 361.

Randall, W. (2008). Getting my stories straight: A narrativist in quest of congruence. *Journal of Aging Studies, 22,* 169–176.

Riediger, M., Li, S-C., & Linderberger, U. (2006). Selection, optimization, and compensation as developmental mechanisms of adaptive resource allocation: Review and preview. In J. E. Birren & K. W. Schaie (Eds.), *Handbook of the psychology of aging* (6th ed., pp. 289–313). Burlington, MA: Elsevier Academic Press.

Ryan, E. B., Anas, A. P., Beamer, M., & Bajorek, S. (2003). Coping with age-related vision loss in everyday reading activities. *Educational Gerontology, 29,* 37–55.

Ryan, E. B., Bieman-Copland, S., Kwong See, S. T., Ellis, C. H., & Anas, A. P. (2002). Age excuses: Conversational management of memory failures in older adults. *Journal of Gerontology: Psychological Services, 57B,* 256–267.

Salthouse, T. A. (2000). Steps towards the explanation of adult age differences in cognition. In T. Perfect & E. Maylor (Eds.), *Models of cognitive aging* (pp. 19–49). Oxford, UK: Oxford University Press.

Schiller, N., Ferreira, V., & Alario, F. (2007). Words, pauses and gestures: New directions in language production research. *Language and Cognitive Processes, 22,* 1145–1150.

Schneider, B., Daneman, M., & Murphy, D. (2005). Speech comprehension difficulties in older adults: Cognitive slowing or age-related changes in hearing? *Psychology and Aging, 20,* 261–271.

Scialfa, C. T. (2002). The role of sensory factors in cognitive aging research. *Canadian Journal of Experimental Psychology, 56,* 153–163.

Shafto, M., Burke, D., Stamatakis, E., Tam, P., & Tyler, L. (2007). On the tip-of-the-tongue: Neural correlates of increased word-finding failures in normal aging. *Journal of Cognitive Neuroscience, 19,* 2060–2070.

Soederberg, L. (1997). The effects of age and expertise on discourse processing. *Dissertation Abstracts International: Section B: The Sciences and Engineering, 58,* 2157.

Spieler, D., & Balota, D. (2000). Factors influencing word naming in younger and older adults. *Psychology and Aging, 15,* 225–231.

Stine-Morrow, E. A. L., Milinder, L. A., Pullara, O., & Herman, B. (2001). Patterns of resource allocation are reliable among younger and older readers. *Psychology and Aging, 16,* 69–84.

Stine-Morrow, E. A. L., Miller, L. M. S., & Hertzog, C. (2006). Aging and self-regulation in language understanding. *Psychological Bulletin, 132,* 582–606.

Thompson, L. A., Aidinejad, M. R., & Ponte, J., (2001). Aging and the effects of facial and prosodic cues on emotional intensity ratings and memory reconstructions. *Journal of Nonverbal Behavior, 25,* 101–135

Thompson, L., Garcia, E., & Mallow, D. (2007). Reliance on visible speech cues during multimodal language processing: Individual and age differences. *Experimental Aging Research, 33,* 373–397.

Thornton, R., & Light, L. L. (2006). Language comprehension and production in normal aging. In J. E. Birren & K. W. Schaie (Eds.), *Handbook of the psychology of aging* (6th ed., pp. 261–287). Burlington, MA: Elsevier Academic Press.

Trunk, D. (2008). The effect of communicative goals on telling two types of autobiographical narratives in young and older adults. *Dissertation Abstracts International: Section B: The Sciences and Engineering, 68,* 6353.

Tun, P. A. (1989). Age differences in processing expository and narrative text. *Gerontology, 44,* 9–15.

Ulatowska, H. K., & Chapman, S. B. (1991). Neurolinguistics and aging. In D. N. Ripich (Ed.), *Handbook of geriatric communication disorders* (pp. 21–37). Austin, TX: PRO-ED.

Verhaeghen, P. (2003, June). Aging and vocabulary score: A meta-analysis. *Psychology and Aging, 18,* 332–339.

Von Eye, A., Dixon, R. A., & Krampen, G. (1989). Text recall in adulthood: The roles of text imagery and orienting tasks. *Psychological Research, 51,* 136–146.

Wierenga, C. E., Perlstein, W. M., Benjamin, M., Leonard, C., Gonzalez Rothi, L., Conway, T., et al. (2009). Neural substrates of object identification: fMRI evidence that category and visual attribute contribute to semantic knowledge. *Journal of the International Neuropsychological Society, 15,* 169–181

Williams, K., Kemper, S., & Hummert, M. L. (2003). Improving nursing home communication: An intervention to reduce elderspeak. *Gerontologist, 43,* 242–247.

Wingfield, A., Prentice, K., Kohl, C. K., & Little, D. (2000). Neural change, cognitive reserve and behavioral compensation in rapid encoding and memory for spoken language in adult aging. In L. T. Connor & L. K. Obler (Eds.), *Neurobehavior of language and cognition: Studies of normal aging and brain damage honoring Martin L. Albert* (pp. 3–21). Boston, MA: Kluwer Academic.

Wingfield, A., Tun, P. A., & McCoy, S. L. (2005). Hearing loss in older adulthood: What it is and how it interacts with cognitive performance. *Current Directions in Psychological Science, 14,* 144–148.

Worrall, L., Hickson, L., Barnett, H., & Yiu, E. (1998). An evaluation of the "Keep on Talking" program for maintaining communication skills into old age. *Educational Gerontology, 24,* 129–140.

Young, A., & Rodriguez, K. (2006). The role of narrative in discussing end-of-life care: Eliciting values and goals from text, context, and subtext. *Health Communication, 19,* 49–59.

Zanini, S., Bryan, K., De Luca, G., & Bava, A. (2005). The effects of age and education on pragmatic features of verbal communication: Evidence from the Italian version of the right hemisphere language battery (IRHLB). *Aphasiology, 19,* 1107–1133.

CHAPTER 10

Language and Aging: Secondary Aging Factors—Language Disorders in Older Adults

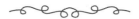

Barbara B. Shadden

IN THIS CHAPTER, SHADDEN focuses exclusively on secondary aging changes in language systems. Aphasia is introduced and defined, with examples provided of the various forms of aphasia. The influence of advanced age on type, severity, and prognosis for recovery is discussed. Shadden provides an overview of aphasia assessment, describing common domains to be observed or tested and emphasizing functionality. Examples of assessment tools for these domains are identified. The remainder of the chapter summarizes approaches to aphasia management, including consideration of computer-based interventions, augmentative and alternative communication, and constraint-induced language treatment. The needs of caregivers are acknowledged. Reimbursement requirements close out the chapter.

Chapter 9 identified the many primary and tertiary aging changes that affect language in aging adults. However, the elderly are also at greater risk for developing a variety of secondary communication disorders. Typically, we differentiate disorders based on both the part of the brain damaged and the underlying cognitive or linguistic processes disrupted. As discussed in Chapter 8, cognitive-communication disorders result from impairments of cognitive skills needed for communication, such as memory, executive function, and attention. The causes of cognitive-communication disorders include the dementias, right-hemisphere damage, and traumatic brain injury.

Other disorders result from damage to various language centers in the brain and their connections to associated brain areas. The many forms of aphasia are the main language disorders experienced by the elderly.

Aphasia: Definition and Characteristics

Definition

Aphasia is an impairment of the ability to understand and use language in all modalities: auditory comprehension, verbal production, reading, and writing. It is an acquired neurogenic disorder typically caused by a single cerebrovascular accident (stroke) affecting language centers and associated pathways in the cortex of the dominant hemisphere of the brain. Strokes may be either *occlusive* (caused by a blockage in an artery) or *hemorrhagic* (due to rupture of an artery in the brain). Other conditions, such as traumatic brain injury, tumors, and infections, may cause aphasic behaviors.

Characteristics

Aphasia characteristics are linked to the nature, extent, and location of neurological damage, and they may be influenced by preexisting cognitive and linguistic skills. Prognosis for recovery of functional language is related to these preexisting factors as well as to general health, personal characteristics (e.g., personality, motivation, emotions), and environmental and interpersonal supports. Core language behaviors affected by aphasia include auditory and reading comprehension, spontaneous discourse (spoken and written), and specific expressive language skills.

Both auditory and reading comprehension can be impaired in aphasia. Comprehension is typically influenced by word characteristics. Shorter words that are familiar and occur commonly in everyday language (e.g., *chair, store*) are easier to understand than multisyllabic abstract words (e.g., *tomorrow, democracy*). Nouns are typically easier to understand than verbs are. Shorter sentences and discourse passages using simple syntax are less challenging to process. In the following example, Sample A is easier for a person with aphasia to follow than is Sample B.

> *Sample A:* John and his girlfriend went to a party. John took her hand. They started dancing.
> *Sample B:* After going to the party, John took his girlfriend by the hand and they began dancing.

Other factors affecting comprehension include rate of speech, use of prosody and emphatic speech, and personal relevance of the topic.

As long as persons with aphasia can understand others and communicate through some modality, basic pragmatic skills are relatively unimpaired. However, a variety of other expressive language behaviors can be affected by aphasia. Impairments may be noted in phonology (or spelling), syntax, semantics and repetition. Each is described briefly.

Phonologic errors are called *paraphasias*. They can be described as the production of unintended syllables or words, sometimes resulting in apparently nonsensical output. A literal or phonological paraphasia occurs when less than half of the target word is altered (e.g., *compuger, pomputer,* or *comduter* for *computer*). A verbal or semantic paraphasia occurs when a different real word is used instead of the target word (e.g. *fork* for *spoon* or *dance* for *dream*). *Neologistic paraphasias* are words that do not exist in the English language, mostly because major portions of the target word have been transposed, substituted for, or otherwise disarranged. Examples of neologistic paraphasias include *widdlesome* for *walking* or *thranter* for *bottle*. As can be seen, neologistic errors are typically too far removed from the target word to be understood by listeners.

Syntactic problems may affect understanding or use of syntax; expressive syntax in aphasia may show agrammatism and paragrammatism. *Agrammatic* or *telegraphic* speech lacks the small connecting words and morphological markers (e.g., articles, auxiliary words, bound morphemes for plurals, verb tense). In contrast, *paragrammatism* refers to use of a wide range of syntactic forms with errors in usage. The following sentences are both attempts to say that people do not always obey the traffic laws when no policeman is present. Sample A is agrammatic and Sample B is paragrammatic.

Sample A: People no law no police.
Sample B: People are not always obey traffic laws when there is no police are present.

Expressive semantic problems are associated primarily with word retrieval or word finding difficulties *(anomia)*. Persons with aphasia deal with word retrieval deficits in different ways. Some simply stop and try to find the word in their mind, whereas others acknowledge the problem. It is very common for a person with aphasia to try to explain: "I know it in here [pointing to head] but it won't come out." In some instances, clients use circumlocution to express the missing word (e.g., "that black stuff you drink in the morning" for *coffee*). Word retrieval problems range from very mild to very severe.

Repetition skills are often impaired in aphasia. Some clients are unable to repeat any word, phrase, or sentence. Others repeat only key words (like saying "the man playing ball his son" for "the man is playing ball with his son") or familiar phrases. Repetition breaks down with longer sentences. Paraphasic errors during repetition tasks are common, as are perseverations (intrusions of previously repeated words).

Classification of Aphasias

Classification systems are helpful in understanding patterns of deficit and prognosis, as well as in developing interventions. Types of aphasia can be described in many ways, using contrasts such as fluent/nonfluent, anterior/ posterior (site of lesion), and receptive/expressive (domain most impaired). In speech–language pathology, aphasia is typically classified by using information about the site of the lesion and each client's pattern of distinctive language deficits. Characteristics of the more common types of aphasia are presented in Table 10.1 (Goodglass, Kaplan, & Barresi, 2001) and described briefly in this section. It should be noted that people rarely display characteristics of only one aphasia type; caution should be exercised when applying diagnostic labels. Further, clients classified initially as having one type of aphasia (e.g., Broca's) may recover over time to look more like they have another classification (e.g., anomic aphasia).

Some contrasts between the aphasia types in Table 10.1 are fairly obvious. A person with *Wernicke's aphasia* has markedly impaired auditory comprehension; fluent, syntactically complex output; frequent paraphasias; severe word retrieval problems; and poor repetition. When asked to describe a picture, this individual may say something like, "Well the thiggle there pointed it to him over the catchair." In contrast, persons with *Broca's aphasia* have only mildly to moderately impaired auditory comprehension, nonfluent (effortful) and telegraphic language output, and limited prosody. Looking at the same picture, this person might say, "Man lady sit . . . uh . . . uh . . . sit . . . chair."

An individual with *conduction aphasia* may have functional comprehension for language and fluent output with numerous paraphasic errors. What is most distinctive about this form of aphasia is a severe impairment in repetition skills. Persons with *anomic aphasia* can repeat anything but struggle primarily with finding the words they want to express themselves. If provided with a choice of words, the individual can typically identify the target readily. In contrast, *global aphasia* refers to severe impairments in both receptive and expressive language, due primarily to strokes that affect both posterior and anterior language centers. Some individuals with global

TABLE 10.1

Characteristics Associated with Common Types of Aphasia

Classification	Possible site of lesion	Auditory comprehension impairment	Verbal expression	Repetition impairment	Fluency	Word retrieval impairment	Paraphasia
Broca's aphasia	Inferior frontal lobe	Mild to moderate	Telegraphic effortful speech, reduced prosody; often accompanied by apraxia of speech	Moderate to severe, depending on apraxia of speech	Nonfluent	Moderate	Variable; if present, typically phonemic
Wernicke's aphasia	Temporal lobe	Severe	Fluent but empty speech, vague terms, often meaningless	Moderate	Fluent	Severe	Multiple, all forms
Anomic aphasia	Variable, although often angular gyrus	Little to none	Primary problem is word finding, so language is grammatically correct but empty or disrupted by word-finding efforts	Mild	Fluent	Variable degree of impairment	Some, usually semantic if present
Mixed nonfluent aphasia	Inferior frontal lobe	Moderate to severe	Like Broca's	Like Broca's	Nonfluent	Moderate	Like Broca's
Conduction aphasia	Arcuate fasciculus	Mild to moderate	Fluent speech with numerous paraphasic errors; fluency disrupted by efforts to self-correct	Severe	Fluent, although fluency disrupted by paraphasias	Moderate to severe	Multiple, all forms

(continues)

TABLE 10.1 (continued)

Classification	Possible site of lesion	Auditory comprehension impairment	Verbal expression	Repetition impairment	Fluency	Word retrieval impairment	Paraphasia
Global aphasia	Major portions of distribution of middle cerebral artery	Severe	Verbal output highly variable, from none to perseverative jargon	Severe	Variable	Severe	Variable
Transcortical sensory aphasia	Posterior watershed regions	Severe	Like Wernicke's	None	Fluent	Moderate to severe	Many
Transcortical motor aphasia	Anterior watershed regions	Mild	Like Broca's	None	Nonfluent	Variable	Like Broca's

Note. Data in the table were adapted from *Boston Diagnostic Aphasia Examination* (3rd ed.), by H. Goodglass, E. Kaplan, and B. Barresi, 2001. Copyright 2001 by PRO-ED, Inc.

aphasia say nothing; others engage in perseverative repetition of meaningless syllables, words, or phrases.

Some forms of aphasia do not match the basic definition as an acquired static disorder resulting from cortical damage. One is *primary progressive aphasia* (PPA). Persons with PPA display language characteristics consistent with definitions of aphasia, but onset is gradual and deficits gradually worsen over time. They may have a coexisting apraxia of speech. In later stages, other cognitive impairments may emerge, often in the form of a frontotemporal dementia. Another atypical disorder is *subcortical aphasia*. While this is a language disorder resulting from one or more strokes, the damage occurs in the thalamus, basal ganglia, or associated white matter pathways. Considerable variability exists in characteristics of subcortical aphasia, partly because the aphasia results from impairment of important neural connections that link language centers to other parts of the brain.

Associated Problems

Because aphasia results from brain damage, it is not surprising to find that other communication disorders may co-occur with aphasia. The most common are the dysarthrias and apraxia of speech described in Chapter 5. Co-existing behavioral consequences also may affect intervention. Persons with brain damage often have impairments in attention and may display perseverative behaviors, getting "stuck" on a word or action. Performance is highly variable within and across days and is susceptible to all of the factors that diminish our resources for cognitive and linguistic functioning. Stroke survivors may experience additional deficits in motor functioning (e.g., hemiparesis), visual acuity and perception (e.g., visual field deficits), and cognition. In fact, impairments in executive functioning may be seen in some individuals with aphasia (Fleming, 2009). Clinicians planning assessment and intervention obviously need to consider more than just language behaviors.

Age does play a role in type, severity, and recovery from aphasia, but care must be taken in interpreting the age factor (Cherney & Robey, 2008). The common causes of aphasia differ across age groups. Younger adults are more likely to have a hemorrhagic stroke or to experience aphasia secondary to other forms of brain damage. In contrast, older persons are more likely to have occlusive strokes, for which prognosis is not as good. The more severe and fluent types of aphasia are more common in older adults than in younger adults, and the pattern of recovery is influenced by age.

Older persons initially diagnosed with global aphasia may improve over time to one of the severe fluent forms of aphasia, whereas younger persons with global aphasia may improve toward a non-fluent Broca's type of aphasia. There is some evidence that younger clients with aphasia show greater overall recovery.

Age is not the only factor contributing to severity of deficits and differences in prognosis. Instead, older clients are more likely to have other health problems, both chronic and acute. They may be struggling with psychosocial challenges like depression or coping with major life alterations. Cognitive skills may be changing, even if they remain within the "normal" range, and these individuals may not have as many resources to focus on recovery of language skills, particularly executive function resources. Clinicians should take care not to let age alone influence prognostic expectations. Many variables potentially affect outcomes in the older individual, including aspects of tertiary aging (see Chapter 9).

Tertiary factors also influence how each person manages the impairment and engages in intervention. Consider 77-year-old John Jones, who is already experiencing memory problems. The onset of secondary aging in the form of a stroke and aphasia may be more challenging for him than the same stroke and aphasia experienced by 78-year-old Nancy Summers, who is "aging well" in the cognitive and linguistic domains. Other factors further complicate the picture. Mr. Jones has been temporarily placed in a long-term-care facility for stroke rehabilitation; unfortunately, the staff in that facility use elderspeak in their interactions with residents. The combination of change in environment, increased dependence, and being treated as incompetent may cause depression and withdrawal, diminishing his sense of self-efficacy and his success in treatment. Meanwhile, Mrs. Summers stayed in her home, doing outpatient speech–language therapy in a community clinic, where her husband was also able to receive support and training to help deal with his wife's aphasia. Her communication recovery was excellent, and her overall quality of life was good. Tertiary factors underscore the importance of understanding aphasia in context, as discussed later in this chapter.

Assessment and Intervention

Many of the primary and tertiary age-related changes experienced by older adults have implications for assessment and intervention. It is relatively simple to make practical accommodations to task, stimuli, or client activities. Examples of these accommodations are provided in Table 10.2

TABLE 10.2

Accommodations and Priorities in Clinical Assessment
and Treatment for Older Clients

System	Age-related accommodations in assessment and intervention
General	• Use testing materials that are appropriately normed for older population. • If depression is suspected, screen before assessment, refer for services, and interpret test results cautiously. • Avoid maximum-effort tasks that tax reserve capacity. • Identify barriers or limitations (psychological, social, environmental, and financial). • Identify actual resources (intrinsic and extrinsic). • Determine which individuals are important in the lives of older clients and include them in clinical management.
Vision	• Make sure client uses glasses and lenses that are clean. • Enlarge print or pictures. • Reduce glare. • Increase illumination or maximize use of available light. • Use a magnifying glass, if needed. • Move pictures or objects to position optimally for individual client.
Hearing	• Ensure that client uses hearing aids (if available). • Provide assistive listening devices. • Gain client's attention first before presenting tasks. • Maximize lighting for face-to-face communication. • Speak loudly (do not shout) and clearly. • Pause for processing. • Reduce ambient noise.
Motor or mobility	• Use larger, more easily manipulated materials. • Explore client ability to manipulate hearing aid, assistive listening device, or AAC. • Accommodate to limitations presented when motor task is timed.
Cognition	• Repeat and simplify instructions. • Provide opportunities for task demonstration and practice. • Present stimuli for longer periods of time. • Allow more time for response. • Extend testing over more than one session. • Use testing materials that are appropriately normed for older population. • Minimize conservative response sets by reducing emphasis upon success. • Allay anxieties about test performance. • Match tasks and environments to attentional capabilities. • Administer MMSE if cognitive impairment is suspected. • See Language section of table.

(continues)

TABLE 10.2 (*continued*)

System	Age-related accommodations in assessment and intervention
Language	• Provide cues when possible or appropriate. • Reduce memory and processing requirements. • Use personally relevant stimuli and tasks. • Use language material that has emotional content. • Use stimuli that are distinctive in some fashion. • Determine and use best modality for language activities. • Use self-paced tasks. • Match therapy to real-life situations as much as possible. • Reduce length and complexity of language used in comprehension or production tasks.
Health	• Schedule testing when person is least likely to be fatigued. • Reduce session length to accommodate fatigue or health problems. • Identify times when medications are administered, and schedule sessions for times of optimal performance. • Schedule multiple short sessions. • Determine the best time of the day to maximize performance.
Environ-mental	• Reduce or eliminate distractions if possible. • Make environment as relaxed and comfortable as possible (not clinically sterile). • See other accommodations noted in the Vision and Hearing sections. • Make recommendations for environmental change if aspects of the environment interfere with communication.
Psycho-social	• Identify and involve significant others as well as those who have the most contact with the client. • Include significant others as much as possible in goal setting and in facilitation of communication. • Allow time for social interaction. • Schedule sessions to avoid conflicts with social activities. • Use materials with age-relevant themes or personal content. • Work with client and significant others to determine functional goals for treatment. • Determine attitudes about needed changes.

Note. AAC = augmentative and alternative communication. MMSE = Mini Mental Status Examination.

Assessment of Aphasia

Basic Considerations and Assessment Goals

Persons with aphasia are usually referred for speech–language evaluation as part of rehabilitation services after a stroke or other neurological incident. Referrals may also come through other healthcare providers, or they may result from the family attending a support group.

Although one would expect referrals to come from physicians, particularly neurologists, this is not always the case. It is still common to find physicians who do not believe speech–language therapy is beneficial to patients with aphasia, despite the fact that efficacy for a number of treatments has been clearly established over the past 20 years (Cherney & Robey, 2008; Simmons-Mackie, Conklin, & Kagan, 2008). This belief may result from the physician expecting language to return to normal, while not recognizing that improvement in communication is a primary treatment target. These same physicians may refer for assessment and treatment of a swallowing disorder. At such times, clinicians must assess linguistic and cognitive skills because those skills influence a client's ability to cooperate in swallowing evaluation and therapy.

Regardless of the reason for referral or referral source, the clinician must be able to identify the basic type and severity of the language disorder, other impairments that may affect treatment, and general prognosis. Ideally, initial evaluation procedures involve significant others and probe how the client and family perceive communicative deficits and their impact on daily life. Common assessment goals include determination of the following:

- presence of aphasia
- type of aphasia (classification)
- related impairments (motor speech)
- nature and severity of deficits in language and cognitive domains
- appropriate treatment priorities
- prognosis
- impact of language deficits on daily activities and interactions and on quality of life

The first goal is particularly important for the elderly. The distinctions between normal aging and mild forms of cognitive and linguistic disorders are not that clear in this age group. Persons with mild cognitive impairment or very early forms of Alzheimer's disease may display word retrieval problems differing only in degree of deficit from those same behaviors in the typical older adult. Word retrieval deficits are also characteristic of aphasia. Older persons may be referred for speech–language evaluation because they or their family members have noted some nonspecific changes in communication. It may be necessary to test other cognitive skills, as well as a mixture of typical left- and right-hemisphere language functions, in order to determine the nature of the underlying deficit. Clinicians must be able to distinguish normal aging changes in language from any of the specific cognitive-communicative and language disorders. Sometimes language changes are the only clues to early dementia.

The last assessment goal is also crucial. Although aphasia is defined by impaired language, language alone does not characterize the experience of living with aphasia. Clinical management of aphasia must consider other factors, such as environment and personal characteristics, as they affect a person's ability to engage in daily activities and participate in desired social contexts and activities. The importance of focusing on daily functioning is highlighted in the life participation approach to aphasia (LPAA) statement of philosophy for service delivery. LPAA defines enhanced life participation as the goal for interventions with persons with aphasia and their significant others (Chapey et al., 2008). This statement acknowledges the chronicity of aphasia and thus the need for services over an extended period of time. If enhanced life participation is the goal, assessment and outcome measures must go beyond language performance to consider quality of life, participation, personal factors, partners, and satisfaction.

During any assessment, the age of a client may influence actual test procedures. Age-related changes in vision, hearing, self-efficacy, and mood can alter test responses, as can primary aging changes in cognitive systems. Other health factors and multiple medications can affect how the elderly respond. It is important to remember how stressful the actual experience of being tested may be. Many older adults have not been asked to complete any kind of formal "test" since they left high school or college. In addition, as noted earlier, some older adults are already fearful about declines in cognition. It is quite common to find that an older client is extremely anxious during initial sessions, and this anxiety can and often does affect performance. Chapter 8 provides clinicians with approaches to minimizing some of these age-related factors.

Assessment Procedures

Given trends in healthcare today, speech–language pathologists rarely have time to complete a battery of aphasia tests. Typically, the emphasis is on providing treatment as quickly as possible using observations and checklists to document status at the beginning of therapy. Choices of initial assessment tests or tasks are influenced primarily by available time, preferred practices in the healthcare setting, and assessment goals.

Case History Information. Ideally, assessment begins with gathering case history information, including medical history related to other health problems or previous neurological events, and information about premorbid cognitive and communicative behaviors. Results of tests such as CT scans and MRIs can provide valuable information about the nature, location, and extent of any brain lesion. Practically, much of this information is not available at the time of initial testing. However, every effort should be made to obtain key history information as early as possible.

Observation and Non-standardized Assessments. Observation is the first and often most important assessment tool available to clinicians. No test is a substitute for observation and reports from the client and significant other. Observations may occur at bedside in acute care or rehabilitation settings, in the therapy room, or in the home. The setting influences performance and should be considered in interpreting outcomes. Speech–language and cognitive domains that should be observed or probed include the following:

- auditory comprehension (different levels of difficulty)
- spontaneous speech (as in conversation and other discourse tasks)
- verbal expression (other elicited behaviors)
- reading and writing
- cognition

Table 10.3 provides examples of behaviors of interest in any assessment observation. When possible, the clinician should make observations unobtrusively and should present specific tasks (such as following commands) in a relaxed, nonthreatening manner.

If comprehensive formal testing is not possible, clinicians can use a combination of observations and administration of a screening test or selected portions of a standardized test to document client status and determine treatment goals. Reimbursement often requires data from a standardized aphasia test battery.

Testing should always have a purpose. Clinician observations of behavior or client or family concerns may guide choice of specific tests to administer. For example, assume hypothetical client John has been evaluated by observation and administration of an aphasia screening test. He and

TABLE 10.3

Assessment Domains for Observation and Probes

Cognitive–linguistic domain	Common assessment tasks
Auditory comprehension (different levels of difficulty)	• Pointing to common environmental objects named or described by the clinician • Answering yes–no questions about personal information, material in the immediate environment, common knowledge, and more abstract content • Following simple and multistep commands • Understanding conversation
Spontaneous speech	• Responding to more open-ended questions (e.g., about stroke, current facility, family) • Performing automatic social behaviors (e.g., greetings and politeness markers) • Participating in conversation (both verbal and nonverbal behaviors; understanding conversational rules about topics and turns, appropriateness, and adequacy of responses) • Sharing a personal story
Verbal expression (elicited)	• Confrontation naming and description of common objects in the environment • Repeating words, phrases, and sentences • Retelling a familiar story (e.g., Cinderella) • Describing a picture (e.g., Cookie Theft)[a] In both spontaneous speech and verbal expression, clinicians should note syntax, fluency, prosody, word retrieval problems, and presence and nature of paraphasias
Written language	• Reading for single words and sentences (demonstrated by selecting correct word based on clinician prompt or by reading aloud) • Reading everyday print material such as a newspaper and then answering questions about the material • Writing name and address, letters, words, and sentences

TABLE 10.3 (*continued*)

Cognitive–linguistic domain	Common assessment tasks
Other cognitive domains: • Attention • Orientation to person, time, and place • Possible visual field deficit or hemispatial neglect • Memory • Visuoperceptual problems • Executive functions (e.g., problem solving)	Language tasks with strong cognitive components: • Answering questions about a short story told by clinician • Telling or retelling a story (with and without delay) • Explaining a joke or figurative phrase Examples of behaviors clinicians should observe to assess cognitive deficits: • Awareness of visual stimuli presented in different parts of the visual field • Observation of effect of ambient noise and interruptions on performance • Memory for information presented at beginning of assessment session

[a]Cookie Theft picture can be found in the *Boston Diagnostic Aphasia Examination* (3rd ed.), by Goodglass, Kaplan, and Baressi (2001).

his family emphasize that reading has been a major priority in his life. The clinician might choose to administer the *Reading Comprehension Battery for Aphasia–2* (RCBA-2; LaPointe & Horner, 1998) to determine where reading comprehension breaks down and to develop focused treatment objectives for reading.

Assessment Instruments. Appendix 10A provides examples of specific test instruments presented in categories based on their primary purpose. A number of assessment tools focus specifically on language. They may be screening tests, comprehensive assessment batteries for aphasia, tests of specific language functions, or tests of language and cognition combined. In addition, functional communication measures are available to explore the impact of language deficits on everyday communication.

However, only functional communication measures provide detailed information about daily activities, interactions, and quality of life. To understand the impact of living with aphasia, clinicians need a framework for determining additional factors of interest. One such framework is the A-FROM (Aphasia: Framework for Outcome Measurement; Kagan & Simmons-Mackie, 2007; Kagan et al., 2007), presented in Figure 10.1.

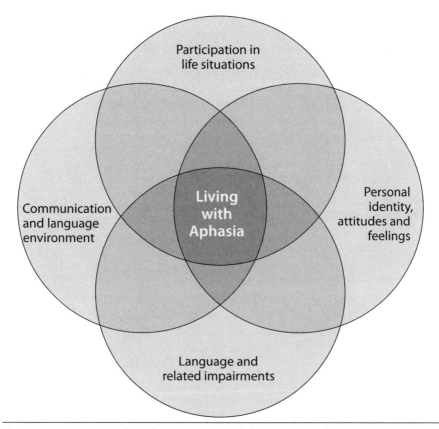

Figure 10.1. Living with Aphasia: Framework for Outcome Measurement (A-FROM). *Note:* From *Aphasia Institute's Living with Aphasia: Framework for Outcome Measurement*, by A. Kagan et al. Copyright 2008 by the Aphasia Institute. Reprinted with permission.

A-FROM was developed to help clinicians understand how life with aphasia is affected by severity of impairment, environment, participation, and personal factors (e.g., identity, feelings, personality). Clinicians can use this framework to determine what should be assessed in order to understand each person's unique experience of living with aphasia. A-FROM is particularly helpful in working with older clients because other primary, secondary, and tertiary age changes are part of the context of a person's life with aphasia.

Based on the A-FROM framework, assessment measures are needed to evaluate quality of life, life satisfaction, well-being, mood and personality, impact of living with aphasia, confidence in communication, activities, participation and barriers to participation, and activities. Caregiver perceptions, needs, burden, and strain should also be examined, as well as the needs and roles played by others in the communication environment. Examples of measures for these domains are included in Appendix 10A. Some instruments are aphasia- or stroke-specific; others are designed for use with a variety of clinical populations. Language difficulties may limit the ability of persons with aphasia to respond on some existing measures of quality of life and daily functioning. It is important to use aphasia-friendly measures or proxy reports of activity, participation, and so on. However, proxy reports are not always accurate barometers of functioning and quality of life. If possible, direct observation of daily activities is helpful.

In evidence-based practice, assessment instruments should be tied directly to desired outcomes. Currently, several Web sites provide clinicians with information on specific assessment tools for various aspects of daily functioning, including psychometric properties such as reliability and validity. One site called Stroke Engine contains information about a variety of stroke-related assessment measures (http://www.medicine.mcgill.ca/Strokengine-assess/).

Aphasia Treatment Approaches

Treatment for aphasia is designed to help clients and significant others communicate as effectively as possible despite language impairment. Interventions may target facilitation of language comprehension and expression, compensation for deficits, or both. In facilitation approaches, the goal is to improve specific skills and the focus is on deficits. Treatment objectives for facilitation are usually framed in terms of improved *accuracy* or *speed* in performing specific language skills like word retrieval or auditory compensation. In contrast, compensation involves using any and all modalities of communication to increase success in communication. The focus is on strengths. For compensation, objectives are framed in terms of *success* with a particular communicative task using available tools such as gesture, drawing, or a communication notebook.

The A-FROM framework makes clear the need to include but go beyond language-specific therapy. Quality of life is the goal. Goal setting is an important aspect of working with individuals living with aphasia. Although clinicians often feel they are best qualified to identify which language systems need to be treated, the goals set by clinicians may be very different from those of the person with aphasia and his or her significant other. Treatment goals should be set collaboratively and should both address client priorities and environmental barriers and include communicative partners (Worrall, Davidson, Hersh, Howe, & Sherratt, 2009). All interventions should be person-centered.

There are numerous approaches for working with people living with aphasia, with considerable overlap in goals across these approaches. Only a few are described briefly here.

Stimulation Approaches

Most clinicians use elements of the stimulation approach to treatment originally developed by Schuell. In these approaches, the clinician manipulates characteristics of stimuli and tasks in order to elicit the best language response from a person with aphasia (Coelho, Sinotte, & Duffy, 2008). Stimulus characteristics that can be manipulated include length, vocabulary (e.g., frequency of occurrence), syntactic complexity, and prosody. Stimuli should be intense, controlled, and typically repetitive; large numbers of responses are desirable. For example, if a client has auditory comprehension problems, the clinician should identify what type of stimulus will allow the client to be successful in a comprehension task, perhaps beginning with short simple commands, presented slowly with key words stressed, and repeated at least once. Once success has been achieved, the clinician reduces one of the supports, such as key word stress, and tries the task again.

Stimulation approaches to aphasia management must take into consideration age-related primary changes in language and cognition. The variables controlled in the stimulation approach to aphasia are those that also affect language performance in the elderly, but aging may have altered the brain's response to cueing, priming, and related processes. Because speed of processing can be reduced for some older adults, less time pressure and slower speaking rates during treatment tasks can facilitate language processing and production. Increased stress on key words should also benefit older clients more than younger. The use of distinctive stimuli (unexpected, unusual) can assist clients experiencing some declines in the ability to inhibit multiple language associations.

Cognitive Interventions

Many aphasia treatment approaches focus primarily on helping the client to understand or use language for basic communication tasks. Therapy activities may not be designed to challenge the client's thinking beyond use of language to label, respond to questions, and so on. In contrast, cognition-based interventions treat the aphasia by working more directly with other cognitive processes that use language systems (Chapey, 2008). The contrast between convergent and divergent thinking illustrates this approach. Convergent operations involve using language in a predictable manner. One example would be a verbal fluency task that asks a client to list animals in a short time interval. The brain is organized around associations like this, and there is no real cognitive challenge beyond the semantic systems. In contrast, a divergent version of that task might involve asking a client to tell all the ways one might use a brick or a baseball bat. This task stimulates other parts of the brain and ties language into other cognitive operations. Cognitive approaches also elicit language for higher order tasks like problem solving or identifying alternatives. Rather than working with a client to develop one way of initiating a conversation, a clinician using cognitive treatment would ask the client to identify as many different ways as possible to accomplish the same task.

Social Approaches

Social approaches to aphasia reflect the shift toward a more functional person-centered perspective on aphasia and its consequences (Simmons-Mackie, 2008). All social approaches share a common emphasis on language functions (information exchange and interaction). Treatment works with language in natural contexts for meaningful purposes, acknowledges the social and personal consequences of aphasia, and accepts and works with the client's perspective (consistent with A-FROM model). Conversation is a primary target. A variety of treatment programs fall under this "social" heading; most involve use of conversation or group interactions, and there is considerable overlap. Many also target the conversational partners of individuals with aphasia. Examples include the following:

- *Partner training and supported conversation* (Kagan, 1998; Lyon, 2000). Supported conversation involves training health professionals, family, friends, and community members to help a person with aphasia to reveal his or her essential communicative competence. The approach involves training in the use of pictures, print, gestures, and other modalities to support communication of a meaningful message to a person with aphasia and to encourage that person to use similar techniques to share his or her thoughts, feelings, and information.
- *Conversational coaching* (Hopper, Holland, & Rewaga, 2002). The clinician takes on the role of coach rather than professional in control. Client objectives and content for conversations are identified, and strategies are developed (some of which involve creating scripts). Interactions are practiced, with the clinician coaching the client through challenges and helping in developing alternative strategies. Coaching

can be particularly helpful in routine activities, where scripts reduce communication failure.

- *Direct conversation therapy* (Simmons-Mackie, 2008). This approach uses conversation as the treatment tool and focuses on developing linguistic and nonverbal behaviors that promote success in meeting a conversation goal. One important component is building confidence through success in natural contexts, which improves well-being and promotes a healthy identity in communicative interactions and relationships.
- *Promoting Aphasics' Communicative Effectiveness* (PACE; Davis, 2005). Many times, language alone cannot achieve the communicative goals of each partner. PACE involves training persons with aphasia and their communication partners to use compensatory strategies in communicative interactions. It is not a treatment program but rather an approach in which the clinician gives up the control that comes with knowing the target language and instead assumes equal responsibility with the client to figure out what strategies work to convey a given message. As with supported conversation, any strategy that leads to successful communication is accepted. PACE can be used with a variety of treatment tasks and stimuli.

Group Treatment Approaches

Group treatment approaches are often considered part of the social approach to aphasia management (Elman, 2007). Group interventions are used to address a variety of outcomes related to living with aphasia. They provide support for persons with aphasia and caregivers, promote strategies for living with aphasia, build conversational and other functional communication skills, and promote empowerment. The social context provided in group settings promotes person-centered life participation goals and activities. Group treatment is particularly valuable once aphasia has become chronic; the interactions that occur in groups allow individuals to improve or modify communicative strategies.

Environmental Intervention

Environment consists of both external and internal physical and social factors that can facilitate or deter communication. Physical factors include inadequate lighting, noise distractions, and inaccessible spaces where interactions occur. Social factors include the people available for communication, their attitudes and interest in communicating, and the activities available as a base for conversation. Environmental interventions begin with assessment of environmental barriers (Lubinski, 2008). Once barriers are identified, clinicians work with persons with aphasia and those in their environment to make needed changes. For example, if family communication typically breaks down in the family room where the TV is always on, an obvious solution is to turn off the TV when communication is attempted. In a nursing home, an environmental barrier might be poor illumination in a resident's room, making it difficult for her or him to process the speech of staff members. Staff could be trained to turn on a brighter light before engaging in any conversation.

Intensive Treatment Approaches

The value of intensive language treatment for aphasia has been debated for many years. More recently, the constraint-induced language treatment (CILT) approach has gained considerable prominence (Raymer, 2009). *Intensive treatment* refers to any intervention that typically involves more than 9 hours (and up to 30 hours) of therapy weekly, although the design of intensive programs varies widely. Both intensive treatment and CILT include massed practice (at least 2–4 hours daily) and daily treatment. CILT adds the use of constraint, requiring the person with aphasia to communicate through verbal channels only (no compensatory strategies). Recent studies provide evidence for the efficacy of intensive treatments and of CILT, although it is not yet clear how important constraint is and which types of aphasia respond best to this treatment (Cherney, Patterson, Raymer, Frymark, & Schooling, 2008).

Language-Specific Interventions

Some treatment approaches target one specific language behavior or set of behaviors. There are treatment programs that systematically address skills such as expressive syntax, word retrieval, reading, writing, and spelling. For example, the anagram and copy treatment for writing starts by presenting clients with cards with the letters needed to form a target word (Beeson & Henry, 2008). Regardless of whether the initial spelling is correct, the client is then asked to copy the word multiple times. Difficulty level is increased by adding foil letters and finally removing all cues. For reading, treatment approaches vary based on the underlying nature and severity of the deficit. One approach targets enhanced attention to improve reading for individuals with mild aphasia (Sinotte & Coehlo, 2007). For word retrieval problems, a semantic features approach has been used extensively

(Boyle & Coehlo, 1995). In this treatment program, clients are helped to generate a variety of semantic features associated with a target word (e.g., category, use, characteristics). These and many other treatments focus on one specific language skill.

Classification-Specific Interventions

Treatments have been developed for specific types of aphasia, like Wernicke's or global. For global aphasia, treatments may begin at the basic level of undifferentiated response (vocalization, eye contact, movement) and then move up a hierarchy of differentiation of response to accurate responses (Peach, 2008). In another approach for global aphasia, Visual Action Therapy (Helm-Estabrooks, Fitzpatrick, & Barresi, 1982), clients are trained systematically to use gestures communicatively by beginning at the level of pairing pictures with objects and moving on to gestural matching.

Behavior-Specific Interventions

Neurological damage brings with it some behaviors that interfere markedly with communicative performance. One such behavior is *perseveration*, the repetition of a previous response when a new one is requested. Because of the disruption caused by perseveration, specific treatment protocols have been designed to reduce its occurrence. One is the Treatment of Aphasic Perseveration (TAP) program, which helps clients bring perseveration to the level of awareness, suppress perseverative responses, and then ask for cues to help in producing more appropriate responses (Helm-Estabrooks, Emery, & Albert, 1987).

Computer-Based Treatments

Computer-based aphasia treatment refers to the use of computers and software to systematically improve communication for persons with aphasia. Katz suggested that there are three broad types of computer interventions (Katz, 2008). The first is computer-only treatment and involves the person with aphasia working alone at a computer, with performance subsequently checked by a supervising clinician who may not be on-site. The second is computer-assisted treatment, during which the clinician and client work together with language software and the clinician provides online guidance. The third form encompasses AAC devices; these are discussed in the next section.

Appendix 10B provides information about the characteristics of each computer-based approach, cautions in using software and products, and examples of specific programs or software. Computer-only and computer-assisted treatments are sometimes delivered through telespeech: The clinician and client are connected by computer via webcam or other form of video hookup. In all of the computer-based approaches, one overriding concern is the familiarity of technology to older clients with aphasia and their families. Other age-related factors, such as sensory impairments, can also adversely affect use of different systems and software.

There are a number of reports of successful efforts to train persons with aphasia to use the Internet and e-mail for communication, support, and information gathering. Although these training initiatives are relatively time and personnel intensive, the outcomes are considered worthwhile. As persons with aphasia become more comfortable with everyday technologies such as the Internet and e-mail, they may also become more receptive to work with treatment and communication software and devices.

Augmentative and Alternative Communication

The third use of computers in aphasia management involves augmentative and alternative communication (AAC). In its broadest sense, AAC includes any technique that supports a person's communication. Appendix 10B provides examples of AAC systems and software currently available for persons with aphasia. An AAC device is sometimes referred to as a *speech generating device*.

Older adults who have acquired aphasia may encounter a number of barriers to use of such a device for communication. The first has already been noted: potential lack of familiarity with computers and technology. The second is specific to aphasia. Aphasia is considered a disorder that affects comprehension and production of language symbols. AAC systems depend on symbols, including not only print words but also pictographs that represent words or messages. Impairments in symbol usage may extend to AAC devices. A third barrier is aphasia's abrupt onset. One minute the person can talk and communicate, the next minute he or she cannot. For most people, the overriding goal in the early stages of recovery is to understand and talk again in a manner comparable to pre-stroke communication. This drive to talk can be a remarkably difficult barrier to overcome. This barrier tends to be even more challenging when the person with aphasia is an older adult with more years of experience talking and limited understanding of the communicative benefits of technology.

Levels or types of communicators have been defined for persons with aphasia (Lasker & Garrett, 2008). These levels describe what a person's AAC needs might be at each level, techniques for providing AAC tools to maximize communication, and strategies for helping the individual become more independent as a communicator. The *Multimodal Communication Screening Test for Aphasia* (MCSTA) can be downloaded and used by clinicians to identify levels (Garrett & Lasker, 2005).

Caregiver Interventions

The abrupt onset of a communication disorder such as aphasia, coupled with other losses of function that may be caused by a stroke, leaves everyone stunned and unsure what to expect. Communication is usually the tool families use to work through difficult situations, share concerns, affirm relationships, and develop strategies to adapt to changes. Aphasia limits the use of that tool. Adjusting to the many life changes that follow, including having to assume the role of caregiver, can be challenging to family members and significant others.

Adjustment to life with aphasia does not happen quickly, and the effects of communication loss are far reaching. Caregivers need education and support for weeks, months, and sometimes years. Their goals change over time, as do the goals of the person with aphasia. Early caregiver goals involve maintaining hope, obtaining some respite, and taking care of their own health (Worrall, 2008; Worrall, Davidson, Ferguson, Hersh, & Howe, 2007). Basic communication is desired at that stage. Later, family members may begin to feel social isolation and express concerns about getting services for the person with aphasia or helping him or her become more independent.

Speech–language pathologists may provide education and individual counseling with respect to the communication changes being experienced, strategies to manage communication breakdown, and validation of feelings and fears of the family member. Sometimes, even the most basic information about aphasia or stroke is not provided during the early days and weeks. Simply referring a caregiver to a Web site or other source of information about aphasia can make a difference.

Caregivers also need support from others who understand their situation. Speech–language pathologists often see clients and their families long after other medical and therapeutic services have ended and can recognize when a family member needs more resources. At that time, referral to some form of support group is appropriate. Some caregivers prefer to join online support forums, while others are willing to participate in a face-to-face support group. It is important to recognize that not all caregivers, particularly older spouses, may feel comfortable with the idea of a support group. Healthcare providers should encourage caregivers to participate without pressuring them. Support groups may be offered for caregivers

only, or for bo   a speech–
language path   𝒴𝒸𝒮 ↓   itator with
someone with

Reimbursement

A physician must write an order for speech–language evaluation and treatment for persons with aphasia and other acquired neurological communication disorders. Under current Medicare provisions, speech–language and physical therapy services combined have an annual benefit cap, although exceptions can be granted if medical necessity for additional services is clearly documented. This cap is a particular challenge with disorders such as aphasia that require more extensive treatment to improve communicative functioning. Many of the interventions described in this chapter are used months and sometimes years after the onset of aphasia. Alternate mechanisms for funding may need to be identified by clients, family members, and clinicians.

Assessment of aphasia has a Current Procedural Terminology (CPT) code (American Medical Association [AMA], 2009a) distinct from the code for the wider range of speech, language, and auditory processing problems. The aphasia CPT code covers formal assessment of expressive and receptive speech and language functions (including reading and writing) with a recognized aphasia test battery. The focus of the evaluation must be on the client's level of functioning, what he or she wants to be able to do, and those factors that may affect performance of desired activities. The evaluation report should state whether treatment is needed. If treatment is recommended, there must be a statement of prognosis for return to pre-morbid status or of maximum anticipated change within a given time frame. There is no code for retesting; any repeat administration of parts of a test should be documented and billed as therapy. Billing is charged per hour and includes interpretation and report writing.

Other CPT codes are available for specialized evaluations:

- *Standardized cognitive assessment.* This code covers administration of standardized cognitive tests (either norm-referenced or criterion-referenced), along with interpretation and report writing. Billing is also per hour for this code.
- *Evaluation for prescription of speech-generating devices.* This code covers evaluation of all language modalities, communication

strategies, and other skills (e.g., motor, visual, hearing) in order to determine the ability to operate and effectively use a speech-generating device or aid. One procedure code is used for the first hour of evaluation, and another code is used for additional 30-minute evaluation sessions on separate days. Evaluation for prescription of a non–speech-generating AAC device should use the basic evaluation code for speech–language, voice, and communication. A separate series of Healthcare Common Procedure Coding System (HCPCS) codes (AMA, 2009b) identifies the actual equipment or devices being considered. The codes differentiate between the type of speech (digitized, synthesized) and presence and duration of prerecorded messages. These codes must be used in any prescription for an AAC device. Therapy services for persons with aphasia must target reduction of impairment or improvement of functions. Documentation of improvement must be specific, measurable, and functional. Progress should be compared to baseline evaluation results and to performance in previous sessions. Defining levels of cueing or factors such as complexity and environmental challenges make it easier to show measurable change. Clinicians should avoid nonspecific wording such as "continue treatment plan." CPT codes that may apply to treatment include the following services:

Speech–language treatment. This is the code for individual therapy sessions and for training for use of a non–speech generating device. The code can also be used for maintenance programs designed to preserve a client's level of functioning or prevent decline. Documentation is critical in maintenance programs, which are typically short-term. Ongoing cycles of termination of therapy and readmission for maintenance typically are not funded.

Group treatment. A group is defined as two to four patients seen at one time. Services must be documented to be reasonable and necessary, and group therapy can be no more than 25% of a patient's total treatment program. Support groups are not reimbursable under this code (or any code).

Cognitive skills development. In some instances, the therapy being provided focuses primarily on cognitive skills

such as attention, memory, and problem solving. This CPT code should be used in those circumstances.
Therapeutic services for use of speech-generating device. This code includes programming and modification services.

Key Points

This chapter described the most common type of secondary aging of language systems: aphasia. The many forms of aphasia, as well as assessment and treatment approaches, were reviewed. The effects of aging on aphasia, as well as tertiary aging influences on functioning post-stroke, were identified. Major themes included the following:

- Subtle normal changes in language may be difficult to differentiate from disorders like mild cognitive impairment or mild aphasia, which is why clinicians must understand normal aging.
- There are many types of aphasia and it is not possible to understand the impact of aphasia without considering the environment, the person's premorbid characteristics, desired activities and level of participation, and significant others.
- It may not be possible to perform a standardized battery of tests to assess a person with aphasia, but observation of key behaviors can provide critical information for treatment and prognosis.
- The goal of aphasia treatment should be improved communication and quality of life, even if language impairment continues.
- Aphasia treatments involve facilitation of language skills or compensation for deficits.
- Aphasia treatments should also target significant others, environmental barriers, and activity limitations. Caregiver interventions are particularly important.

References

American Medical Association. (2009a). *Current procedural terminology 2010*. Chicago: Author.

American Medical Association. (2009b). *Healthcare common procedure coding system 2010: Level II*. Chicago: Author.

Babbitt, E., & Cherney, L. R. (2009, March). *Aphasia treatment research at RIC: Clinical application*. Presentation at the annual conference of the Mississippi Speech-Language-Hearing Association, Jackson, MS.

Beeson, P. M., & Henry, M. L. (2008). Comprehension and production of written words. In R. Chapey (Ed.), *Language intervention strategies in aphasia and related neurogenic communication disorders* (6th ed., pp. 654–686). Philadelphia: Lippincott Williams & Wilkins.

Blackstone, S., & Berg, M. (2003). *Social networks: A communication inventory for individuals with complex communication needs and their communication partners.* Monterey, CA: Augmentative Communication.

Boyle, M., & Coelho, C. A. (1995). Application of semantic features analysis as a treatment for aphasic dysnomia. *American Journal of Speech-Language Pathology, 4,* 94–98.

Brookshire, R. H., & Nicholas, L. E. (1997). *The discourse comprehension test.* Minneapolis, MN: BRK.

Burns, M. (1979). *Burns brief inventory of communication and cognition.* San Antonio, TX: Psych Corp.

Caserta, M. S., Lund, D. A., & Wright, S. D. (1996). Exploring the Caregiver Burden Inventory: Further evidence for a multidimensional view of burden. *International Journal of Aging and Human Development, 43,* 21–34.

Chapey, R. (2008). Cognitive stimulation: Stimulation of recognition/comprehension, memory and convergent, divergent, and evaluative thinking. In R. Chapey (Ed.), *Language intervention strategies in aphasia and related neurogenic communication disorders* (6th ed., pp. 469–506). Philadelphia: Lippincott Williams & Wilkins.

Chapey, R., Duchan, J. F., Elman, R. J., Garcia, L. J., Kagan, A., Lyon, J G., et al. (2008). Life-participation approach to aphasia: A statement of values for the future. In R. Chapey (Ed.), *Language intervention strategies in aphasia and related neurogenic communication disorders* (6th ed., pp. 279–289). Philadelphia: Lippincott Williams & Wilkins.

Cherney, L. R., Patterson, J. P., Raymer A., Frymark, T., & Schooling, T. (2008). Evidence-based systematic review: Effects of intensity of treatment and constraint-induced language therapy with stroke-induced aphasia. *Journal of Speech, Language, and Research, 51,* 1282–1299.

Cherney, L. R., & Robey, R. R. (2008). Aphasia treatment: Recovery, prognosis, and clinical effectiveness. In R. Chapey (Ed.), *Language intervention strategies in aphasia and related neurogenic communication disorders* (6th ed., pp. 186–202). Philadelphia: Lippincott Williams & Wilkins.

Coelho, C. A., Sinotte, M. P., & Duffy, J. (2008). Schuell's stimulation approach to rehabilitation. In R. Chapey (Ed.), *Language intervention strategies in aphasia and related neurogenic communication disorders* (6th ed., pp.403–449). Philadelphia: Lippincott Williams & Wilkins.

Davis, G. A. (2005). PACE revisited. *Aphasiology, 19,* 21–38.

Doyle, P., McNeil, M., Hula, W., & Mikolic, J. (2003). The burden of stroke scale: Validating patient-reported communication difficulty and associated psychological distress in stroke survivors. *Aphasiology, 17,* 291–304.

Duncan, P. W., Wallace, D., Lai, S. M., Dallas, J., Embretson, S., & Laster, L. J. (1999). The stroke impact scale version 2.0: Evaluation of reliability, validity, and sensitivity to change. *Stroke, 30,* 2131–2140.

Elman, R. J. (Ed.) (2007). *Group treatment of neurogenic communication disorders: The expert clinician's approach.* San Diego, CA: Plural.

Enderby, P., Wood, Y., & Wade, D. (2006). *Frenchay aphasia screening test* (2nd ed.). Hoboken, NJ: John Wiley & Sons.

Fitch-West, J., & Sands, E. S. (1998). *Bedside evaluation screening test* (2nd ed.). Austin, TX: PRO-ED.

Fleming, V. B. (2009, May). *Comprehension and aging: The mediating effects of executive function.* Paper presented at the annual Clinical Aphasiology Conference, Keystone, CO.

Folstein, M. F., & Luria, R. (1973). Reliability, validity, and clinical application of the Visual Analogue Mood Scales. *Psychological Medicine, 3,* 479–486.

Frattali, C., Holland, A. L., Thompson C. K., Wohl, C. B., & Ferketic, M. M. (1995). *American Speech-Language-Hearing Association functional assessment of communication skills for adults.* Rockville, MD: American Speech-Language-Hearing Association.

Garrett, K. L., & Lasker, J. P. (2005). *The multimodal communication screening test for persons with aphasia.* Retrieved August 1, 2009, from http://aac.unl.edu/screen/screen.html

Goodglass, H., Kaplan, E., & Baressi, B. (2001). *Boston diagnostic aphasia examination* (3rd ed.). Baltimore: Lippincott Williams & Wilkins.

Helm-Estabrooks, N. (2001). *Cognitive linguistic quick test.* San Antonio, TX: Psych Corp.

Helm-Estabrooks, N., Emery, P., & Albert, M. L. (1987). Treatment of aphasic perseveration program: A new approach to aphasia therapy. *Archives of Neurology, 4,* 1253–1255.

Helm-Estabrooks, N., Fitzpatrick, P., & Barresi, B. (1982). Visual action therapy for global aphasia. *Journal of Speech and Hearing Disorders, 47,* 385–389.

Hilari, K., Byng, S., Lamping, D., & Smith, S. (2003). Stroke and aphasia quality of life scale–39: Evaluation of acceptability, reliability, and validity. *Stroke, 34,* 1944–1950.

Holbrook, M., & Skilbeck, C. E. (1983). An activities index for use with stroke patients. *Age and Aging, 12,* 166–170.

Holland, A. L., Frattali, C. M., & Fromm, D. (1999) *Communication activities of daily living* (2nd ed.). Austin, TX: PRO-ED.

Hopper, T., Holland, A., & Rewaga, M. (2002). Conversational coaching: Treatment outcomes and future directions. *Aphasiology, 16,* 745–762.

Kagan, A. (1998). Supported conversation for adults with aphasia: Methods and resources for training conversation partners. *Aphasiology, 12,* 816–830.

Kagan, A., & Simmons-Mackie, S. (2007). Beginning with the end: Outcome-driven assessment and intervention with life participation in mind. *Topics in Language Disorders, 27,* 309–317.

Kagan, A., Simmons-Mackie, N., Rowland, A., Huijbregts, M., Shumway, E., McEwen, S., et al. (2007). Counting what counts: A framework for capturing real-life outcomes of aphasia intervention. *Aphasiology, 22,* 258–280.

Kaplan, E., Goodglass, H., & Weintraub, S. (2001). The Boston naming test (2nd ed.). Philadelphia: Lippincott Williams & Wilkins.Katz, R. C. (2008). Computer applications in aphasia treatment. In R. Chapey (Ed.), *Language intervention strategies in aphasia and related neurogenic communication disorders* (6th ed., pp. 852–876). Philadelphia: Lippincott Williams & Wilkins.

Keenan, J., & Brassell, E. G. (1975). *Aphasia language performance scales.* Murfreesboro, TN: Pinnacle Press.

Kertesz, A. (1982). *Western aphasia battery.* New York: Grune and Stratton.

Kertesz, A. (2006). *Western aphasia battery* (Enhanced). San Antonio, TX: Psych Corp.

LaPointe, L. L., & Horner, J. (1998). *Reading comprehension battery for aphasia* (2nd ed.). Austin, TX: PRO-ED.

Lasker, J. P., & Garrett, K. L. (2008). Aphasia and AAC: Enhancing communication across health care settings. *The ASHA Leader, 13*, 10–13.

Lawton, M. P., Kleban, M. H., Moss, M., Rovine, M., & Glicksman, A. (1989). Measuring caregiving appraisal. *Journal of Gerontology: Psychological Sciences, 44*, 61–71.

Lazarus, R., & Folkman, S. (1984). *Stress, appraisal, and coping.* New York: Springer.

Lomas, J., Pickard, L., Bester, S., Elbard, H., Finlayson, A., & Zoghaib, C. (1989). The communication effectiveness index: Development and psychometric evaluation of a functional communication measure for adult aphasia. *Journal of Speech and Hearing Disorders, 54*, 113–124.

Lubinski, R. (2008). Environmental approach to adult aphasia. In R. Chapey (Ed.), *Language intervention strategies in aphasia and related neurogenic communication disorders* (6th ed., pp. 319–348). Philadelphia: Lippincott Williams & Wilkins.

Lyon, J. (2000). Finding, defining, and refining functionality in real-life for people confronting aphasia. In L. Worrall & C. Frattali (Eds.), *Neurogenic communication disorders: A functional approach* (pp. 137–161). New York: Thieme.

McNeil, M. R., & Prescott, T. E. (1978). *Revised token test.* Austin, TX: PRO-ED.

Novak, M., & Guest, C. (1989). Application of a multidimensional caregiver burden inventory. *The Gerontologist, 29*, 798–803.

Peach, R. K. (2008). Global aphasia: Identification and management. In R. Chapey (Ed.), *Language intervention strategies in aphasia and related neurogenic communication disorders* (6th ed., pp. 565–594). Philadelphia: Lippincott Williams & Wilkins.

Porch, B. E. (1967). *Porch index of communicative ability: Theory and development.* (Vol. 1). Palo Alto, CA: Consulting Psychologists Press.

Radloff, L. S. (1977). The CES-D scale: A self-report depression scale for research in the general population. *Applied Psychological Measurement, 1*, 385–401.

Raymer, A. (2009). Constraint-induced language therapy: A systematic review. *The ASHA Leader, 14*, 26–27.

Ryff, C. D., & Singer, B. (1998). The contours of positive human health. *Psychological Inquiry, 9*, 1–28.

Schuell, H. (1965). *The Minnesota test for differential diagnosis of aphasia.* Minneapolis: University of Minnesota Press.

Shewan, C. N. (1979). *Auditory comprehension test for sentences.* Chicago: Biolinguistics Institutes.

Simmons-Mackie, N. (2008). Social approaches to aphasia. In R. Chapey (Ed.), *Language intervention strategies in aphasia and related neurogenic communication disorders* (6th ed., pp. 290–318). Philadelphia: Lippincott Williams & Wilkins.

Simmons-Mackie, N., Conklin, J., & Kagan, A. (2008). Think tank deliberates future directions for the social approach to aphasia. *Perspectives on Neurophysiology and Neurogenic Speech and Language Disorders, 18*, 24–32.

Sinotte, M. P., & Coelho, C. A. (2007). Attention training for reading impairment in mild aphasia. *NeuroRehabilitation, 22*, 303–310.

Stern, R. A. (1997). *Visual analog mood scales.* Lutz, FL: Psychological Assessment Resources.

Sutcliffe, L. M., & Lincoln, N. B. (1998). The assessment of depression in aphasic stroke patients: The development of the Stroke Aphasic Depression Questionnaire. *Clinical Rehabilitation, 12*, 506–513.

Swinburn, K., & Byng, S. (2006). *Communication disability profile*. London, England: Connect Press.

Swinburn, K., Porter, G., & Howard, D. (2004). *Comprehensive aphasia test*. Hove, East Sussex, UK: Psychology Press.

Van der Meulen, I., Van de Sandt-Koenderman, W., Duivenvoorden, H. J., & Ribbers, G. M. (2010). Measuring verbal and non-verbal communication in aphasia: Reliability, validity, and sensitivity to the Scenario Test. *International Journal of Language and Communication Disorders, 45,* 424–435.

Vitaliano, P. P., Russo, J., Carr J. E., Maiuro, R. D., & Becker, J. (1985). The ways of coping checklist: Revision and psychometric properties. *Multivariate Behavioral Research, 20,* 3–26.

Williams, L. S., Weinberger, M., Harris, L., Clark, D., & Biller, J. (1999). Development of a stroke-specific quality of life scale. *Stroke, 30,* 1362–1369.

Worrall, L. (1999). *The everyday communication needs assessment*. London: Winslow Press.

Worrall, L. (2008, November). *Principal principles of the social model in aphasia: Our research and clinical tools*. Mini-seminar presented at the Annual Convention of the American Speech-Language-Hearing Association, Chicago, IL.

Worrall, L., Davidson, B., Ferguson, A., Hersh, D., & Howe, T. (2007, November). *What people with aphasia want: Goal-setting in aphasia rehabilitation*. Mini-seminar presented at the Annual Convention of the American Speech-Language-Hearing Association, Boston, MA.

Worrall, L., Davidson, B., Hersh, D., Howe, T., & Sherratt, S. (2009, May). *What do people with aphasia and their families want? Introducing the Goals in Aphasia Protocol*. Workshop presented at the 2009 Advancing Speech Pathology Innovation, Research, and Excellence Speech Pathology Australia National Conference, Adelaide, South Australia.

Yesavage, J. A., Brink, T. L., Rose, T. L., Lum, O., Huang, V., Adey, M. B., et al. (1983). Development and validation of a geriatric depression screening scale: A preliminary report. *Journal of Psychiatric Research, 17,* 37–49.

Zarit, S. H., Reever, K. E., & Bach-Peterson, J. (1980). Relatives of the impaired elderly: Correlates of feelings of burden. *The Gerontologist, 20,* 649–655.

Examples of Standardized and Non-standardized Assessment Instruments to Assess Living with Aphasia

Language and related cognitive impairment instruments	Examples
Bedside or screening tests of aphasia	• *Aphasia Language Performance Scales* (Keenan & Brassell, 1975) • *Bedside Evaluation Screening Test–2* (Fitch-West & Sands, 1998) • *Frenchay Aphasia Screening Test–2* (Enderby, Wood, & Wade, 2006)
Comprehensive aphasia assessment instruments	• *Western Aphasia Battery and Western Aphasia Battery–Enhanced* (Kertesz, 1982, 2006) • *Boston Diagnostic Aphasia Examination–3* (Goodglass, Kaplan, & Baressi, 2001) • *Porch Index of Communicative Ability* (Porch, 1967) • *Minnesota Test for Differential Diagnosis of Aphasia* (Schuell, 1965)
Tests of specific language functions:	
Auditory comprehension of sentences	• *Auditory Comprehension Test for Sentences* (Shewan, 1979)
Reading comprehension from words to paragraphs	• *Reading Comprehension Battery for Aphasia–2* (LaPointe & Horner, 1998)
Single-word picture naming	• *Boston Naming Test* (Kaplan, Goodglass, & Weintraub, 2001)
High-level auditory comprehension	• *Revised Token Test* (McNeil & Prescott, 1978)
Discourse understanding	• *Discourse Comprehension Test* (Brookshire & Nicholas, 1997)
Tests of language and cognition combined	• *Burns Brief Inventory of Communication and Cognition* (Burns, 1979) • *Western Aphasia Battery–Enhanced* (Kertesz, 2006) • *Cognitive Linguistic Quick Test* (Helm-Estabrooks, 2001) • *Comprehensive Aphasia Test* (Swinburn, Porter, & Howard, 2004).

Examples of Standardized and Non-standardized
Assessment Instruments to Assess Living with Aphasia (*continued*)

Language and related cognitive impairment instruments	Examples
Functional communication measures	• *ASHA-Functional Assessment of Communication Skills for Adults* (Frattali, Holland, Thompson, Wohl, & Ferketic, 1995) • *Communication Activities of Daily Living–2* (Holland, Frattali, & Fromm, 1999) • *Communication Effectiveness Index* (Lomas et al., 1989)

Additional assessment domains	Examples of assessment tools
Living with stroke or aphasia (impact, disability, functioning)	• *Communication Disability Profile* (Swinburn & Byng, 2006) • *Burden of Stroke Scale* (Doyle, McNeil, Hula, & Mikolic, 2003) • *Stroke Impact Scale Version 2.0* (Duncan et al., 1999) • *Assessment of Living with Aphasia* (Kagan & Simmons-Mackie, 2007) • *Communication Confidence Rating Scale for Aphasia* (Babbitt & Cherney, 2009)
Quality of life	• *Stroke Specific Quality of Life Scale* (Williams, Weinberger, Harris, Clark, & Biller, 1999) • *Stroke and Aphasia Quality of Life Scale* (Hilari, Byng, Lamping, & Smith, 2003).
Mood (depression or other)	• *Center for Epidemiologic Studies Depression Scale* (Radloff, 1977) • *Geriatric Depression Scale* (Yesavage et al., 1983) • *Visual Analog Mood Scales* (Folstein & Luria, 1977; Stern, 1997) • *Stroke Aphasic Depression Questionnaire* (Sutcliffe & Lincoln, 1998)
Well-being (caregiver or person with aphasia)	• *Ryff Scales of Psychological Well-Being* (Ryff & Singer, 1998)
Communication partners and participation	• *Social Networks: A Communication Inventory for Individuals with Complex Communication Needs and Their Communication Partners* (Blackstone & Berg, 2003)

(*continues*)

Examples of Standardized and Non-standardized
Assessment Instruments to Assess Living with Aphasia (*continued*)

Additional assessment domains	Examples of assessment tools
Communicative needs	• *Everyday Communication Needs Assessment* (Worrall, 1999)
Communication activities	• *Frenchay Activities Index* (Holbrook & Skilbeck, 1983)
Communication goals	• *Goals in Aphasia Protocol* (Worrall, Davidson, Hersh, Howe, & Sherratt, 2009)
Participation	• *Rijndam Scenario Test* (van der Meulen, van de Sandt-Koenderman, Mieke, Duivenvoorden, & Ribbers, 2010)

Caregiver:
   Stress and strain
   Burden
   Physical and emotional well-being
	• *Caregiver Appraisal Measure* (Lawton, Kleban, Moss, Rovine, & Glicksman, 1989)
	• *Zarit Burden Interview* (Zarit, Reever, & Bach-Peterson, 1980)
	• *Ways of Coping Checklist* (Lazarus & Folkman, 1984; Vitaliano, Russo, Carr, Maiuro, & Becker, 1985)
	• *Caregiver Burden Inventory* (Novak & Guest, 1989; Caserta, Lund, & Wright, 1996)

Computer-Based Aphasia Treatments

Type of computer-based treatment	Description of approach and caveats	Software programs or companies
Computer-only treatment	Client works alone at computer (typically at home), with clinician checking performance at different times. Ideally, software is selected by the clinician and all changes are made with clinician guidance. Common language skills targeted include reading, writing, auditory comprehension, and expressive language, if client can imitate and repeat. Users typically download or purchase software or buy a license to use. Caveats: • All aspects of language cannot be practiced on a computer (e.g., spoken word retrieval). • Programs are not always purchased or used with guidance from an SLP. Lack of SLP monitoring may lead to client frustration, loss of motivation, and sense of failure.	Companies producing software for cognitive and linguistic deficits: • Parrot Software (www.parrotsoftware.com) • Bungalow Software (www.bungalowsoftware.com) • Aphasia Therapy Products (CHAT or Computerized Home Aphasia Therapy program; www.aphasia-therapy.com) • Crick Software (www.cricksoftware.com) • BrainTrain (www.braintrain.com)
Computer-assisted treatment	Clinician and client work together with language software. Clinician provides online guidance to ensure that treatment is flexible and responsive to client responses. Caveats: • Computer-assisted treatment programs are not appropriate for all clients. Clinicians must adhere to described criteria for program and levels of difficulty within programs. • Other age-related considerations include familiarity and comfort with computers, visual or hearing problems, and motivation. Basic training with computers and technology may be needed before a client can work with specific software.	Software programs: • MossTalk Words—Naming deficits (include virtual therapist as part of software) • AphasiaScripts (or Computerized Conversational Script Training)—Development/practice with scripts used in daily conversations (includes virtual therapist) • Sentactics—Targets comprehension and production of complex syntactic forms • Oral Reading for Language in Aphasia (ORLA) —For reading comprehension using phonological and semantic reading pathways (includes virtual therapist)

(continues)

Computer-Based Aphasia Treatments (*continued*)

Type of computer-based treatment	Description of approach and caveats	Software programs or companies
Alternative and augmentative communication (AAC)	AAC is any technique that supplements or replaces spoken language for communication purposes. In the context of computer-based treatment, AAC refers to use of computerized devices or software programs to help the client communicate with others. Caveats: • Older adults may not be familiar or comfortable with computers and technology. • AAC systems may be difficult to use easily because they depend on symbols (e.g., print, pictographic icons). • Use of AAC may be seen as giving up on verbal communication.	All major manufacturers of AAC technology report systems beneficial for persons with aphasia. Devices and software designed specifically for aphasia include the following: • Computer-Aided Visual Communication (C-ViC)—Basic communication software for persons with severe aphasia. Success depends heavily on nature and extent of underlying lesions. • Lingraphica—AAC system. Facilitates use of phrases and selection of key content in everyday communication. It was also designed as a treatment tool with multiple levels of speech exercises for rehearsal and repetition.

End-of-Life Planning and Care Considerations

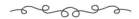

Gillian Woods, Mary Ann Westphal,
and Alan D. Gluth

CHAPTER 11 ADDRESSES END-OF-LIFE care from the perspective of legal planning and actual end-of-life services and needs. Written by a clinical psychologist and two attorneys, the chapter begins with an overview of legal precedents for end-of-life decision making and the right to die. Westphal and Gluth describe advanced directives and other legal documents used in estate planning and for empowering legal representatives. Healthcare professionals must understand these legal documents; an example of the failure to understand or comply with the legal wishes of an older person is provided. The chapter closes with Woods's discussion of the needs of individuals who are dying, as well as their loved ones and healthcare professionals. Types of available services, including hospice, are described. Emphasis is placed on the role of speech–language pathologists (SLPs) in end-of-life care and on the emotional challenges some healthcare providers may experience.

Legal Considerations for Medical Decisions

Any textbook on aging should address issues related to end-of-life care. The aging process inherently generates the need for individual decision making with respect to a number of complex end-of-life issues. The potentially difficult and controversial nature of some of these issues is such that strong legal implications have evolved to ensure that the lawful wishes of each individual are clearly outlined and honored. Knowledge of these issues is particularly relevant to the practice of clinicians who care for the aging population. In the first portion of this chapter, a concise discussion of key end-of-life legal topics is undertaken.

Background: End-of-Life Decisions and the Right to Die

As medical knowledge and technology advance, doctors are increasingly able to prolong the process of dying through the use of drugs, medical equipment, and medical procedures. The question that has inevitably surfaced is, "Does the dying person have the right to refuse medical treatment designed to prolong life?" Stated another way, do we have a right to die?

It is only within the last 40 years that the courts have addressed this issue. Historically, the first "right to die" case to reach national prominence was that of Karen Ann Quinlan in 1975. Ms. Quinlan was placed on a ventilator after falling into a coma. Her parents eventually asked the hospital to remove the ventilator. The hospital refused. Her parents filed suit to have the life support removed. When the case reached the New Jersey Supreme Court, the court agreed with Ms. Quinlan's parents, finding that Ms. Quinlan's constitutionally guaranteed right of privacy included a right to have the ventilator removed (*Quinlan*, 1976).

Fifteen years later, the first case on this issue reached the United States Supreme Court. In 1983, Nancy Cruzan was involved in an automobile accident that left her in a permanent vegetative state. Her life was maintained by a tube that provided nutrition and hydration. After 4 years, her parents, believing their daughter would not have wanted to live in this condition, filed suit to have her life support removed. After 3 years of litigation in the lower courts, the case reached the U.S. Supreme Court (*Cruzan v. Dir., MO Dept. of Health*, 1990). The Supreme Court refused to grant the parents' wishes because it found insufficient evidence concerning Ms. Cruzan's wishes on the withdrawal of artificial hydration and nutrition. The case was, however, historic because in its discussion our highest court recognized a legal right to die. To exercise that right, the court required "clear and convincing evidence" of the dying person's wishes, made at a time when the individual is competent to express them. The court also recognized the right of an agent to act in these matters on behalf of an incapacitated person.

The law set out in the Cruzan case was reinforced in the more recent case involving Terri Schiavo (*Schiavo v. Schiavo*, 2005). This case had its beginnings in Florida in 1990 when Ms. Schiavo, seemingly healthy and in the prime of her life at age 27, suffered a heart attack that left her severely brain damaged. She never regained consciousness, and over the next 8 years her condition deteriorated to what is commonly referred to as a "persistent vegetative state." She had no cognition or awareness of her surroundings, much of the cerebral cortex of her brain was gone, and her movements were reflexive. No known medical treatment existed to reverse her condition.

Her husband, acting as her court-appointed guardian, petitioned the court in May 1998 to have her feeding tube removed. He presented evidence, through the testimony of family and friends, that his wife had not wanted her life to be maintained in this way. Despite the vigorous objection of Ms. Schiavo's parents, the trial judge found that clear and convincing evidence had been presented of Ms. Schiavo's desires. In 2000, the judge ordered the tubes be removed, and Ms. Schiavo's parents appealed.

This case is important not only because it ultimately reinforced the law previously set out in Cruzan but also because it highlights the emotional and legal turmoil that may surround end-of-life decisions. In 2003, when all appellate avenues had been exhausted and the decision of the trial court to remove the feeding tube was affirmed, it was removed. End of story? No. The Florida legislature got involved and immediately passed a law that allowed Governor Jeb Bush to order the feeding tube reinserted, which he did. The parties went back to court, this time over the constitutionality of the new Florida law. After 2 more years and a trip to the United States Supreme Court, the Florida law was determined to be unconstitutional and the decision of the original Florida trial court was implemented. On March 18, 2005, Ms. Schiavo's feeding tube was disconnected and she died 13 days later.

The following sections discuss specific legal documents individuals should consider executing as a part of their personal estate planning. Most of the documents relate to medical matters; therefore, healthcare practitioners should be knowledgeable of the restrictions they place on the services provided. It is important to note that laws vary from state to state and that the terms, conditions, and forms used by each state may differ for the documents discussed. An individual should consult with an attorney in his or her state who specializes in estate planning law to ensure that the proper documents are prepared and executed in order to cover all medically related decision making.

Advanced Directives

People usually cannot predict when they will be unable to make decisions for themselves or when end-of-life care decisions will be necessary.

It makes many people uncomfortable to think about these issues, so they may be reluctant to discuss the issues with family members or healthcare providers. *Advanced directives* are the legal documents that convey the person's wishes regarding the medical care they do or do not want if they become unable to make those decisions.

Living Will

The three cases discussed previously—Quinlan, Cruzan, and Schiavo—have one important element in common. In each of them, the court wanted "clear and convincing evidence" of the desires of the dying person. To address this need, after the Quinlan case in 1975, many state legislatures enacted "right to die" laws that establish the framework for a written expression of an individual's wishes. The document that sets out these provisions is often called a *living will*. Because each state has its own laws in this area, it is best to consult the laws of the state of residence before executing a living will. It is important to remember that a living will does not replace the actual wishes of a person competent to state them. It serves only to state the wishes of a person who is no longer able to communicate them, when the decision has to be made by someone else on the patient's behalf.

Although the laws differ, in general, they give individuals the right to refuse medical treatment that would prolong the process of dying in the event of "imminent death" or "permanent unconsciousness." Such treatment generally includes the use of mechanical or artificial means to restore, sustain, or replace a bodily function without which the person would die. Two of the previously described cases centered on provision of nutrition and hydration through a feeding tube. Feeding tubes do not support life in the same way as other mechanisms, such as ventilation. Removal of artificial ventilation results in death within minutes; removal of a feeding tube may take days or weeks. Due to the unique issues posed by feeding tubes, individuals should specifically designate their wishes regarding artificial nutrition.

Healthcare Power of Attorney

A different medical situation presents itself when a person who is *not* facing imminent death or a persistent vegetative state is nonetheless incapable of making medical decisions when they must be made. A person in a coma or a person who has suffered a stroke, heart attack, or other debilitating condition, or someone with advanced dementia, may be unable to make and communicate medical decisions. To address this possibility, state legislatures have enacted laws authorizing an individual to appoint an agent to act for him or her in these circumstances. The document that puts this into place is alternately called a *healthcare power of attorney, healthcare directive, medical power of attorney, healthcare proxy,* or *durable power of attorney for healthcare.*

The healthcare power of attorney must be established when the person is competent. Healthcare professionals should be aware that it becomes effective *only* during incapacity. The healthcare power of attorney is designed to serve a variety of functions. Primarily, the designated agent has the power and authority to make all decisions involving medical and healthcare treatment. The agent can hire and fire healthcare personnel and authorize them to do—or not to do—all types of medical procedures. Medications may be given or withheld based on the directives of the agent. Mechanical procedures that affect the body's function may be authorized or refused by the agent.

The power of the agent may also extend to selecting the proper venue for care—hospital, nursing home, residential care facility, or assisted living facility. The authority to hire medical, social service, and other support personnel is generally made a part of the healthcare power of attorney. At times, it also includes the right to make anatomical gifts of all or part of the patient's body for medical purposes.

HIPAA Authorization

Integral to all of these powers is the ability of the agent to obtain the individual's medical information and documentation. In 1996, Congress passed a law that is commonly referred to by its initials: HIPAA (Health Insurance Portability and Accountability Act of 1996). This law, based on the individual's right to privacy, has effectively cut off access to medical information without an individual's consent. A healthcare power of attorney *must* address this issue. Agents should not only be given access to the individual's medical information and records but should also be given the right to disclose the contents to others. In some states, it is customary for an individual to sign a HIPAA Authorization form separate and apart from a living will and healthcare power of attorney.

Do Not Resuscitate Order

A first cousin to the living will is a *do not resuscitate order*. Usually referred to as a DNRO or DNR, this document confirms an individual's wish that no resuscitation efforts should be made if respiratory failure or cardiac arrest is sustained. In many states, this document applies when the individual has respiratory failure or cardiac arrest outside of a hospital setting. It is directed to healthcare personnel and emergency medical services staff. Each state has specific regulations and sometimes even required language for the DNRO. In some states, it may *only* be executed by a patient in a terminal condition. In all states, it is signed by the patient's physician.

Estate Planning

The focus until now has been on medical decision making. Equally significant is the need to designate someone to handle *non-medical* issues that arise. This person may have to make decisions regarding financial issues when a person is still alive, as well as decisions that must be made after death.

Financial Power of Attorney

Financial activities may involve selling and managing property, executing contracts of all types, operating a business, signing tax returns, and handling tax and legal matters. The simplest document designed for this purpose is the power of attorney. The person who executes the power of attorney must be competent and is called the *principal*. As with the medical power of attorney, the person receiving the authority to act for the principal is generally referred to as an *attorney-in-fact* or *agent*.

In a power of attorney, the principal authorizes another individual or entity to act in his or her place and on his or her behalf. This authorization can be broad (a general power of attorney) or limited (a special power of attorney). The power of attorney can go into effect as soon as it is executed, or it may be designed to become effective only after the onset of incapacity. If properly drafted, it can continue throughout any period of the principal's incapacity, but keep in mind that it *always* ends at its maker's death. A power of attorney may *not* be used to distribute property or take other action on behalf of a deceased person.

In an estate-planning context, the power of attorney is usually general, but it must always be a durable power of attorney. The *durable* power of attorney allows the agent to continue to act after the principal has become disabled or incapacitated. What makes a power of attorney durable is a statement contained directly in the document such as "This power of attorney will continue to be effective even if I become disabled, incapacitated, or incompetent." Without this language, the power of attorney ceases to be usable when it is needed most: at the onset of incapacity.

Before executing a durable power of attorney, individuals should consult the laws of the state in which they reside or see an attorney who specializes in estate-planning law. It is always essential that the document be drafted in conformity with state requirements. However, it is equally important that the individual selected to serve as attorney-in-fact is responsible, trustworthy, and competent to handle the wide array of decision making that may arise. A well-drafted durable power of attorney in the hands of an effective attorney-in-fact generally negates the need for a court-appointed guardian of the estate or conservator of the incapacitated person.

Last Will and Testament

The will defines who is to be in charge of administering the estate, commonly referred to as an *executor* or *personal representative*, the powers and responsibilities of that person, and the directions for distributing the assets of the deceased person. Once again, this is all carried out under the supervision of a court of law.

There are alternatives to passing property through a will, many of which focus on avoiding the probate process. Under certain circumstances, a beneficiary designation will be the preferred strategy. Other times, PODs (payable on death) and TODs (transfer on death) are used. For passing real estate, joint tenancy with rights of survivorship and tenancy by the entirety designations may be useful. Some states have also enacted laws that allow for the use of beneficiary deeds to transfer real estate without the need for probate. The revocable living trust is another popular non-probate vehicle used for transferring property at death. The discussion of when it is appropriate to use a revocable trust as opposed to a last will and testament is beyond the scope of this book and is better conducted with an experienced estate planning attorney. However, in almost all cases where an individual elects to use a revocable trust, he or she still executes what is referred to as a *pourover* last will and testament, which transfers any assets that were not transferred to the revocable trust during lifetime to the revocable trust upon death. This pourover will, not the revocable trust instrument, typically provides for guardianship for any minor children.

If an individual dies without having a last will and testament or revocable trust, the person is considered to have died intestate, and the laws of the state in which the person had a legal residence control how his or her personal property assets pass. For real property, the intestacy laws of the state in which the real property is located control its passage. The intestacy statutes of each state cover every family situation and are designed to be logical concerning the testamentary wishes of the decedent. One of the primary roles of the judge of a court that handles an intestate estate is to determine who the decedent's heirs are under the intestacy statutes. Depending upon the procedure used to determine the heirs, it is typically more expensive and time consuming to administer an estate for an individual who dies without a will, as compared to administering an estate where the decedent left a last will and testament.

The important thing to remember is that all estate-planning documents are intended to reflect the wishes of the maker. The foundation for understanding those wishes and having them effectively transferred to the proper legal document is communication.

Appointment of Agent to Control Disposition of Remains

In some states, an individual may also sign a document that appoints a person to be in control of how the decedent's remains are handled. The most common direction contained in this type of document is whether the individual wishes to be cremated or buried. However, the document may go into as much detail as necessary or desirable regarding the timing, method, and location of the cremation or burial. While these types of instructions are sometimes incorporated into an individual's last will and testament, it can typically take 2 to 4 weeks to have a last will and testament admitted to probate by a court of competent jurisdiction after a person dies. Until a last will and testament is admitted to probate, its terms are not effective, including instructions regarding the decedent's remains. Therefore, it is typically recommended that instructions regarding the disposition of an individual's remains be set forth in a separate document. As with all of the other documents discussed in this chapter, one should consult with an estate-planning attorney who is knowledgeable regarding the state laws applicable to the disposition of one's remains after death.

Role of Healthcare Professionals

If healthcare professionals are not cognizant of the types of advanced directives available and the specific requirements and limitations of each, patients' lives and healthcare professionals' careers are at risk. A frightening example of what could happen concerned Mrs. W., an 81-year-old woman who was hospitalized for an aortic dissection.

Prior to entering the hospital, Mrs. W. had established a living will, which stated that she should be denied nutrition and hydration only if she was in a coma or persistent vegetative state. In another document, a financial power of attorney, she named her granddaughter as her agent but did not grant her medical power of attorney.

When the elderly woman fell ill, her granddaughter had her transferred to a hospice center, although she was not considered terminally ill. The granddaughter claimed to have the legal authority to make healthcare decisions for her grandmother and requested that her grandmother not be given food or water. According to one report, the granddaughter's reason for this decision was that her grandmother was old and sick and would not want to live with the disabilities she would have. Mrs. W. was sedated and no means of nutrition or hydration was provided.

The granddaughter's decision was in direct conflict with the wishes expressed by the elderly woman. Unfortunately, the professionals involved did not realize that the granddaughter was misrepresenting her legal powers, and they were not diligent in examining and following the legal documents. By the time relatives with the legal right to make healthcare decisions became involved, Mrs. W.'s physical condition was precarious. Further, because of dehydration, malnutrition, and medication, she was no longer lucid. She was not competent at that point to express her wishes.

Does Aging Play a Role in End-of-Life Care Decisions?

It would be reassuring to believe that making and documenting the legal decisions described in previous sections of this chapter would resolve all end-of-life care issues. Unfortunately, chronological age and age-related physical and mental changes can influence care decisions, as Mrs. W.'s story demonstrates. The critical question in the previous scenario is, would this have happened if the patient was not an elderly individual? The answer is, probably not.

The simple fact of being old and increasingly dependent can influence care. There is a tendency to assume that the elderly are "ready to go" or "have had a full life." In reality, each older person has specific wishes for end-of-life care, and these wishes need to be stated in legally binding documents and made known to friends and family. With younger adults, physical illness is seen as very distinct from mental incompetence. With older adults, however, the lines between physical and cognitive impairment become blurred. Healthcare providers should take responsibility for understanding and clearly describing a person's competence and being an advocate when necessary. When a health problem leaves an older adult with a communication disorder, SLPs should clearly explain the distinction between being unable to communicate verbally and being mentally incompetent.

The elderly are more likely to face terminal illness. Even with advanced age, they may not be prepared for such a prognosis. While they may have had many friends who required end-of-life services, the elderly are no more prepared than are younger persons in terms of being aware of the obstacles they will confront or the assistance that might be available.

Perspectives on the End-of-Life Experience: Needs and Services

A number of end-of-life (EOL) issues confront both elderly individuals and their loved ones. In some instances, EOL concerns arise because an aging person is dealing with a chronic, progressive disease that is ultimately fatal. In other instances, the simple reality of becoming older raises questions and concerns about dying and preparing for death. Previous sections of this chapter have discussed planning for the later years and, more specifi- cally, healthcare rights and legal responsibilities during illness and dying.

The following sections describe both the issues that may arise when an older person is dying and the services available to address the needs of that person and the family members. Healthcare providers should be aware of these EOL issues and knowledgeable about resources. They should also have a basic understanding of common barriers to service utilization. Nor- mal age-related changes, chronic diseases, and socio-emotional stressors affect end-of-life communication at the very time when communication is most needed for meeting EOL needs and accessing services. Speech– language pathologists can play a specific role in helping family members and other professionals use more effective communication strategies with an older person experiencing age-related primary or secondary changes in communication.

Supportive Services at the End of Life

Services

The emerging senior healthcare industry recognizes the importance of ho- listic, interdisciplinary team (IDT) services to meet the needs of the ag- ing population and specifically those facing the end of life. The goal of care should be treatment of the entire person, addressing physical, mental, emotional, social, and spiritual needs. Further, healthcare should be tai- lored to the unique needs of each individual. While the primary client is the patient, elderly patients are often dependent on family members for some or all support; therefore, families should be included in healthcare conversations, treatment planning, and decision making.

Hospice programs are examples of holistic end-of-life healthcare. A key hospice concept is that hospice care neither prolongs life nor hastens death. Hospice care focuses on death with dignity for patients and families dealing with terminal illnesses. *Terminal* is defined as a life expectancy of 6 months or less. Patients are reevaluated at each 6-month period to assess the appropriateness of hospice. Patients can be discharged from hospice services if after 6 months their physical or mental condition has improved and the prognosis is no longer limited to 6 months or less. Patients also can remain on hospice services with a physician certification. Because the goal of hospice is not to cure but rather to provide holistic comfort care, patients can revoke hospice services for any reason, including a desire to seek aggressive treatment for their conditions (e.g., chemotherapy to treat cancer).

Hospice care is a specialized medical service, tending to the disease processes, pain management, and comfort care. Members of a hospice IDT work together to address patient and family needs throughout the end-of-life and bereavement processes. Interdisciplinary team members include physicians, nurses, home health aides, social workers, chaplains, grief counselors, a trained cadre of volunteers, and music and art therapists. Other healthcare professionals, such as SLPs, are consulted either individually or through hospitals and long-term care units in which the patients reside.

Patients and family members can request an information visit from hospice staff to address questions and concerns. If a patient is considered hospice-appropriate based on self-, family, or physician referrals, a functional assessment is conducted prior to admission. Once a person receives hospice services, individual care plans are developed and evaluated by the IDT, usually weekly or bi-weekly. Care plans include the type, purpose, and frequency of IDT visits, and a goal of the IDT is to make sure that patients have been visited at least within 24 hours of death, based on patient and family preferences. Team members, including 11th-hour volunteers, are available 24 hours a day and will remain at the bedside per request.

Hospice care can be provided in one's place of residence (e.g., private home or apartment, assisted-living, independent-living facility, nursing home), hospital, or at a hospice facility. Hospice is a benefit available through Medicare and Medicaid, private insurance, and military health coverage. All hospice-related services, equipment, and medication are provided through these benefits. Medicare policies dictate that educational and outreach programs, such as grief counseling or support groups, should be available to community members, regardless of hospice use.

Most hospices provide community education and outreach to enhance awareness and understanding of hospice support services. Community education is needed because it is still common to find that patients are not admitted to hospice until only hours or days before death. While comfort care is important up until the moment of death, families and patients all too often voice regret for not having used hospice support earlier.

As has already been noted, placement under care of hospice typically means that only palliative measures will be used. For example, Medicare will not pay for an augmentative communication device for a person with amyotrophic lateral sclerosis (ALS) who is under care of hospice. Hospice programs vary in policies and procedures for palliative care, so older adults and their families need to be informed consumers when selecting a hospice program.

While hospice services are broad-reaching and comprehensive, elderly individuals and their families do not need to be in a hospice program to take advantage of the range of socio-emotional support services that may be available in the community. For example, psychotherapy and other counseling services are available to assist with the reconciliation of preexisting family troubles, existential concerns, loss and grief, and skills training (e.g., social, communication, coping, and problem-solving skills). Virtual or telephone support services are readily available and can assist in garnering further education, information, and support, especially for those who are isolated or perceive limited social support.

Respite services are extremely important for caregivers of older adults to prevent burnout. *Respite* refers to any program that gives caregivers temporary relief from caregiving activities. Such services are provided in-home by individuals or through agencies, as well as at adult daycare or skilled nursing facilities. Often, older persons show improvement during respite because they receive additional attention and care from the professionals. The caregiver's mood, attitude, and behaviors also are positively affected because of the respite time.

Legal and financial planning services are important tools for older adults and caregivers. Discussions about these services may facilitate dialogue between patients and their loved ones, in order to ensure that personal wishes about EOL care are met.

Generational or Cohort Challenges

Challenges in accessing and using services are often generation-specific. The elderly are not a homogenous group. In fact, older adults are sometimes considered in three age groups that reflect cohort differences (e.g., WWII versus Vietnam generations). These groups include the young-old, middle-old, and the old-old. There is no standard agreement on the chronological ages that are described by these group labels, with the most variation being seen in when the label "old" is first applied—55? 60? 65? Depending on choice of chronological age, the baby boomers include young-old as well as middle-age adults. Most people agree that individuals above 85 fit into the old-old category. In many instances, the young-old are the adult children of some of today's old-old.

The WWII old-old generation tends to view professionals as authorities rather than healthcare partners. This attitude, along with other healthcare beliefs, means that today's old-old may have trouble communicating with healthcare professionals about symptoms, fears, concerns, and needs. This particular generation is less likely than younger generations to initiate conversations about their healthcare concerns, particularly in the socioemotional domain. Those who are 85 years or older may be less familiar than other elderly persons are with the advances in and expansion of healthcare services to meet not only their needs but their families' needs as well. The old-old generation is most likely to live with multiple chronic illnesses, to live in healthcare facilities, and to be in need of services geared toward end of life. In contrast, middle-old and baby boomers are more educated, active, and living independently with fewer illnesses than are their older counterparts. The baby boomers are more likely to seek support, share concerns, and expect answers.

Healthcare providers should know what services are available in the community, understanding that age or cohort differences affect health communication and healthcare needs. Professionals should help older adults and families navigate the healthcare system as efficiently as possible in order to best meet care recipients' needs.

Communication in Service Delivery

Information about diagnosis, prognosis, and treatment options must always be provided in a clear fashion, and questions and requests for clarification should be encouraged. When the channels for communication are strong, healthcare professionals have a greater understanding of patient and family wishes, experiences, reasons for behaviors, and decisions. Consequently, care recipients experience greater satisfaction and confidence with respect to their care, and all parties benefit by defining and pursuing agreed-upon goals. This health communication interaction is an ongoing process, with contexts, preferences for care, and goals changing over time. Healthcare providers need to be aware of generational differences and tailor communications and interventions according to the generation and the individual.

SLP Role in Bridging Communication Gaps

While health communication is a crucial piece of the healthcare experience for everyone, there is a unique subset of the older population that may need additional help in communicating. These older adults are already experiencing cognitively based communication problems or specific speech–language disorders. Persons with cognitive challenges may not be able to participate fully in end-of-life decisions although SLPs can provide guidance about communication strategies. In contrast, those with a specific speech–language disorder like dysarthria or aphasia need assistance expressing their wishes about care and comfort, even as those wishes and needs evolve over time. The SLP can identify the communication needs and provide tools and strategies to support aging individuals in both categories.

In order to do so, the SLP must be knowledgeable about the types of conversations that may need to occur, as well as the possibility of other socio-emotional barriers to communicate. Dying individuals and their families may need to be able to come together to share and celebrate past experiences, confirm feelings, ask forgiveness, and say goodbyes. As noted earlier, SLPs also need to understand the legal ramifications of documents such as healthcare directives and should be able to explain the dying person's communicative competence.

SLPs are sometimes in the unique position of being the person with whom a dying individual can communicate most easily. In some instances, this means the SLP hears feelings not shared with family members and other professionals, or may be asked questions that are not within the SLP's scope of practice to answer. It is important to establish clearly what information can be shared and with whom; for example, it is important to identify which people are allowed access to medical information. Professional and personal boundaries can be difficult to maintain, as discussed later in this chapter.

SLPs may also be asked to provide swallowing intervention to terminally-ill patients who insist on continuation of oral feeding contrary to all medical opinion. The balance between quality of life and threat to life is delicate in these cases. The patient should be made aware of the real implications of the decision. Obviously, a person with dysphagia experiences more than a loss in the enjoyment of food. Inability to swallow also results in reduced social interaction and a decline in physical comfort due to factors such as a dry mouth and throat or unmanaged secretions. Continuing to eat, however, can speed death and cause discomfort in response to coughing, choking, stasis of food in the mouth and throat, and infections. These difficulties reduce the enjoyment of the food and the enjoyment of social interactions that the person is attempting to maintain. In these cases, the clinician must make the appropriate recommendations for health and safety and try to ensure that the patient and family have the information needed to understand the recommendations and the probable consequences if those recommendations are not followed.

During the final days of life, even people who were not previously identified as dysphagic may experience occasional difficulty triggering a swallow. This trouble can alarm both the patient and the family. Instructions in ways to improve oral hydration, provide oral stimulation, and trigger a swallow may help provide some measure of comfort during the final days of the person's life.

Common End-of-Life Concerns and Challenges

Individuals facing the end of life have many specific concerns. Awareness of the more common ones makes it possible for healthcare professionals to provide opportunities for discussing them and for showing support.

Fear of the Unknown

One of the most common concerns of dying patients and families is fear of the unknown. Ambiguity and uncertainty about what to expect lead to a sense of dread, thus increasing fear and anxiety. Patients and families need to create meaning out of their EOL experiences. This meaning-making fosters a sense of control and can serve as a cognitive–behavioral coping mechanism.

The primary fears expressed by dying patients relate to experiencing a painful death, burdening their loved ones, and how their loved ones will cope with the caregiver role and the death processes. Often, elderly patients are more comfortable with the EOL experience than are their family members. This difference is due in part to the sense of purpose that comes from the natural life review or meaning-making processes engaged in by some older adults. These processes can reduce fear of the unknown. For family members, however, it may be more difficult to find a sense of meaning, and fear of the unknown can be a greater issue for them than for the dying individual.

Based on clinical practice, dying care recipients have expressed a desire for ongoing education about a variety of topics, including

- prognosis, disease, and dying processes (e.g., what to expect, what is normal aging versus the disease process);
- interventions to improve communication with loved ones;
- additional support services;
- purpose and expected outcomes of interventions; and
- common experiences of those in similar circumstances.

Families have similar needs. Education and information enhance one's sense of control and self-efficacy when confronting unknown and potentially frightening EOL experiences.

Anticipatory Loss and Grief

Anticipatory loss and grief are natural reactions to losses prior to death. These feelings actually allow people to prepare emotionally for the inevitable, the unacceptable. Families routinely state that the most difficult part of the aging and dying process is the sense of losing the person they have known and loved. Despite advanced age, families often express the sense that they "never feel fully prepared to lose Mother, even if she is 92."

Emotional reactions to anticipated loss can negatively affect important conversations about topics such as change and deterioration, supportive interventions (e.g., hospice or home health services), and difficult treatment decisions (e.g., placing a feeding tube). These discussions require acknowledgement of real and anticipated losses and ultimately death. Care recipients and family members may also struggle to create a sense of control in the face of the inevitable and emotionally unacceptable outcomes. These struggles may interfere with accepting and receiving services.

Anticipatory loss and grief can affect all aspects of functioning: cognitive, social, behavioral, emotional, spiritual, and physical. Unfortunately, healthcare professionals sometimes feel frustrated by patients' and families' apparent difficulty comprehending details and making decisions. It is important to recognize that care recipients may simply be overwhelmed, making it difficult to listen to and process information. Loss and stress can also impair cognitive abilities such as concentration, attention, and problem solving, all of which are involved in decision making. Of course, other factors can also influence decision making. In some instances, a patient or family member may not agree with advice but remains uncertain about other options.

Caregivers face multiple losses that may be compounded by additional life stressors. The typical caregiver is a married female in her forties who works outside of the home, has children in the home, and provides care for a loved one, most often a widowed elderly mother (National Alliance for Caregiving and AARP, 2004). Despite being at higher risk for psychological and physical illnesses, caregivers underutilize services. Many factors influence service utilization. Cost is a problem for some caregivers. Others feel it takes too much time and effort to prepare the patient to leave the home. Healthcare providers need to know about community resources and make appropriate referrals as needed.

Sociocultural Pressures

Throughout the EOL process, beliefs, expectations, and roles can change based on the sociocultural context. Patients and families internalize cultural, religious, and family messages or beliefs about what defines aging, caregiving, and the dying (along with stigmas and stereotypes about these processes). These beliefs and stigmas greatly affect care and communication between patients, families, and healthcare professionals. Examples of beliefs that may influence behavior include the following:

- "Don't be selfish; always put others first."
- "I should be able to cope with this on my own."
- "I shouldn't complain or have a pity party."
- "Don't let anyone down, especially family."
- "Be the dutiful child [or partner, etc.], despite negative history."
- "Always go the extra mile."
- "Why can't you be more like …?" "Why can't I be more like …?"

Beliefs and expectations can place tremendous pressures on the dying person and caregivers to perform in ways that may not be possible under the circumstances. Often people experience a disconnect between real and ideal performance, with *ideal* being defined by culture, religion, or family standards—things we "should" do. Failure to live up to expectations can lead to guilt and shame, and these emotions can impair daily functioning, treatment adherence, and support utilization. Feelings of resentment about the caregiver role or anger directed toward the care recipient may also be perceived as socially unacceptable; the caregiver may be reluctant to express such feelings.

Healthcare professionals should be sensitive to these issues. Some pressures may be reduced if professionals recognize and acknowledge conflicting expectations, pressures, and fears. Education about some of the EOL topics described earlier can help people sort what is realistic and practical from what is culturally expected. Openness to conversations about concerns and pressures is also critical, although no caregiver should be pressured to talk about sensitive personal issues. Discussions of patient and caregiver strengths, skills, and limitations may be helpful. If healthcare providers feel there are issues that require additional support, referrals can be made to a mental health professional.

Case Example

The following case example illustrates the complex interaction among beliefs, pressures, fears, and support needs for both elderly parents with chronic progressive disorders and their adult daughter, who is their caregiver. The basic elements of the EOL story here are all too common, although the reality of dealing with two parents with dementia may be less so.

Susie is a 42-year-old married woman who has an adolescent child. Susie provides in-home care for both of her parents, each of whom has dementia and comorbid chronic diseases. Susie's father is in the later stages of Alzheimer's and is not expected to live much longer. Susie quit her job to provide care for her parents, which has created financial strain on the family.

Susie's father is unable to communicate his preferences for care, although he exhibits disruptive behaviors anytime his care routine is altered, especially when Susie places her parents in a long-term-care facility for respite purposes. While Susie's mother expresses a desire to stay in her own home, she has been deemed incompetent to make her own decisions. Susie has looked into long-term-care facilities for her parents; however, she is not emotionally prepared to make that decision, despite urges from healthcare professionals. Susie expresses the belief that she "should take care of [her] parents" and "should be doing more to help them, since they took such good care of [her]."

Susie visits with a counselor weekly and also attends a support group. Her primary concerns are losing her best friends (i.e., her parents), not knowing what to expect, and fear of "ruining" her marriage and relationship with her child due to her demanding caregiver role. Susie reports feeling as if she is "going crazy," "getting dementia," and arriving at her "breaking point" watching her parents "slip away."

Susie is seeking help through many available channels; however, the burden is heavy and there are no simple solutions. Healthcare providers should be sensitive to the stresses she is experiencing and should be realistic in terms of their expectations for her involvement in care.

Barriers to Providing Support and Effective Health Communication

Cultural Barriers

Sociocultural pressures on individuals were acknowledged in the previous section, but they are described further here in the broader context of service delivery. America is a death-denying, youth-obsessed culture that offers few authentic images about aging and the EOL experiences. Instead, the American culture has shaped and promoted negative attitudes about aging and end-of-life experiences, thus affecting the triad of patient, family, and professional, all of whom are involved with end-of-life care. Existential awareness is avoided by isolating the sick, aged, bereaved, and even geriatric healthcare workers. Industrialization has led to the geographical separation and isolation of families, which further limits personal exposure to aging, illness, caregiving, and death. All of these factors perpetuate the experience of the isolated "invisible elder" and can lead to misinformation and myths, inaccurate stereotypes, and negative attitudes and expectations. Negative cultural attitudes about death and dying probably contribute to the fact that there are insufficient resources available for EOL organizations, professionals, and care recipients (e.g., financial resources, ancillary supportive services).

End-of-life and death experiences vary by culture, based on customs and mores. Social, religious, and ethnic cultures, as well as cohorts, can affect health communication and receptiveness to key information. Key information and related decisions may include treatment options and prognosis, whether the patient will be told about the prognosis, who will be the contact professionals, whether advanced planning decisions will be made (e.g., living wills, power of attorney), and whether treatment recommendations will be followed. In conveying this information, IDT members providing EOL care must be sensitive to fundamental issues concerning whether members of different cultures or groups seek, trust, and accept medical care. Some examples of issues that may affect healthcare for minorities, in addition to other cultural, institutional, and professional barriers, are listed in Appendix 11A.

Despite the varied effects of group culture on EOL care, ultimately each patient and family is a "culture of one," with their own rules for relating and issues about healthcare. The context for understanding families is dynamic, and healthcare providers must continually assess and remain sensitive to cultural beliefs and cohort differences. When the beliefs of patients or families seem to contradict the beliefs prominent in healthcare, practitioners must find some way to work within the context of the care recipient's beliefs, not change them.

Cultural Case Example

The following case example illustrates the fact that culture comes in many forms, one of which is religion. In this scenario, the patient's religious beliefs were in opposition to her adult child's beliefs, and to the hospice philosophy. Further, those beliefs affected her EOL experience and care options. The communication barriers between the patient, her family, and IDT members were only resolved when team members were helped to accept Mrs. A.'s choices, which were based on her religious beliefs.

Mrs. A. was an 80 year-old widow living in an assisted-living facility. After being diagnosed with a malignant melanoma, she was admitted to hospice services. The cancer had spread through her chest cavity, literally decaying the tissue until all that remained was a bleeding hole. Mrs. A.'s cause of death was expected to be bleeding out through this wound.

Mrs. A. refused all treatments, including pain medication, based on her Christian Scientist religious beliefs. She allowed the hospice workers to visit in order to change the wound dressings and to provide social support services. The hospice IDT members regularly visited with Mrs. A.'s adult children, who disagreed with their mother's decisions not to receive treatment and especially pain medication. Mrs. A. reported experiencing intense physical pain.

The IDT members, especially the nurses, found it difficult to respect Mrs. A.'s religious cultural beliefs, as they saw a dying woman in pain who easily could have been comforted physically. In fact, the philosophy of hospice is focused primarily on comfort care for the dying. Mrs. A.'s primary hospice nurse expressed the unethical desire to provide pain medication in a topical form, by telling Mrs. A. that the purpose of the powder was to eliminate the odor from her necrotic tissue. There was disagreement amongst the IDT about how to define and provide comfort care for this patient. Ultimately, the IDT chaplains provided the other team members with repeated education about respect for religious cultural beliefs. Mrs. A. was not in spiritual pain, which was more important to her religious cultural belief system than was physical pain due to her cancer.

Institutional Barriers

The Medical Model of Healthcare. Traditionally, the medical model of healthcare has been relied upon for end-of-life and long-term care. This model does not acknowledge the holistic care needs of the elderly population or indeed of any chronically ill population. Illness is seen as the only target and is approached solely as a diagnosable and treatable physical disease process. Needs outside of the physical domain, while potentially of equal importance in EOL care, are not readily acknowledged within the medical model.

Awareness about holistic care needs at the end of life has increased in the last few decades, and the current EOL institutional culture is shifting from a medical model to a biopsychosocial model of care (e.g., hospice). However, complex medical institutions continue to have limitations that affect access to and delivery of services. Limitations, for instance, may be placed on reimbursement for services through the managed care system. Insufficient numbers of geriatric healthcare providers means that acute, long-term, and EOL organizations are understaffed. While state and federal regulations are in place to maintain quality care, unfortunately, the paperwork required to document compliance with regulations often reduces time spent providing direct patient care. Each of these barriers limits the quality of healthcare communication and service provision. Two important institutional barriers will be discussed in-depth in the following sections.

Lack of Geriatric Healthcare Education. There is not enough geriatric healthcare education about normal aging and EOL experiences. Just as pediatric professionals require specialized education and training, so too do geriatric professionals. Professionals cannot meet the unique needs of this population without a basic understanding of age-related changes and of the effects of chronic disease processes on EOL and caregiver experiences.

Practitioners with training in geriatrics and end-of-life practices strive to provide education for community members and healthcare professionals. However, even with appropriate knowledge, medical institutions and systems are complex and difficult to navigate. Lack of education and understanding of aging and EOL experiences can lead to communication breakdown, patient and family dissatisfaction with care, and healthcare professional burnout due to overwhelming job demands and associated feelings of inadequacy in meeting patient needs. Such negative effects are magnified by the fact that many elderly patients have some form of communication limitation. In recent years, healthcare institutions have made improvements in EOL education. However, professionals should actively seek continued education about aging, end-of-life, dying, death, and bereavement.

Like healthcare institutions, the EOL healthcare *culture* has also changed tremendously in the last few decades and will continue to evolve. In the meantime, professionals must remain aware of institutional barriers to service utilization and provision, and be willing to maintain open communication about these issues in order to improve geriatric and EOL healthcare.

Healthcare Professional Barriers

Healthcare professionals have their own cultures, values, and personal beliefs about EOL processes. Care must be taken to avoid imposing one's beliefs on patients and family members. An IDT can provide the balance of perspectives that may help clinicians maintain perspective on their work. However, it is important to recognize the types of personal barriers that may affect service delivery to those dealing with EOL.

Boundaries. End-of-life healthcare professionals work within both adaptive and maladaptive family and medical systems, with a wide array of beliefs that affect behavior and communication. In some instances, it can be difficult not to pass judgment and attempt to improve the family dynamics. Healthcare providers must continually strive to maintain a balance between respect for different family and medical systems while facilitating communication among all parties. This balance is achieved in part by reminding oneself of professional roles and boundaries, as well as ethical duties.

Boundaries exist between patient preferences and a professional's perspectives on what is best for that patient. These boundaries can be difficult to maintain during EOL service provision. Dying individuals and their families have the right to make decisions about end-of-life care. Often these decisions are made in advance (as described earlier in this chapter), but cognitively competent patients continue to have autonomy in choosing what they do and do not want in terms of healthcare services. The bottom line is that EOL care may not always be provided or used. For some health-care professionals, this can be difficult to accept.

Healthcare professionals are caregivers who have chosen the medical field in order to help people. When professionals feel unable to assist clients effectively because of choices made by clients or family members, dissonance occurs and boundaries blur. Clinicians may be grappling with their own issues of mortality or may bring too much of their own personal histories into the professional interaction. For speech–language patholo-gists, as noted earlier, boundaries may also be unclear if a dying individual shares feelings, desires, and other personal information only with the SLP, with whom it is easiest to communicate.

Increased Existential Awareness. A common, although not universal, effect of working in EOL healthcare can be increased existential aware-ness. Chronic illness, death, and grief surround EOL professionals. Work with dying patients can be sad and overwhelming; healthcare professionals have personal limits and often need time and support to unwind or debrief after complicated cases. A professional's experiences with EOL care can challenge beliefs about the world, healthcare best practices, and personal purpose or meaning. At the same time, reminders of existential concerns may allow practitioners to focus more on personal health and wellness, family and friends, and the value of supporting those in need during one of the most difficult times in life.

Personal History. Just as the cultural experiences of patients are var-ied and fluid, so too are a professional's culture and values. With each new patient, belief systems can be challenged and ultimately can change. An ethically responsible professional is aware of personal beliefs about the end-of-life process and associated best practices and recognizes how such beliefs might affect care. The healthcare provider's personal history also can influence care. There are always certain diseases, patients, or settings that trigger discomfort, anxiety, or a desire to cross professional boundaries (e.g., the hospice nurse for Mrs. A.).

Education does not prepare clinicians fully for the emotional experi-ence of being professional caregivers. You cannot help all patients all the time. You will not feel comfortable working with all patients. You will not like all patients. You will become emotionally attached to some patients. You will struggle at times, especially when experiencing compounded stress from your own personal life challenges. You will not have all the answers.

You will need support, and that is okay. Despite being trained professionals, you are human, with personal histories and physical, cognitive, and emotional limits that will affect services. Healthcare workers, especially those working within end-of-life healthcare, are at risk for burnout due to the aforementioned cultural and institutional barriers, the emotionally demanding job duties, as well as compounded personal stress.

Communication Considerations in End-of-Life Care

Throughout this discussion of end-of-life care, the importance of communication has been highlighted. For all healthcare providers, basic guidelines to effective communication for end-of-life care are as follows:

- Establish rapport and trust.
- Be direct, honest, and empathetic when reporting bad news.
- Be realistic and honest, but provide hope when appropriate.
- Listen. Allow patients and families to share their stories in order to find deeper meaning.
- Tailor communication content and form to the needs of the individual and family.
- Respect differences in care choices and communication styles that result from differences in cultures, values, or perceived roles.
- Give patients and families permission to express themselves openly; painful feelings expressed, acknowledged, and validated will diminish.
- Educate patients.
- Encourage reminiscence.
- Facilitate communication.

For speech–language pathologists, there are additional professional roles and responsibilities in working with dying clients and families. SLPs may be called on to assist in a variety of ways, all of which are designed to help dying individuals and their family members and healthcare providers communicate about choices, feelings, and needs. SLP roles include the following:

- Assess the communication skills and any deficits of the dying individual.

- Evaluate swallowing functioning, identify factors that inter-fere with quality of life, and make recommendations that will facilitate quality of life.
- Identify the presence of any cognitive-communication disor-der or other age-related problems that may interfere with communication (like visual and auditory sensory issues).
- If there is cognitive impairment, determine what the dying individual can and cannot process and how others can inter-act most effectively in the context of cognitive deficits.
- If there is a specific communication disorder like aphasia, develop communication strategies to be used in all commu-nicative interactions.
- Educate and train family members and healthcare providers to use these strategies effectively.
- Provide tools for communication about unique end-of-life care preferences.

Speech–language pathologists working with older adults should take responsibility for understanding the legal issues surrounding end-of-life care and decisions. They should also be knowledgeable about available com-munity services and sensitive to evolving needs and cultural differences.

Key Points

Legal Considerations

Estate and healthcare planning are discussed and specific legal documents are defined. The following important factors were addressed:

- Advanced directives are legal documents that establish a per-son's wishes for medical care at times when they are unable to make decisions.
- Living wills are advanced directives for end-of-life care when a person is unable to make decisions and is in the end stages of a terminal disease or a permanent coma or vegetative state. Artificial nutrition wishes should be designated specifi-cally.
- Healthcare power of attorney is an advanced directive that provides for an agent to make medical decisions when a per-son is incapacitated and unable to make decisions but is not facing imminent death or in a persistent vegetative state.

- HIPAA authorization is needed to allow an agent named in a healthcare power of attorney to effectively manage healthcare.
- A DNRO states that a person does not wish to be resuscitated in the event of cardiac arrest or respiratory failure.
- A financial power of attorney designates an agent to manage a person's estate in the event of incapacitation.
- A last will and testament describes the person's wishes regarding distribution of assets following death.
- After death, wishes for burial or cremation may be facilitated by appointment of an agent to control distribution of remains.
- Even with all appropriate legal documents completed, end-of-life care decisions may not be honored if those around the dying individual do not take responsibility for ensuring wishes are followed.

End-of-Life Care

Services for dying patients and their caregivers are described. The role of communication disorders professionals in providing end-of-life care is discussed. The following are primary points:

- A variety of services are available to individuals and families who are facing end-of-life challenges.
- Hospice is one of the better known services, although most people do not understand what is and is not provided as part of hospice care.
- A number of challenges may be faced during end-of-life healthcare, including cultural and generational differences and problems with communication.
- Persons facing the end of life have concerns about the unknown nature of what is to come and may already be experiencing a sense of loss and grief.
- Cultural expectations about roles (e.g., being a caregiver) may place additional stress on all persons dealing with EOL.
- There are cultural, institutional, and professional barriers to effective service delivery for those facing EOL. Healthcare providers must be aware of their own values and beliefs in order to make sure they do not interfere with the delivery of care.

- Speech–language pathologists may become involved professionally in assessing communication and cognitive skills and deficits, and in recommending appropriate communication strategies.
- Speech–language pathologists may also be involved in evaluating swallowing and making recommendations based on quality-of-life issues.

References

Cruzan v. Dir., MO Dept of Health, 497 U.S. 261 (1990).

Health Insurance Portability and Accountability Act of 1996, Public Law 104-191.

National Alliance for Caregiving & AARP. (2004). *Caregiving in the U.S.* Washington, DC: Author.

Quinlan, 70 N.J. 10, 355 A.2d 647 (1976), cert. denied, 429 U.S. 92 (1976).

Schiavo v. Schiavo, 358 F Supp 2d 1161 (M.D. Fla. 2005) aff'd by Schiavo v. Schiavo, 403 F.3d 1289 (11th Cir. 2005).

Multicultural Issues in End-of-Life Healthcare

Care domain	Barrier or issue
Support services	• Limited availability • Decreased awareness of and accessibility to services • Inadequate outreach materials (not addressing unique cultural concerns or not framed in the primary language of the cultural group)
Healthcare experiences and perceptions	• Decreased likelihood of trusting and understanding mainstream healthcare professionals and institutions • Tendency in some cultural groups to utilize alternative rather than mainstream forms of treatment • Greater tendency to rely on extended family rather than health professionals for care
Other considerations	• Lower socioeconomic status and educational levels in some groups • Insurance coverage inequities

CHAPTER 12

Counseling and Clinical Interactions With Older Clients and Caregivers

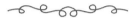

Barbara B. Shadden and Mary Ann Toner

SHADDEN AND TONER RETURN the reader to the broader consideration of counseling and clinical interactions with older clients and their families. Guidelines are provided for both counseling and clinical interactions in general.

Communication requires interaction. Good therapy requires good interaction skills. Without those skills, the best treatment techniques in the world will probably have limited effectiveness.

While these seem to be basic premises, it may not be that simple—particularly with the elderly. Communication disorders professionals are busy people. We know what we need to get done and often develop set procedures for completing our tasks. Much of our clinical training focuses on the nature of specific disorders and on use of assessment and treatment tools and techniques. We learn how to take a case history, administer a test, make observations, draw conclusions, and make recommendations. During the remediation process, we learn to identify goals and objectives, implement appropriate therapy strategies, take data, and report progress. Too often in the training of communication disorders professionals, the term *counseling* is used in a manner that restricts it to the last part of an evaluation session or to a specific portion of intervention. What is termed "counseling" in those cases is often "instruction." The clinician *tells* the client and caregiver what the problem is and what can be done. The client and caregiver contribution may be limited to the time when the clinician wraps up by saying, "Do you have any questions?" During therapy, the clinician *tells* the client and caregiver what the objectives are, how they will be approached, how the client is progressing, and maybe what the client or caregiver should be doing outside of therapy. There is very little *inter*action.

Clinical interaction and counseling should begin when the first contact is made with a client or a caregiver and ends with the last contact. A successful start helps achieve a successful result. Counseling opportunities—often feared by clinicians and rarely understood—are present throughout the intervention process.

Some principles of clinical interaction apply to all people of all ages; others are particularly relevant to older adults and their families. With children, clinical education involves understanding normal development of communication skills along with associated behaviors and interaction techniques appropriate to various age groups. With adults, however, there is limited attention to changes people experience as they move through the lifespan and to the implications of these changes for clinical interactions. This is unfortunate because therapeutic relationships are built on these clinical interactions. Clinical relationships evolve as clients and their significant others adapt to communication disorders.

This chapter addresses basic principles of interacting clinically with older clients. As suggested, counseling is an important component of those interactions, not a separate process. In fact, if clinicians see counseling as a discrete objective for a particular assessment or treatment session, counseling is doomed to failure. Counseling interactions must take into consideration the unique circumstances, needs, and life experiences of older clients and their family members.

Since counseling should be embedded in the therapeutic interaction, this chapter begins with a brief overview of basic definitions of counseling. The rest of the chapter discusses guidelines for interactions with older adults and their significant others.

Counseling and the Elderly

Counseling is part of the scope of practice of speech–language pathologists and audiologists. Despite this fact, practitioners continue to struggle with defining how and when to engage in counseling.

Shipley and Roseberry-McKibbin's (2006) definitions of counseling, guidance, and psychotherapy are helpful in defining professional roles. Counseling relates primarily to personal adjustment rather than to major personality and psychiatric issues. In communication disorders, counseling might include discussion of changes in daily communication related to the person with aphasia being unable to engage easily in conversational small talk (everyday chitchat) and how that makes everyone feel. The key here is support for and validation of the feelings of all concerned parties.

Guidance is an educational process in which advice, suggestions, and information are used to influence another person's thoughts and behaviors in a positive direction. For example, a clinician providing ideas about how to support the verbal expression of a person with aphasia might be considered guidance. Guidance is particularly evident when the clinician provides a positive framework for understanding the client's or family member's behaviors. If a client becomes irritated by a spouse's constant finishing of his sentences, the clinician might provide the client with ideas about how to request a change in the spouse's behavior or perhaps suggestions about when to request a change and when to let the spouse's behavior go.

In contrast, *psychotherapy* is seen as the province of specially trained professionals who deal with individuals with chronic life problems and serious emotional disorders. A stroke patient with a premorbid diagnosis of bipolar disorder may need help from professional counselors as well as a speech–language pathologist. Some clients or significant others experience profound depression that interferes with carrying out of everyday tasks, such as shopping for food or following up on medical appointments. If a clinician becomes aware of these problems, a referral to a mental health professional or physician may be appropriate. If there are true emotional impairments that require mental health intervention, clinicians should consider referrals carefully. Not every mental health professional feels comfortable or qualified to deal with a client who has a significant communication impairment. Clients or family members may be prepared to tackle only one challenge, and the emotional problems may outweigh the communication disorders. There is no room here for "judging" clients or significant others based on their choices of intervention.

Beyond basic clinical competencies, the healthcare professional must have the skills and attitudes that allow successful counseling. According to Shipley and Roseberry-McKibbin (2006), the characteristics of good counselors include flexibility, openness, honesty, emotional stability, trustworthiness, self-awareness, belief in the client's ability to change, and commitment to helping people change. Some of these characteristics are particularly important in working with older clients and their families. For example, self-awareness includes recognition of any personal attitudes about aging and the elderly. Similarly, belief in the client's ability to change may be influenced by age biases. If you are unsure about your attitudes and biases, refer to the opening sections of Chapter 1.

Webster and Newhoff (1981) described four elements of family counseling by speech–language pathologists and audiologists: receiving information that families wish to share; providing information to family members; helping individuals clarify ideas, attitudes, and emotions; and providing family members with options for changing their behaviors and the behaviors of the person with the impairment. These four counseling elements apply equally to counseling with older clients with communication disorders.

Counseling challenges vary depending on the specific communication disorder as well as numerous premorbid personal and family characteristics. With older adults, clinicians sometimes assume that the client cannot be an active participant in the counseling process. As a result, the emphasis is on helping family members learn about the disorder and manage the emotions they experience in dealing with the "impaired" family member. Adjustment is sometimes made around the person with the disorder. This is inappropriate. Instead, counseling should be seen as part of the ongoing clinical interaction process with all parties.

Exchange of information is fundamental to successful counseling. The key word is *exchange*, which is not to be confused with *instructing* clients or family members. To be effective, a balance of control must exist between the client, the caregivers, and the professional. Throughout the therapeutic process, each of these participants must be given opportunities to provide and receive information. This information can then be used to set goals, identify resources, facilitate the therapeutic process, and promote successful communication.

Exchange of information is not as simple as it sounds. Older adults may not always provide complete information to physicians. In some instances, the patient may assume that if the doctor does not ask about a behavior or problem, it is not important. Many elderly patients are hesitant to take up too much of the doctor's time. In contrast, patients and their families are sometimes more comfortable bringing up a variety of issues with someone like the speech–language pathologist, whom they may see regularly over a period of time. The speech–language pathologist should not attempt to answer medical questions but might be able to facilitate the client's or family's interaction with the physician. For example, questions could be written down and presented to the physician at the next visit. Such preparation allows the physician to optimize valuable counseling minutes.

Despite these challenges, counseling is a key element in treating the whole person (Luterman, 2008). Successful counseling with older adults depends, in part, on the clinician's understanding of both aging and counseling dynamics and on the quality of clinical interactions.

Guidelines for Clinical Interactions With Older Adults

Guidelines for clinical interactions with the elderly and their families include the following:

- Use clinical interaction time wisely.
- Know what's normal (from everyone's perspectives).
- Learn about the individuals involved.
- Create a therapeutic partnership.
- Develop and maintain trust.
- Adapt to evolving needs and concerns.
- Adjust and support communication appropriately.

Use Clinical Interaction Time Wisely

Clinicians need to learn to use clinical interaction time wisely. Admittedly, in today's healthcare system, there is never enough time to do what needs to be done in working with older clients and their families. Clinicians are faced with the challenge of conducting a comprehensive assessment, identifying personally relevant treatment goals, and actually treating the swallowing or communication disorder. They also need to work with families and provide counseling about strategies and outcomes. Further, older clients require additional time either to interact and discuss personal concerns or to complete treatment tasks. To accomplish all of this, clinicians are allowed only brief units of assessment or treatment time, and a limited number of such units.

Clinicians can find ways to address more than one treatment goal during clinical interactions. Assessment, treatment, and counseling can be ongoing and co-occurring processes. For example, while a client is learning to use an augmentative communication device, the clinician is continuing to assess visual, motor, and cognitive skills and also gathering information that will guide further treatment.

Part of time management involves clinician flexibility. Older clients need to be allowed to provide information in their preferred style. Many individuals are most comfortable relating information in stories. Although this method of information gathering is time consuming, it may be essential to gaining important facts and perceptions. Stories provide a wealth of personal life detail that can be helpful in designing interventions and suggesting strategies for communication work outside of the clinical setting.

Another way to optimize clinical time is to build treatment activities around personal history and interests. If a client is experiencing moderate word-finding problems, a treatment session might include discussion of a favorite hobby or an interesting life experience. The client and significant others can prepare materials to bring to the session to support word finding, and the actual discussion may provide the clinician with insights into client preferences, premorbid interests, and priorities in terms of treatment goals.

Treatment should not be restricted to one-on-one therapy with a clinician. If a client works on communication deficits only during treatment sessions, the odds of success are poor. Part of using clinician time wisely involves finding ways to engage the client and family in ongoing communication activities outside of the treatment session. There may also be advantages to involving clients and families in support groups or other community-based activities. If a client is discharged from therapy before maximizing communicative performance, clinicians should take responsibility for identifying other community resources for additional services and support.

Know What's Normal

This text has provided descriptions of normal or primary aging changes in various systems, as well as tertiary factors that include environments and social networks. The assumption has been that understanding what constitutes normal behavior provides guidance in working with elderly individuals with communication disorders. Clinicians who do not fully understand the effects of aging run the risk of confusing signs of normal aging with symptoms of disorders.

As issues of primary aging emerge in clinical interactions, speech–language pathologists may need to help older clients and families make successful adjustments to the normal aging process. The clinician should be able to provide reassurance regarding primary aging processes while not discounting concerns regarding these changes and their effects. Unfortunately, many speech–language pathologists feel most comfortable when dealing with secondary aging disorders and their consequences. They may discourage discussions of other age-related changes and concerns.

Clinical interactions must also address the effects of tertiary aging factors on treatment. Tertiary factors often determine the degree to which the individual and family are able to make successful adjustments. Clinicians should have a basic understanding of family systems, the dynamics of family equilibrium, and family roles (Norlin, 1986). Some of the family issues faced in counseling may be concerns about power, roles, intimacy, and conflict management. These same issues are central to the adaptation of the older client and caregivers. In counseling exchanges, clinicians should monitor their behavior carefully for signs of loss of personal objectivity. At the very least, reduced objectivity and increased personal involvement should signal the need for an outside perspective.

It is critical to identify what clients and families perceive as normal. For example, some aging adults may perceive changes in swallowing as part of the normal aging process and may not describe them to a physician. An adult child of an aging client may assume that increasing daily difficulties with memory are to be expected and warrant no further assessment. In each case, the individual may not be referred initially for assessment or treatment. However, if either of these older persons eventually sees a clinician, it will be important to understand when and how changes in these systems began.

Learn About the Individuals Involved

To achieve a balanced exchange of information and develop management strategies, the client, primary caregiver, and speech–language pathologist must all be involved in ongoing clinical interactions that allow for information exchange. Characteristics of each "player" will influence therapeutic outcomes.

Clinician

As already established in Chapter 1, clinicians often have biases and stereotypes about aging and the elderly. Whether positive or negative, those biases influence clinical interaction and expectations for treatment outcomes. Clinicians should not work with older clients before they have examined their own perceptions. Before working with the elderly, clinicians should also assess their knowledge of primary, secondary, and tertiary aging.

Caregivers

The challenges faced by caregivers were described in Chapter 1 and acknowledged in other chapters in this text. Caregiver adjustment has a direct impact on the well-being and progress of the client. Stress is reduced when the caregiver knows what to expect—an outcome of adequate counseling (Shadden, Raiford, & Shadden, 1983). Caregivers can learn to adapt to their new roles, adjust to the requirements of their new lifestyle, and accept the changes in their plans for the future. Families may be helped to establish closer ties, develop new respect for each other, and realize greater self-worth.

While there are many tools for measuring caregiver stress and burden, most clinicians do not have the time or resources to pursue such assessments. However, during clinical interactions, healthcare providers should try to understand the unique stresses that exist and the problems confronting individual caregivers. Speech–language pathologists should identify needs and available resources, develop communication strategies, and provide appropriate support, thus reducing the negative impact of caregiving and preventing a crisis in care. Clinicians must be sensitive to caregiver stress and burden. It is unrealistic and unfair to ask already overwhelmed caregivers to take on major responsibilities in communication intervention.

Client

To understand a client's communication problems, speech–language pathologists have access to a variety of tools, including case history questionnaires, medical records, interviews, standardized tests, and behavioral checklists. Current communication partners, settings, and environments can also be evaluated. Unfortunately, time does not always allow administration of various assessment tools.

Before making recommendations or engaging in goal setting, speech–language pathologists should try to determine if the client has any particular negative feelings about specific interventions. One obvious example would be when a client rejects augmentative and alternative communication (AAC) because anything short of speech is unacceptable. If feelings like these are recognized early, the clinician can avoid alienating the client by introducing AAC gradually along with other speech interventions (if appropriate). Other factors influence acceptance of clinical recommendations, including the client's premorbid communication style, social roles, and conversational preferences.

When communication impairment is severe, the client may not always be able to complete attitude scales or provide information about interests, attitudes, motivations, and preferences. Different ways of eliciting information from such clients are discussed later in this chapter. When clinicians are forced to rely primarily on family input in these cases, it is important to remember that family members are not always an unbiased source, and different family members may present contradictory information about the client. For example, a spouse may indicate, "I don't understand why he wants to talk now; he never wanted to talk before," whereas an adult child may see the parent as a storyteller. One family member may describe the client's reaction to problems as calm and thoughtful, whereas another reports it as demanding and impatient. Even when communication is severely impaired, it is possible to obtain some idea of the client's expectations, desires, and frustrations through careful observation of behaviors—how the client interacts with various communication partners, how he or she responds to assessment or therapy stimuli, and how he or she performs in different settings.

Create a Therapeutic Partnership

One of the secrets of success in working with older clients and caregivers involves creating a genuine sense of partnership in planning goals, strategies, and communication activities. Partnerships grow out of shared knowledge of each individual and of aging. The speech–language pathologist should facilitate, not control. Clinical advice should be tailored to the specific client, based on his or her history, lifestyle, financial resources, value system, and stage of emotional adjustment. Clinicians must recognize that a client or caregiver may not be ready to accept certain recommendations at particular stages of treatment.

Clinicians can make the client and caregiver feel valued early on by actively seeking input. It may be helpful to begin the process by encouraging the caregiver or client to prepare lists of background information, issues and concerns, questions, and any other information he or she believes the clinician should be provided. Conversations should begin informally, with casual or familiar topics that set up an environment of shared control and balanced exchange. The clinician can move on to other critical information after the interaction has been comfortably established. Once information has been obtained, it is crucial to demonstrate that it has been used in treatment.

Some clients may be willing to write down observations and questions throughout the treatment process, as a form of clinic log or journal. Clinicians should provide opportunities for review of this material. This "journal" format can be helpful for long-term counseling and monitoring of behaviors. Some older clients or caregivers may need little or no direction in maintaining such a journal once they realize that the information is valued and is used productively. Others may require some guidance in focusing their written observations; for example, the clinician may need to ask the person to record specific observations about a single behavior, such as ordering in a restaurant.

If the clinician controls most of the information content and flow, there may be a breakdown in the clinical interaction. To avoid this dilemma, the clinician should provide open-ended opportunities for the sharing of issues and raising of questions. Rather than assuming what the participants need to know, it might be better to begin by asking, "What are some of your questions about what's happened?" or "What do you need to know?"

Speech–language pathologists should provide clients with the tools needed to participate in the therapeutic partnership. Some clients may want to convey a great deal of information but may be unable to do so verbally. The speech–language pathologist should be attentive to nonverbal cues and use techniques to facilitate the client's communication. Techniques might involve asking questions with restricted response choices, using a 20-question format, and encouraging communication through all modalities.

The speech–language pathologist often becomes a negotiator between caregiver and client in setting goals. The client may want something the family cannot afford or demand more than the caregiver can provide. Occasionally, caregivers are more reluctant than clients to accept communication limitations and may set unrealistic goals and challenges. Further, it can be difficult for some clients to define treatment goals because most people take communication for granted. Assistance should be provided as needed.

If the clinicians find themselves in the middle of such negotiations, a few simple rules may be helpful.

- Present options, citing the pros and cons of particular alternatives.
- Avoid becoming attached to your recommendations and taking things personally.
- Explain a recommendation; do not argue with the client or family member.
- Demonstrate the value of recommendations by showing their application to the lives of the participants.

Ultimately, decisions about actions and goals are in the hands of the client and caregivers. It is particularly important to avoid taking sides. Clients often recognize that the speech–language pathologist understands their problems best, and so they may want support for their efforts and issues. Spouses frequently try to enlist the speech–language pathologist to tell the client to do, or stop doing, something. It can be difficult to avoid getting caught up in what Norlin (1986) called the "rescue triangle" roles of victim, rescuer, and persecutor. Needless to say, speech–language pathologists tend to gravitate toward the rescuer role. When the perspective of one participant begins to be favored over another, clinicians should reevaluate their roles and actions.

One way to build a therapeutic partnership is to develop a written plan of care that uses input from all parties. At the heart of a care plan is the setting of functional, mutually agreed-upon goals for treatment. This plan should be revisited frequently and revised as needed. Thus, it is an ongoing component of treatment. In some instances, having a plan of care that targets functional outcomes also increases the likelihood of success in obtaining insurance funding.

Develop and Maintain Trust

A therapeutic partnership involves the development and maintenance of trust through clinical interactions. All participants, including speech–language pathologists and audiologists, need to be valued and to feel that they are making a contribution to the process. Unfortunately, professionals sometimes devalue input from the elderly. When this occurs, the message can be conveyed by nonverbals, tone of voice, or seemingly harmless well-intended remarks, such as, "I hope I'm doing as well when I'm your age."

A professional is not automatically a trusted source of information for all elders. Even when older clients are uncertain about the clinician's advice and opinions, their reactions may not be obvious. The client may seem somewhat disengaged in clinical interactions or may appear unwilling to follow through on recommendations. Devaluing the opinions of the professional is particularly problematic if the clinician is young. A relatively young clinician may have to "demonstrate" professional competence more than an older, more experienced clinician would. It is particularly important for younger practitioners to dress in appropriate professional attire and behave respectfully. Clinicians of all ages must find and build common ground with the client in terms of topics of interest in conversation. As noted in Chapter 7, personally relevant material is most likely to engage an older adult. Nothing can be more destructive to building trust and a therapeutic partnership than statements like, "So you are interested in politics. I don't really know much about that," or "I don't know anything about that. It happened before I was born."

Sometimes, it may be reasonable for an older adult *not* to trust a professional. As has been mentioned throughout this text, many healthcare providers know relatively little about aging and the elderly. Unfortunately, that lack of knowledge leads to a tendency to assume all elderly people are the same, with damaging consequences for healthcare. Older adults and their families should be cautious when healthcare providers talk in terms of "all old people." Communication disorders professionals should never assume that they have acquired some global understanding about what all older adults do or don't do. If clinicians make statements of this sort, the therapeutic relationship will be damaged.

Other factors affect the development of trust. Elderly persons from higher socioeconomic classes typically value "expert" opinions and trust professionals. In contrast, elders from lower socioeconomic classes often place more trust in information obtained from friends and acquaintances. Some attributes appear to qualify one as a "trusted source" for all people, regardless of age or social class. For example, we tend to trust someone who has been through the same life experience, but the experience must be truly equivalent. Many clients and caregivers have an extremely negative reaction to comments that they feel trivialize their situation, such as, "I know how you feel; I forget things all the time." Professionals who have really "been there" often find that clients accept their advice more readily when they are aware of the common experience. There is greater confidence that the professional has a clear understanding of the issues involved, an awareness of solutions and resources, and investment in resolving the problem. Obviously, trust is earned when professional recommendations consider the needs of the client and caregiver, support their current beliefs, and result in improved communication.

Trust is enhanced when the speech–language pathologist demonstrates empathy, not sympathy. This may be an attitude that is difficult to fake. Sympathy is often revealed in casual comments, such as, "I feel so bad for you." Empathy may be expressed through earnest attempts to understand the problem, genuine expressions of concern, and a sincere desire to assist the client and caregiver. Trust is also encouraged when participants feel that the professional is a long-term partner. If some follow-up is promised and provided after the client is discharged, the family feels that they have a continuing source of support and advice.

Any trust that is built can be rapidly destroyed if the clinician is not careful to maintain confidences. Clients may share information that they do not want the spouse to know; conversely, the spouse may request that the clinician not share concerns with the client. Occasionally, this lack of sharing may seem to inhibit progress and the openness of the counseling process, but violating confidences can cause irreparable damage to the established relationships.

Development of an atmosphere of trust and mutual respect often begins in the first encounter through observance of appropriate conversational conventions. The speech–language pathologist should remember that many of today's older adults come from a generation that emphasizes formality and convention. Clinicians do not need to be stiff, but they do need to convey an understanding of these conventions. First names or nicknames should not be used unless a relationship has already been established and permission has been given to do so. In fact, some older individuals prefer to address the clinician in a more formal manner. Clinicians should be sensitive to the fact that some older clients (and caregivers) have difficulty responding to questions about feelings or psychological state because discussions of this sort are uncommon in their age or cultural group. Once again, trust must be built before clients are willing to share some personal information.

Adapt to Evolving Needs and Concerns

Building trust in a therapeutic relationship is a necessary element in guiding clients and families as they adapt to the changes brought about by the swallowing or communication disorder. Once again, the process is ongoing. Many elderly individuals are already dealing with feelings of loss due to normal aging when a communication disorder develops. Each may be in a different stage of coping. The communication disorder itself, with its associated disruptions in interpersonal processes, becomes yet another loss to be managed. Clinicians should be aware of a client's or family member's current stage of adjustment and its relationship to his or her available coping strategies. Each individual experiences communication disorders differently, and clinicians must be aware of these unique experiences.

There are many models for defining timelines and cycles in coping with communication disorders, including Tanner and Gerstenberger's (1988) framework for the "grief response," which reflects coping with perceived or real losses of person, self, and object (skill). It is important to recognize that there are considerable differences among the common communication disorders that affect older individuals. These differences affect personal and familial coping responses. For example, an acquired disorder such as aphasia secondary to stroke appears abruptly and unexpectedly. Clients and families are unprepared and ill-equipped for understanding and adapting to the resulting life changes. In contrast, dysarthria secondary to Parkinson's disease is gradual in onset. Clients and significant others have time to adapt but also must cope with the knowledge that communication skills will continue to deteriorate. One would expect major differences in the way these two disorders are experienced.

Other factors influence adaptations. Obviously the severity of a swallowing or communication disorder is related to the effects of the disorder on daily functioning. Adaptation is also affected by the degree to which the disorder is perceived to be just another aspect of normal aging. It may be easier to accept a problem if it is considered part of growing old. In fact, some older clients may start at a point of acceptance because they believe changes are normal, but they end up moving away from acceptance as they recognize they are experiencing a specific disorder. The relative importance of a particular speech–language skill to a client will also define how great the loss appears and how difficult the challenges of coping will be.

Tanner and Gerstenberger (1988) described four stages in adaptation: denial, frustration, depression, and acceptance. Not all people go through every stage, and they may not experience them in the same order.

Denial

Most models of coping with grief and loss describe a stage of *denial*. Denial serves primarily as a buffer, buying time to confront the impact of a speech–language disorder at some later time. The individual may adopt one of the following stances with respect to the disorder:

- I don't have a problem, but the listener does.
- I have a problem, but it's minor.
- I have a significant problem, but it's temporary because God (or something else) will fix it (external locus of control, passive stance).
- I have a significant problem, but I can overcome it (internal locus of control).

During denial, it may be difficult, if not impossible, for clients and caregivers to process detailed information. In fact, some information (e.g., prognosis) may be unwelcome. Information provided at this time may be ignored, or it may simply confuse the individual. Clinical conversations and counseling during this stage should focus on immediate issues and concerns identified by the client or caregiver. Additional brief written information about the disorder should be provided, but extensive educational efforts and complicated recommendations are not appropriate.

Frustration

Frustration can encompass elements of helplessness and anger. When clients are frustrated, they may reject clinician suggestions and treatment activities or find it impossible to work on certain behaviors. Frustration tends to be directed at someone or something, and the target may vary from moment to moment. If the clinician is the target, client frustrations should not be taken personally. However, it is also important for clinicians to recognize that other aging factors may be contributing to a client's frustration. If a family member has just told a client that he will have to be moved to a nursing home because he cannot care for himself physically, speech therapy may not be a priority. In contrast, there may be times when frustrations about communication failures in a client's personal life are carried over into a treatment activity.

Depression

Depression is a common response to a loss in communicative or swallowing functions. Several factors can contribute to depression. At any age, depression can leave the client or caregiver passive and unmotivated, and progress may be limited. Clinicians are often uncomfortable with depressed clients and try to avoid depressing topics or ignore the behaviors associated with depression. However, as part of the clinical interaction, clients or caregivers may sometimes need to talk briefly about what is causing their depression. It is not appropriate to ignore such topics, attempt to "cheer up" the client or caregiver, or suggest that the person should feel better because "things could be worse." Instead, possible reasons for depression can be acknowledged, and then the clinician can attempt to move forward with treatment when possible.

Acceptance

In many models of loss and grief, the last stage is *acceptance*, a term often used synonymously with adaptation, adjustment, and accommodation. As usually defined, when acceptance has been achieved, the client or caregiver acknowledges the full extent of the communication disorder and is willing to move forward. However, there can be a fine line between acceptance and resignation. *Resignation* suggests passive toleration of what has happened; clinicians may find resigned clients or caregivers unwilling or unable to engage in clinical interactions effectively. They have given up and truly believe that nothing more can be done. If older people are experiencing numerous life changes, it may be difficult for them to find the inner resources to continue to move forward with treatment.

Strategies for long-term adaptation and coping are influenced by many factors. Coping responses are dynamic, not static. Speech–language pathologists must constantly monitor the emotional state of clients and caregivers, focusing on their reactions to the communication disorder and its impact on life events. It is important to avoid a simplistic view of these cycles of emotional adaptation (e.g., thinking "It's no big deal. Mrs. Jones is just in the anger stage right now"). Feelings should be acknowledged and accepted by the clinician unless they seem severe enough to warrant referral to a mental health professional.

Adjust and Support Communication Appropriately

This chapter and this text end with guidelines for communicating with older clients and their caregivers. Many of these recommendations result from points highlighted in previous sections. Together, they underscore the fact that the quality of clinical interactions and counseling involving older clients may be the single most important factor in productive treatment.

Elderspeak and Related Speech Style Accommodations

Throughout this text, elderspeak has been alluded to as a factor in the success or failure of communication with older adults. Those who talk with the elderly often modify the way they communicate in an unproductive and almost insulting fashion (Harwood & Giles, 1996; Hummert, Shaner, Garstka, & Henry, 1998). These modifications, also called *speech style accommodations*, occur partly because we are unconsciously changing our communication style based on stereotypes about older persons, as opposed to the real characteristics of a client or caregiver. Common changes seen in elderspeak include exaggerated intonation patterns, higher pitch, simpler vocabulary and grammar, frequent repetitions or redundancies, slower speaking rate, and use of additional controlling devices such as pet names or tag questions ("We're going to take our bath now, aren't we?").

There are a number of forms of "talking down"; distinct types can be characterized in terms of how *caring* and *controlling* they are (Ryan, Hummert, & Boisch, 1995). Because both caring and controlling are issues in clinical interactions and counseling, each of these communication styles is described briefly.

- *Baby talk* is both caring and controlling. It involves many of the basic elderspeak characteristics and includes generic terms of endearment (e.g., Sweetie, Honey) and "cutesy" phrases such as one might use with a small child.
- *Overly personal* is high in caring but low in controlling. Older adults are spoken to as though they are a treasured toy (e.g., "I just love how cute you look today"). This type of overly personal speech is often accompanied by touch or other positive nonverbal behaviors.

- *Directive talk* is primarily controlling with little or no caring, a kind of institutional speech register. The goal appears to be getting through the communication exchange with as little effort as possible. Directive talk involves telling elders what they should or should not do, typically with a cold or angry tone and an implied message that the person is noncompliant.
- *Superficial talk* is neither caring nor controlling. The best example is when a speaker discusses an older person as though he or she was not present, or when the health professional abruptly changes topics when the elder is expressing strong feelings or needs.

Elderspeak and other versions of "talking down" can be triggered unconsciously by a variety of cues, such as an old-sounding voice, gray hair, wrinkles, or use of a walker. Sometimes, simply knowing the chronological age of a person is enough to trigger elderspeak. The effects of elderspeak and talking down vary considerably based on setting, task, and characteristics of older and younger conversational partners. In general, when mentally competent aging adults are talked to in a demeaning way, they feel less competent. In contrast, use of exaggerated inflection with dementia patients may reduce problem behaviors. Speaking more slowly with careful intonation and using short simple sentences may be helpful to normal older adults when they need to process detailed information, like instructions about taking medicines (Gould, Saum, & Belter, 2002).

Chapter 1 encouraged readers to identify their stereotypes and attitudes about aging and the elderly. We end this text with the same request. Clinicians must examine their own communication patterns and tendencies in talking with older adults and attempt to recognize what older client characteristics may trigger elderspeak. It is not always easy to identify the fine line between appropriate speech style accommodations (e.g., talking slower for a person with receptive aphasia) and talking down to that same individual.

Appropriate speech style accommodation is the first recommendation for effective communication in health care interactions with older adults and their families. The following section provides additional guidelines for verbal and nonverbal communication with older individuals.

Other Accommodations for Communication in Clinical Interactions

- Provide an environment that is as communication friendly and age-sensitive as possible. Consider the arrangement of furniture to ensure safety, comfort, and ease of access. Ensure adequate lighting and eliminate glare, fluorescent lighting, and backlight if possible. Use contrasting colors to highlight room features. Reduce background noises that may be distracting (e.g., radio, television, hallway or external noises). See Chapter 10 for additional recommendations.

- Be an active listener. Don't just pretend to be listening. Listen to the words and the underlying thoughts, connections, and concerns. Clarify or ask questions if you are not sure you understand what is being said. Be attentive. Demonstrate your attention by facing the person, using an open posture, leaning toward the person, maintaining eye contact, and avoiding distractions. Part of being attentive is appearing to be relaxed and giving your focus to the individual.
- "Listen" to more than the words—all behavior is communication. Pay particular attention to nonverbal clues, including tone of voice, eye contact, body language, dress, and personal care. Observe nonverbal exchanges between the client and the caregiver for suggestions of concerns or problem areas.
- Be aware of your own nonverbal messages. Touch has been described as particularly important in communicative interactions, although not all older adults appreciate physical contact from a relative stranger. Gestures and facial expressions may be particularly important in communicating with an older adult with a hearing impairment.
- Allow time for conversation as well as other information gathering. Try to avoid the question-and-answer interaction that suggests that all the power is in the hands of the questioner. Provide opportunities for the older person to initiate topics or questions. Do not do all the talking.
- Allow the older person extra time to respond. Do not leap in if there is a pause.
- Stick to a topic for a while, rather than constantly shifting. If there are several people involved in the interaction, try to restate the topic periodically to help maintain continuity.

Clinicians need to understand these distinctions and monitor their own communications and stereotypical responses when counseling older individuals. Successful counseling exchanges can *only* occur when the clinician adjusts his or her communication style based on each individual client's attributes and life circumstances.

Reimbursement

Counseling is an essential and ongoing part of the services provided by communication disorders professionals. This service is typically integrated into assessment and intervention services and not billed separately. If a speech–pathologist or audiologist participates in a conference that includes an interdisciplinary medical team, reimbursement may be obtained using Current Procedural Terminology (CPT; American Medical Association, 2009) codes that indicate either a face-to-face conference with the patient and the patient's family or a team conference for which the patient or family is not present. Conferences must last at least 30 minutes to be eligible for reimbursement.

Communication disorders professionals may be involved in end-of-life services as discussed in Chapter 11. For example, a speech–language pathologist may be asked to facilitate the older person's communication with professionals and family members during estate planning. This type of service is not covered by a CPT code available to communication disorders practitioners. Professional participation in services not covered by CPT codes may be reimbursed through a consultation fee charged to the requesting party, such as an attorney.

Summary

The basic premises of this text are simple. Clinicians must understand the effects of primary, secondary, and tertiary aging on communication and swallowing. This knowledge can be used to distinguish normal behaviors from disordered ones, and to understand the many aging factors that can affect assessment and intervention outcomes. In this chapter, these basic premises were applied to understanding clinical interactions with elderly clients and their significant others.

All of the guidelines provided in this chapter can be translated into one overriding theme. Clinicians are responsible for understanding not only aging in general, but also the unique aging experiences and life circumstances of each client. This understanding is the foundation for developing clinical interactions that will lead to successful treatment of older adults with communication and swallowing disorders.

Key Points

Without appropriate personal interaction skills, clinical service delivery will not be effective. The following themes were highlighted in this chapter:

- Good clinical interaction is at the heart of successful treatment.
- Counseling is part of the scope of practice of speech–language pathologists and audiologists and should be a component of the ongoing process of interacting with older clients.
- Counseling includes receiving information that families wish to share; providing information to family members; helping individuals clarify ideas, attitudes, and emotions; and providing family members with options for changing their behaviors and the behaviors of the impaired person.
- Guidelines for successful clinical interaction and counseling include the following:
  - Use clinical interaction time wisely.
  - Know what's normal (from everyone's perspective).
  - Learn about the individuals involved.
  - Create a therapeutic partnership.
  - Develop and maintain trust.
  - Adapt to evolving needs and concerns.
  - Adjust and support communication appropriately.

Acknowledgment

Portions of this chapter were adapted from "Counseling Challenges: Working with Older Clients and Caregivers," by M. A. Toner and B. B. Shadden, 2002, in *Contemporary Issues in Communication Sciences and Disorders,* 29, 68–78. Adapted with permission of the National Student Speech-Language-Hearing Association.

References

American Medical Association. (2009). *Current procedural terminology* (CPT) 2010. Chicago: Author.

Gould, O. N., Saum, C., & Belter, J. (2002). Recall and subjective reactions to speaking styles: Does age matter? *Experimental Aging Research, 28,* 199–213.

Harwood, J., & Giles, H. (1996). Reactions to older people being patronized: The roles of response strategies and attributed thoughts. *Journal of Language and Social Psychology, 15,* 395–412.

Hummert, M. L., Shaner, J. L., Garstka, T. A., & Henry, C. (1998). Communication with older adults: The influence of age stereotypes, context, and communicator age. *Human Communication Research, 25,* 124–151.

Luterman, D. (2008). *Counseling persons with communication disorders and their families* (5th ed.). Austin, TX: PRO-ED.

Norlin, P. F. (1986). Familiar faces, sudden strangers: Helping families cope with the crisis of aphasia. In R. Chapey (Ed.), *Language intervention strategies in adult aphasia* (2nd ed., pp. 174–186). Baltimore: Williams & Wilkins.

Ryan, E. G., Hummert, M. L., & Boisch, L. H. (1995). Communication predicaments of aging: Patronizing behavior toward older adults. *Journal of Language and Social Psychology, 14,* 144–166.

Shadden, B. B., Raiford, C. A., & Shadden, H. S. (1983). *Coping with communication disorders in aging.* Portland, OR: C.C. Publications.

Shipley, K. G., & Roseberry-McKibbin, C. (2006). *Interviewing and counseling in communicative disorders: Principles and procedures* (3rd ed.). Austin, TX: PRO-ED.

Tanner, D. C., & Gerstenberger, D. I. (1988). The grief response in neuropathologies of speech and language. *Aphasiology, 2,* 79–84.

Toner, M. A., & Shadden, B. B. (2002). Counseling challenges: Working with older clients and caregivers. *Contemporary Issues in Communication Sciences and Disorders, 29,* 68–78.

Webster, E., & Newhoff, M. (1981). Intervention with families of communicatively impaired adults. In D. S. Beasley & G. A. Davis (Eds.), *Aging communication processes and disorders* (pp. 229–240). New York: Grune and Stratton.

Subect Index

mealtime and eating strategies, 130–131
post-feeding strategies, 131
prefeeding strategies, 130
FEES (flexible endoscopic evaluation of swallowing), 122
FEESST, 122
Financial power of attorney, 276–277
Flaccid dysarthria, 79, 81
FLCI (*Functional Linguistic Communication Inventory*), 202
Flexible endoscopic evaluation of swallowing (FEES), 122
Fluid intelligence, 149
FM system, 49–50
Food. *See* Feeding strategies; Nutrition
Frazier Water Protocol, 127, 129
Frenchay Activities Index, 268
Frenchay Aphasia Screening Test-2, 266
Frenchay Dysarthria Assessment (FDA), 86
Frontotemporal dementia (FTD), 174–175
Frustration, counseling and, 312–313
FTD. *See* Frontotemporal dementia (FTD)
Functional ability, assessment of, 23
Functional Linguistic Communication Inventory (FLCI), 202
Functional speech disorders, 82

Gastro-intestinal system
dysphagia and, 115
primary aging changes and diseases associated with, 21
Gastroesophageal reflux disease (GERD), 123–124, 139–140
GDS (Geriatric Depression Scale), 24
GERD (gastroesophageal reflux disease), 123–124, 139–140
Geriatric Depression Scale, 267
Geriatric Depression Scale (GDS), 24
Geriatric healthcare education, 290–291
Global aphasia, 238, 240, 241. *See also* Aphasia
Glottis, 59
Goals and discourse behaviors, 213–214
Goals in Aphasia Protocol, 268
Grade, Roughness, Breathiness, Aesthenia, Strain Scale (GRBAS), 88
Granulomas, 63, 69
GRBAS (Grade, Roughness, Breathiness, Aesthenia, Strain Scale), 88
Grief
acceptance and, 313–314
anticipatory loss and grief and end-of-life (EOL) care, 285–286
responses to, and counseling, 311–314
Group therapy
for aphasia, 254
for cognitive communication disorders, 195
Gugging Swallowing Screen (GUSS), 119
Guidance, 301. *See also* Counseling and clinical interactions
GUSS (*Gugging Swallowing Screen*), 119

Author Index

AARP, 286
Abrahamowicz, M., 120
Abrams, L., 223, 226
Adams, C., 215
Aidinejad, M. R., 222
Alario, F., 217
Albert, M. L., 256
Albert, M. S., 158
Alderman, N., 203
Allen-Burge, R., 189
Alpert, N., 226
Altman, M., 101
AMA. *See* American Medical Association (AMA)
American Academy of Otolaryngology–Head & Neck Surgery, 46
American Association of Retired Persons, 26
American Medical Association (AMA), 13, 46, 52, 53, 97, 98, 132, 133, 259, 260, 317
American Psychiatric Association (APA), 171
American Speech-Language-Hearing Association (ASHA), 88
Amerman, J., 77
Aminzadeh, B., 24
Anas, A. P., 221, 223
Anstey, K. J., 150
Antuono, P., 175
APA. *See* American Psychiatric Association (APA)
Apert, N. M., 158
Arbuckle, T. A., 220
Aronson, A., 78, 94
ASHA. *See* American Speech-Language-Hearing Association (ASHA)
Atkinson, R. C., 151
Austin, A., 220

Babbitt, E., 267
Bach-Peterson, J., 268
Backman, L., 158
Baddeley, A., 203
Baijens, L., 126
Baines, K. A., 202
Bajorek, S., 223
Baldwin, C. T., 42
Ball, K., 229
Balota, D., 211
Baltes, P. B., 155, 164
Barber, R., 175
Baressi, B., 238–240, 249, 256, 266
Barlow, J. A., 77
Barnett, C., 177
Barnett, H., 229
Bava, A., 222
Bayles, K., 202, 215
Beaman, A., 195, 214
Beamer, M., 223
Becker, D., 127
Becker, J., 268
Beers, M. H., 23–24
Beeson, P., 215, 255
Behlau, M., 61
Bell, R., 227
Belter, J., 315
Berg, E., 71, 91
Berg, M., 267
Berkow, R., 23–24
Bernstein, J. H., 202
Beukelman, D., 89
Bieman-Copland, S., 221
Biller, J., 267
Bird, T., 175
Blackstone, S., 267
Bloom, J. E., 217
Boczko, F., 195